AEQUANIMITAS

AEQUANIMITAS

With other Addresses to Medical Students, Nurses and Practitioners of Medicine

By

Sir WILLIAM OSLER, Bt., M.D., F.R.S.

Late Regius Professor of Medicine, Oxford
Honorary Professor of Medicine, Johns Hopkins University

THIRD EDITION

The Blakiston Division

McGraw-Hill, Inc.
New York   St. Louis   San Francisco   Auckland   Bogotá
Caracas   Lisbon   London   Madrid   Mexico City   Milan
Montreal   New Delhi   San Juan   Singapore
Sydney   Tokyo   Toronto

PRINTED IN THE UNITED STATES OF AMERICA

33 34 35 36 37 BKMBKM 9 9

0-07-047915-1

To

DANIEL C. GILMAN,

Ex-President of the Johns Hopkins University.

Dear Dr. Gilman,

Please accept the dedication of this volume of addresses, in memory of those happy days in 1889 when, under your guidance, the Johns Hopkins Hospital was organized and opened; and in grateful recognition of your active and intelligent interest in medical education.

Yours sincerely,

William Osler.

PREFACE TO THE SECOND EDITION

DELIVERED at sundry times and in divers places in the course of a busy life, it was not without hesitation that I collected these addresses for publication. That the simple message they contain has not been unacceptable is shown by the exhaustion of three impressions within eighteen months. I have to thank my friends, lay and medical, for their kind criticisms of the volume; but above all I have been deeply touched that many young men on both sides of the Atlantic should have written stating that the addresses have been helpful in forming their life ideals. Loyalty to the best interests of the noblest of callings, and a profound belief in the gospel of the day's work are the texts, with variations here and there, from which I have preached. I have an enduring faith in the men who do the routine work of our profession. Hard though the conditions may be, approached in the right spirit—the spirit which has animated us from the days of Hippocrates—the practice of medicine affords scope for the exercise of the best faculties of the mind and heart. That the yoke of the general practitioner is often galling cannot be denied, but he has not a monopoly of the worries and trials in the meeting and conquering of which he fights his life battle; and it is a source of inexpressible gratification to me to feel that I may perhaps have helped to make his yoke easier and his burden lighter.

To this edition I have added the three Valedictory addresses delivered before leaving America. One of these —The Fixed Period—demands a word of explanation.

"To interpose a little ease," to relieve a situation of singular sadness in parting from my dear colleagues of the Johns Hopkins University, I jokingly suggested for the relief of a senile professoriate an extension of Anthony Trollope's plan mentioned in his novel, *The Fixed Period.* To one who had all his life been devoted to old men, it was not a little distressing to be placarded in a world-wide way as their sworn enemy, and to every man over sixty whose spirit I may have thus unwittingly bruised, I tender my heartfelt regrets. Let me add, however, that the discussion which followed my remarks has not changed, but has rather strengthened my belief that the real work of life is done before the fortieth year and that after the sixtieth year it would be best for the world and best for themselves if men rested from their labours.

OXFORD, *July*, 1906.

CONTENTS

ix

x CONTENTS

I
AEQUANIMITAS

Thou must be like a promontory of the sea, against which, though the waves beat continually, yet it both itself stands, and about it are those swelling waves stilled and quieted.

MARCUS AURELIUS.

> I say: Fear not!   Life still
> Leaves human effort scope.
> But, since life teems with ill,
> Nurse no extravagant hope;
> Because thou must not dream, thou need'st not then despair!

MATTHEW ARNOLD, *Empedocles on Etna.*

1

AEQUANIMITAS[1]

TO many the frost of custom has made even these imposing annual ceremonies cold and lifeless. To you, at least of those present, they should have the solemnity of an ordinance—called as you are this day to a high dignity and to so weighty an office and charge. You have chosen your Genius, have passed beneath the Throne of Necessity, and with the voices of the fatal sisters still in your ears, will soon enter the plain of Forgetfulness and drink of the waters of its river. Ere you are driven all manner of ways, like the souls in the tale of Er the Pamphylian,[2] it is my duty to say a few words of encouragement and to bid you, in the name of the Faculty, God-speed on your journey.

I could have the heart to spare you, poor, careworn survivors of a hard struggle, so "lean and pale and leaden-eyed with study;" and my tender mercy constrains me to consider but two of the score of elements which may make or mar your lives—which may contribute to your success, or help you in the days of failure.

In the first place, in the physician or surgeon no quality takes rank with imperturbability, and I propose for a few minutes to direct your attention to this essential bodily virtue. Perhaps I may be able to give those of you, in whom it has not developed during the critical scenes of the past month, a hint or two of its importance, possibly a suggestion for its attainment. Imperturbability means

[1] Valedictory Address, University of Pennsylvania, May 1, 1889.
[2] *The Republic,* Book X.

3

coolness and presence of mind under all circumstances, calmness amid storm, clearness of judgment in moments of grave peril, immobility, impassiveness, or, to use an old and expressive word, *phlegm*. It is the quality which is most appreciated by the laity though often misunderstood by them; and the physician who has the misfortune to be without it, who betrays indecision and worry, and who shows that he is flustered and flurried in ordinary emergencies, loses rapidly the confidence of his patients.

In full development, as we see it in some of our older colleagues, it has the nature of a divine gift, a blessing to the possessor, a comfort to all who come in contact with him. You should know it well, for there have been before you for years several striking illustrations, whose example has, I trust, made a deep impression. As imperturbability is largely a bodily endowment, I regret to say that there are those amongst you, who, owing to congenital defects, may never be able to acquire it. Education, however, will do much; and with practice and experience the majority of you may expect to attain to a fair measure. The first essential is to have your nerves well in hand. Even under the most serious circumstances, the physician or surgeon who allows "his outward action to demonstrate the native act and figure of his heart in complement extern," who shows in his face the slightest alteration, expressive of anxiety or fear, has not his medullary centres under the highest control, and is liable to disaster at any moment. I have spoken of this to you on many occasions, and have urged you to educate your nerve centres so that not the slightest dilator or contractor influence shall pass to the vessels of your face under any professional trial. Far be it from me to urge you, ere Time has carved with his hours those fair brows, to quench on all occasions the blushes of ingenuous shame,

but in dealing with your patients emergencies demanding
these should certainly not arise, and at other times an
inscrutable face may prove a fortune.   In a true and perfect
form, imperturbability is indissolubly associated with wide
experience and an intimate knowledge of the varied aspects
of disease.   With such advantages he is so equipped that
no eventuality can disturb the mental equilibrium of the
physician; the possibilities are always manifest, and the
course of action clear.   From its very nature this precious
quality is liable to be misinterpreted, and the general accusation of hardness, so often brought against the profession,
has here its foundation.   Now a certain measure of insensi-
bility is not only an advantage, but a positive necessity in
the exercise of a calm judgment, and in carrying out delicate
operations.   Keen sensibility is doubtless a virtue of high
order, when it does not interfere with steadiness of hand or
coolness of nerve; but for the practitioner in his working-day
world, a callousness which thinks only of the good to be
effected, and goes ahead regardless of smaller considerations,
is the preferable quality.

Cultivate, then, gentlemen, such a judicious measure of
obtuseness as will enable you to meet the exigencies of
practice with firmness and courage, without, at the same
time, hardening "the human heart by which we live."

In the second place, there is a mental equivalent to this
bodily endowment, which is as important in our pilgrimage
as imperturbability.   Let me recall to your minds an
incident related of that best of men and wisest of rulers,
Antoninus Pius, who, as he lay aying, in his home at Lorium
in Etruria, summed up the philosophy of life in the watch
word, *Aequanimitas*.   As for him, about to pass *flammantia
moenia mundi* (the flaming ramparts of the world), so for
you, fresh from Clotho's spindle, a calm equanimity is the

desirable attitude. How difficult to attain, yet how necessary, in success as in failure! Natural temperament has much to do with its development, but a clear knowledge of our relation to our fellow-creatures and to the work of life is also indispensable. One of the first essentials in securing a good-natured equanimity is not to expect too much of the people amongst whom you dwell. "Knowledge comes, but wisdom lingers," and in matters medical the ordinary citizen of to-day has not one whit more sense than the old Romans, whom Lucian scourged for a credulity which made them fall easy victims to the quacks of the time, such as the notorious Alexander, whose exploits make one wish that his advent had been delayed some eighteen centuries. Deal gently then with this deliciously credulous old human nature in which we work, and restrain your indignation, when you find your pet parson has triturates of the 1000th potentiality in his waistcoat pocket, or you discover accidentally a case of Warner's Safe Cure in the bedroom of your best patient. It must needs be that offences of this kind come; expect them, and do not be vexed.

Curious, odd compounds are these fellow-creatures, at whose mercy you will be; full of fads and eccentricities, of whims and fancies; but the more closely we study their little foibles of one sort and another in the inner life which we see, the more surely is the conviction borne in upon us of the likeness of their weaknesses to our own. The similarity would be intolerable, if a happy egotism did not often render us forgetful of it. Hence the need of an infinite patience and of an ever-tender charity toward these fellow-creatures; have they not to exercise the same toward us?

A distressing feature in the life which you are about to enter, a feature which will press hardly upon the finer spirits among you and ruffle their equanimity, is the uncertainty which pertains not alone to our science and art, but to the very hopes and fears which make us men. In seeking absolute truth we aim at the unattainable, and must be content with finding broken portions. You remember in the Egyptian story, how Typhon with his conspirators dealt with good Osiris; how they took the virgin Truth, hewed her lovely form into a thousand pieces, and scattered them to the four winds; and, as Milton says, "from that time ever since, the sad friends of truth, such as durst appear, imitating the careful search that Isis made for the mangled body of Osiris, went up and down gathering up limb by limb still as they could find them. We have not yet found them all,"[1] but each one of us may pick up a fragment, perhaps two, and in moments when mortality weighs less heavily upon the spirit, we can, as in a vision, see the form divine, just as a great Naturalist, an Owen or a Leidy, can reconstruct an ideal creature from a fossil fragment.

It has been said that in prosperity our equanimity is chiefly exercised in enabling us to bear with composure the misfortunes of our neighbours. Now, while nothing disturbs our mental placidity more sadly than straightened means, and the lack of those things after which the Gentiles seek, I would warn you against the trials of the day soon to come to some of you—the day of large and successful practice. Engrossed late and soon in professional cares, getting and spending, you may so lay waste your powers that you may find, too late, with hearts given away, that there is no place in your habit-stricken souls for those gentler influences which make life worth living.

It is sad to think that, for some of you, there is in store disappointment, perhaps failure. You cannot hope, of

[1] *Areopagitica.*

course, to escape from the cares and anxieties incident to professional life.   Stand up bravely, even against the worst. Your very hopes may have passed on out of sight, as did all that was near and dear to the Patriarch at the Jabbok ford, and, like him, you may be left to struggle in the night alone.   Well for you, if you wrestle on, for in persistency lies victory, and with the morning may come the wished-for blessing.   But not always; there is a struggle with defeat which some of you will have to bear, and it will be well for you in that day to have cultivated a cheerful equanimity.   Remember, too, that sometimes "from our desolation only does the better life begin."   Even with disaster ahead and ruin imminent, it is better to face them with a smile, and with the head erect, than to crouch at their approach.   And, if the fight is for principle and jus-tice, even when failure seems certain, where many have failed before, cling to your ideal, and, like Childe Roland before the dark tower, set the slug-horn to your lips, blow the challenge, and calmly await the conflict.

It has been said that "in patience ye shall win your souls," and what is this patience but an equanimity which enables you to rise superior to the trials of life?   Sowing as you shall do beside all waters, I can but wish that you may reap the promised blessing of quietness and of assurance forever, until

> Within this life,
> Though lifted o'er its strife,

you may, in the growing winters, glean a little of that wisdom which is pure, peaceable, gentle, full of mercy and good fruits, without partiality and without hypocrisy.

The past is always with us, never to be escaped; it alone is enduring; but, amidst the changes and chances which succeed one another so rapidly in this life, we are apt to live too much for the present and too much in the future. On such an occasion as the present, when the *Alma Mater* is in festal array, when we joy in her growing prosperity, it is good to hark back to the olden days and gratefully to recall the men whose labours in the past have made the present possible.

The great possession of any University is its great names. It is not the "pride, pomp and circumstance" of an institution which bring honour, not its wealth, nor the number of its schools, not the students who throng its halls, but the *men* who have trodden in its service the thorny road through toil, even through hate, to the serene abode of Fame, climbing "like stars to their appointed height." These bring glory, and it should thrill the heart of every alumnus of this school, of every teacher in its faculty, as it does mine this day, reverently and thankfully to recall such names amongst its founders as Morgan, Shippen, and Rush, and such men amongst their successors as Wistar, Physick, Barton, and Wood.

Gentlemen of the Faculty—*Noblesse oblige.*

And the sad reality of the past teaches us to-day in the freshness of sorrow at the loss of friends and colleagues, "hid in death's dateless night." We miss from our midst one of your best known instructors, by whose lessons you have profited, and whose example has stimulated many. An earnest teacher, a faithful worker, a loyal son of this University, a good and kindly friend, Edward Bruen has left behind him, amid regrets at a career untimely closed, the memory of a well-spent life.

We mourn to-day, also, with our sister college, the grievous loss which she has sustained in the death of one of her most distinguished teachers, a man who bore with honour an honoured name, and who added lustre to the profession of this city. Such men as Samuel W. Gross can ill be spared. Let us be thankful for the example of a courage which could fight and win; and let us emulate the zeal, energy, and industry which characterized his career.

Personally I mourn the loss of a preceptor, dear to me as a father, the man from whom more than any other I received inspiration, and to whose example and precept I owe the position which enables me to address you to-day. There are those present who will feel it no exaggeration when I say that to have known Palmer Howard was, in the deepest and truest sense of the phrase, a liberal education—

> Whatever way my days decline,
> I felt and feel, tho' left alone,
> His being working in mine own,
> The footsteps of his life in mine.

While preaching to you a doctrine of equanimity, I am, myself, a castaway. Recking not my own rede, I illustrate the inconsistency which so readily besets us. One might have thought that in the premier school of America, in this Civitas Hippocratica, with associations so dear to a lover of his profession, with colleagues so distinguished, and with students so considerate, one might have thought, I say, that the Hercules Pillars of a man's ambition had here been reached. But it has not been so ordained, and to-day I sever my connexion with this University. More than once, gentlemen, in a life rich in the priceless blessings of friends, I have been placed in positions in which no words could express the feelings of my heart, and so it is with me now. The keenest sentiments of gratitude well up from my innermost being at the thought of the kindliness and goodness which have followed me at every step during the past five years. A stranger—I cannot say an alien—among you,

I have been made to feel at home—more you could not have done. Could I say more? Whatever the future may have in store of success or of trials, nothing can blot the memory of the happy days I have spent in this city, and nothing can quench the pride I shall always feel at having been associated, even for a time, with a Faculty so notable in the past, so distinguished in the present, as that from which I now part.

Gentlemen,—Farewell, and take with you into the struggle the watchword of the good old Roman—*Aequanimitas.*

II
DOCTOR AND NURSE

There are men and classes of men that stand above the common herd: the soldier, the sailor, and the shepherd not infrequently; the artist rarely; rarelier still, the clergyman; the physician almost as a rule. He is the flower (such as it is) of our civilization; and when that stage of man is done with, and only to be marvelled at in history, he will be thought to have shared as little as any in the defects of the period, and most notably exhibited the virtues of the race. Generosity he has, such as is possible to those who practise an art, never to those who drive a trade; discretion, tested by a hundred secrets; tact, tried in a thousand embarrassments; and what are more important, Heraclean cheerfulness and courage. So that he brings air and cheer into the sick room, and often enough, though not so often as he wishes, brings healing.

ROBERT LOUIS STEVENSON, Preface to *Underwoods*.

Think not Silence the wisdom of Fools, but, if rightly timed, the honour of wise Men, who have not the Infirmity, but the Virtue of Taciturnity, and speak not out of the abundance, but the well-weighed thoughts of their Hearts. Such Silence may be Eloquence, and speak thy worth above the power of Words.

SIR THOMAS BROWNE.

II

DOCTOR AND NURSE[1]

THERE are individuals—doctors and nurses, for
example—whose very existence is a constant reminder
of our frailties; and considering the notoriously irritating
character of such people, I often wonder that the world
deals so gently with them. The presence of the parson
suggests dim possibilities, not the grim realities conjured up
by the names of the persons just mentioned; the lawyer
never worries us—in this way, and we can imagine in the
future a social condition in which neither divinity nor law
shall have a place—when all shall be friends and each one a
priest, when the meek shall possess the earth; but we cannot
picture a time when Birth and Life and Death shall be
separated from the "grizzly troop" which we dread so much
and which is ever associated in our minds with "physician
and nurse."

Dread! Yes, but mercifully for us in a vague and misty
way. Like schoolboys we play among the shadows cast by
the turrets of the temple of oblivion, towards which we
travel, regardless of what awaits us in the vale of years
beneath. Suffering and disease are ever before us, but life
is very pleasant; and the motto of the world, when well, is
"forward with the dance." Fondly imagining that we are
in a happy valley, we deal with ourselves as the King did
with the Gautama, and hide away everything that suggests

[1] Johns Hopkins Hospital, 1891.

15

our fate.   Perhaps we are wise.   Who knows?   Mercifully, the tragedy of life, though seen, is not realized.   It is so close that we lose all sense of its proportions.   And better so; for, as George Eliot has said, "if we had a keen vision and feeling of all ordinary human life, it would be like hearing the grass grow, or the squirrel's heart beat, and we should die of that roar which lies on the other side of silence."

With many, however, it is a wilful blindness, a sort of fool's paradise, not destroyed by a thought, but by the stern exigencies of life, when the "ministers of human fate" drag us, or—worse still—those near and dear to us, upon the stage.   Then, we become acutely conscious of the drama of human suffering, and of those inevitable stage accessories —doctor and nurse.

If, Members of the Graduating Class, the medical profession, composed chiefly of men, has absorbed a larger share of attention and regard, you have, at least, the satisfaction of feeling that yours is the older, and, as older, the more honourable calling.   In one of the lost books of Solomon, a touching picture is given of Eve, then an early grandmother, bending over the little Enoch, and showing Mahala how to soothe his sufferings and to allay his pains. Woman, "the link among the days," and so trained in a bitter school, has, in successive generations, played the part of Mahala to the little Enoch, of Elaine to the wounded Lancelot.   It seems a far cry from the plain of Mesopotamia and the lists of Camelot to the Johns Hopkins Hospital, but the spirit which makes this scene possible is the same, tempered through the ages, by the benign influence of Christianity.   Among the ancients, many had risen to the idea of forgiveness of enemies, of patience under wrong doing, and even of the brotherhood of man; but the spirit of Love only received its incarnation with the ever memorable reply to the ever memorable question, Who is my neighbour?—a reply which has changed the attitude of the world. Nowhere in ancient history, sacred or profane, do we find pictures of devoted heroism in women such as dot the annals of the Catholic Church, or such as can be paralleled in our own century. Tender maternal affection, touching filial piety were there; but the spirit abroad was that of Deborah not Rizpah, of Jael not Dorcas.

In the gradual division of labour, by which civilization has emerged from barbarism, the doctor and the nurse have been evolved, as useful accessories in the incessant warfare in which man is engaged. The history of the race is a grim record of passions and ambitions, of weaknesses and vanities, a record, too often, of barbaric inhumanity, and even to-day, when philosophers would have us believe his thoughts had widened, he is ready as of old to shut the gates of mercy, and to let loose the dogs of war. It was in one of these attacks of race-mania that your profession, until then unsettled and ill-defined, took, under Florence Nightingale—ever blessed be her name—its modern position.

Individually, man, the unit, the microcosm, is fast bound in chains of atavism, inheriting legacies of feeble will and strong desires, taints of blood and brain. What wonder, then, that many, sore let and hindered in running the race, fall by the way, and need a shelter in which to recruit or to die, a hospital, in which there shall be no harsh comments on conduct, but only, so far as is possible, love and peace and rest? Here, we learn to scan gently our brother man, judging not, asking no questions, but meting out to all alike a hospitality worthy of the *Hôtel Dieu*, and deeming ourselves honoured in being allowed to act as its dispensers. Here, too, are daily before our eyes the problems which have ever perplexed the human mind; problems not presented in the dead abstract of books, but in the living concrete of some poor fellow in his last round, fighting a brave fight, but sadly weighted, and going to his account "unhousell'd, disappointed, unanel'd, no reckoning made." As we whisper to each other over his bed that the battle is decided and Euthanasia alone remains, have I not heard in reply to that muttered proverb, so often on the lips of the physician, "the fathers have eaten sour grapes," your answer, in clear accents—the comforting words of the prayer of Stephen?

But our work would be much restricted were it not for man's outside adversary—Nature, the great Moloch, which exacts a frightful tax of human blood, sparing neither young nor old; taking the child from the cradle, the mother from her babe, and the father from the family. Is it strange that man, unable to dissociate a personal element from such work, has incarnated an evil principle—the devil? If we have now so far outgrown this idea as to hesitate to suggest, in seasons of epidemic peril, that "it is for our sins we suffer"—when we know the drainage is bad; if we no longer mock the heart prostrate in the grief of loss with the words "whom the Lord loveth He chasteneth"—when we know the milk should have been sterilized—if, I say, we have, in a measure, become emancipated from such teachings, we have not yet risen to a true conception of Nature. Cruel, in the sense of being inexorable, she may be called, but we can no more upbraid her great laws than we can the lesser laws of the state, which are a terror only to evildoers. The pity is that we do not know them all; in our ignorance we err daily, and pay a blood penalty. Fortunately it is now a great and growing function of the medical profession to search out the laws about epidemics, and these outside enemies of man, and to teach to you, the public—dull, stupid pupils you are, too, as a rule—the ways of Nature, that you may walk therein and prosper.

It would be interesting, Members of the Graduating Class, to cast your horoscopes. To do so collectively you would not like; to do so individually—I dare not; but it is safe to predict certain things of you, as a whole. You will be better women for the life which you have led here. But what I mean by "better women" is that the eyes of your souls have been opened, the range of your sympathies has been widened, and your characters have been moulded by the events in which you have been participators during the past two years.

Practically there should be for each of you a busy, useful, and happy life; more you cannot expect; a greater blessing the world cannot bestow. Busy you will certainly be, as the demand is great, both in private and public, for women with your training. Useful your lives must be, as you will care for those who cannot care for themselves, and who need about them, in the day of tribulation, gentle hands and tender hearts. And happy lives shall be yours, because busy and useful; having been initiated into the great secret— that happiness lies in the absorption in some vocation which satisfies the soul; that we are here to add what we can *to*, not to get what we can *from*, life.

And, finally, remember what we are—useful supernumeraries in the battle, simply stage accessories in the drama, playing minor, but essential, parts at the exits and entrances, or picking up, here and there, a strutter, who may have tripped upon the stage. You have been much by the dark river—so near to us all—and have seen so many embark, that the dread of the old boatman has almost disappeared, and

When the Angel of the darker Drink
At last shall find you by the river brink,
And offering his cup, invite your soul
Forth to your lips to quaff—you shall not shrink:

your passport shall be the blessing of Him in whose footsteps you have trodden, unto whose sick you have ministered, and for whose children you have cared.

III
TEACHER AND STUDENT

A University consists, and has ever consisted, in demand and supply in wants which it alone can satisfy and which it does satisfy, in the communication of knowledge, and the relation and bond which exists between the teacher and the taught. Its constituting, animating principle is this moral attraction of one class of persons to another; which is prior in its nature, nay commonly in its history, to any other tie whatever; so that, where this is wanting, a University is alive only in name, and has lost its true essence, whatever be the advantages, whether of position or of affluence, with which the civil power or private benefactors contrive to encircle it.

JOHN HENRY NEWMAN.

It would seem, Adeimantus, that the direction in which education starts a man will determine his future life.

PLATO, *Republic*, iv.—Jowett's Translation.

III

TEACHER AND STUDENT[1]

I

TRULY it may be said to-day that in the methods of teaching medicine the old order changeth, giving place to new, and to this revolution let me briefly refer, since it has an immediate bearing on the main point I wish to make in the first portion of my address. The medical schools of the country have been either independent, University, or State Institutions. The first class, by far the most numerous, have in title University affiliations, but are actually devoid of organic union with seats of learning. Necessary as these bodies have been in the past, it is a cause for sincere congratulation that the number is steadily diminishing. Admirable in certain respects—adorned too in many instances by the names of men who bore the burden and heat of the day of small things, and have passed to their rest amid our honoured dead—the truth must be acknowledged that the lamentable state of medical education in this country twenty years ago was the direct result of the inherent viciousness of a system they fostered. Something in the scheme gradually deadened in the professors all sense of the responsibility until they professed to teach (mark the word), in less than two years, one of the most difficult arts in the world to acquire. Fellow teachers in medicine, believe me that when fifty or sixty years hence some historian traces the development of the profession in this country, he will dwell on the notable achievements, on the

[1] University of Minnesota, 1892.

great discoveries, and on the unwearied devotion of its members, but he will pass judgment—yes, severe judgment —on the absence of the sense of responsibility which permitted a criminal laxity in medical education unknown before in our annals. But an awakening has come, and there is sounding the knell of doom for the medical college, responsible neither to the public nor the profession.

The schools with close university connexions have been the most progressive and thorough in this country. The revolution referred to began some twenty years ago with the appearance of the President of a well-known University at a meeting of its medical faculty with a peremptory command to set their house in order.[1]   Universities which teach only the Liberal Arts remain to-day, as in the middle ages, Scholæ minores, lacking the technical faculties which make the Scholæ majores. The advantages of this most natural union are manifold and reciprocal. The professors in a University medical school have not that independence of which I have spoken, but are under an influence which tends constantly to keep them at a high level: they are urged by emulation with the other faculties to improve the standard of work, and so are given a strong stimulus to further development.

To anyone who has watched the growth of the new ideas in education it is evident that the most solid advances in methods of teaching, the improved equipment, clinical and laboratory, and the kindlier spirit of generous rivalry— which has replaced the former debased method of counting heads as a test of merit—all these advantages have come from a tightening of the bonds between the medical school and the University.

[1] See Holmes on President Eliot in *Life and Letters of O. W. Holmes*, 1896, ii, 187, 188, 190.

And lastly there are the State schools, of which this college is one of the few examples. It has been a characteristic of American Institutions to foster private industries and to permit private corporations to meet any demands on the part of the public. This idea carried to extreme allowed the unrestricted manufacture—note the term—of doctors, quite regardless of the qualifications usually thought necessary in civilized communities—of physicians who may never have been inside a hospital ward, and who had, after graduation, to learn medicine somewhat in the fashion of the Chinese doctors who recognized the course of the arteries of the body, by noting just where the blood spurted when the acupuncture needle was inserted. So far as I know, State authorities have never interfered with any legally instituted medical school, however poorly equipped for its work, however lax the qualifications for license. Not only has this policy of non-intervention been carried to excess, but in many States a few physicians in any town could get a charter for a school without giving guarantees that laboratory or clinical facilities would be available. This anomalous condition is rapidly changing, owing partly to a revival of loyalty to higher ideals within the medical profession, and partly to a growing appreciation in the public of the value of physicians thoroughly educated in modern methods. A practical acknowledgment of this is found in the recognition in three States at least of medicine as one of the technical branches to be taught in the University supported by the people at large.

But it is a secondary matter, after all, whether a school is under State or University control, whether the endowments are great or small, the equipments palatial or humble; the fate of an institution rests not on these; the inherent, vital element, which transcends all material interests, which may give to a school glory and renown in their absence, and lacking which, all the "pride, pomp and circumstance" are vain—this vitalizing element, I say, lies in the men who work in its halls, and in the ideals which they cherish and teach. There is a passage in one of John Henry Newman's Historical Sketches which expresses this feeling in terse and beautiful language: "I say then, that the personal influence of the teacher is able in some sort to dispense with an academical system, but that system cannot in any way dispense with personal influence. With influence there is life, without it there is none; if influence is deprived of its due position, it will not by those means be got rid of, it will only break out irregularly, dangerously. An academical system without the personal influence of teachers upon pupils, is an Arctic winter; it will create an ice-bound, petrified, cast-iron University, and nothing else."

Naturally from this standpoint the selection of teachers is the function of highest importance in the Regents of a University. Owing to local conditions the choice of men for certain of the chairs is restricted to residents in the University town, as the salaries in most schools of this country have to be supplemented by outside work. But in all departments this principle should be acknowledged and acted upon by trustees and faculties, and supported by public opinion—that the very best men available should receive appointments. It is gratifying to note the broad liberality displayed by American colleges in welcoming from all parts teachers who may have shown any special fitness, emulating in this respect the liberality of the Athenians, in whose porticoes and lecture halls the stranger was greeted as a citizen and judged by his mental gifts alone. Not the least by any means of the object lessons taught by a great University is that literature and science know no country, and, as has been well said, acknowledge "no sovereignty but that of the mind, and no nobility but that of genius." But it is difficult in this matter to guide public opinion, and the Regents have often to combat a provincialism which is as fatal to the highest development of a University as is the shibboleth of a sectarian institution.

II

To paraphrase the words of Matthew Arnold, the function of the teacher is to teach and to propagate the best that is known and taught in the world. To teach the current knowledge of the subject he professes—sifting, analyzing, assorting, laying down principles. To propagate, i.e., to multiply, facts on which to base principles—experimenting, searching, testing. The best that is known and taught in the world—nothing less can satisfy a teacher worthy of the name, and upon us of the medical faculties lies a bounden duty in this respect, since our Art, co-ordinate with human suffering, is cosmopolitan.

There are two aspects in which we may view the teacher —as a worker and instructor in science, and as practitioner and professor of the art; and these correspond to the natural division of the faculty into the medical school proper and the hospital.

In this eminently practical country the teacher of science has not yet received full recognition, owing in part to the great expense connected with his work, and in part to carelessness or ignorance in the public as to the real strength of a nation. To equip and maintain separate laboratories in Anatomy, Physiology, Chemistry (physiological and pharmacological), Pathology and Hygiene, and to employ skilled teachers, who shall spend all their time in study and instruction, require a capital not to-day at the command of

any medical school in the land.   There are fortunate ones
with two or three departments well organized, not one
with all.   In contrast, Bavaria, a kingdom of the German
Empire, with an area less than this State, and a population
of five and a half millions, supports in its three University
towns flourishing medical schools with extensive laboratories, many of which are presided over by men of world-
wide reputation, the steps of whose doors are worn in many
cases by students who have crossed the Atlantic; seeking
the wisdom of methods and the virtue of inspiration not
easily accessible at home.   But there were professors in
Bavarian medical schools before Marquette and Joliet had
launched their canoes on the great stream which the intrepid
La Salle had discovered, before Du Lhut met Father
Hennepin below the falls of St. Anthony; and justice compels us to acknowledge that while winning an empire from
the back-woods the people of this land had more urgent
needs than laboratories of research.   All has now changed.
In this State, for example, the phenomenal growth of which
has repeated the growth of the nation, the wilderness has
been made to blossom as the rose, and the evidences of
wealth and prosperity on every side almost constrain one
to break out into the now old song, "Happy is that people
that is in such a case."

But in the enormous development of material interests
there is danger lest we miss altogether the secret of a nation's
life, the true test of which is to be found in its intellectual
and moral standards.   There is no more potent antidote
to the corroding influence of mammon than the presence in
a community of a body of men devoted to science, living
for investigation and caring nothing for the lust of the eyes
and the pride of life.   We forget that the measure of the
value of a nation to the world is neither the bushel nor the

barrel, but *mind;* and that wheat and pork, though useful and necessary, are but dross in comparison with those intellectual products which alone are imperishable. The kindly fruits of the earth are easily grown; the finer fruits of the mind are of slower development and require prolonged culture.

Each one of the scientific branches to which I have referred has been so specialized that even to teach it takes more time than can be given by a single Professor, while the laboratory classes also demand skilled assistance. The aim of a school should be to have these departments in the charge of men who have, first, *enthusiasm*, that deep love of a subject, that desire to teach and extend it without which all instruction becomes cold and lifeless; secondly, *a full personal knowledge of the branch taught;* not a second-hand information derived from books, but the living experience derived from experimental and practical work in the best laboratories. This type of instructor is fortunately not rare in American schools. The well-grounded students who have pursued their studies in England and on the Continent have added depth and breadth to our professional scholarship, and their critical faculties have been sharpened to discern what is best in the world of medicine. It is particularly in these branches that we need teachers of wide learning, whose standards of work are the highest known, and whose methods are those of the masters in Israel. Thirdly, men are required who have a *sense of obligation*, that feeling which impels a teacher to be also a contributor, and to add to the stores from which he so freely draws. And precisely here is the necessity to know the best that is taught in this branch, the world over. The investigator, to be successful, must start abreast of the knowledge of the day, and he differs from the teacher, who, living in the present, expounds only what is current, in that his thoughts must be in the future, and his ways and work in advance of the day in which he lives. Thus, unless a bacteriologist has studied methods thoroughly, and is familiar with the extraordinarily complex flora associated with healthy and diseased conditions, and keeps in touch with every laboratory of research at home and abroad, he will in attempting original work, find himself exploring ground already well-known, and will probably burden an already over-laden literature with faulty and crude observations. To avoid mistakes, he must know what is going on in the laboratories of England, France and Germany, as well as in those of his own country, and he must receive and read six or ten journals devoted to the subject. The same need for wide and accurate study holds good in all branches.

Thoroughly equipped laboratories, in charge of men, thoroughly equipped as teachers and investigators, is the most pressing want to-day in the medical schools of this country.

The teacher as a professor and practitioner of his art is more favoured than his brother, of whom I have been speaking; he is more common, too, and less interesting; though in the eyes of "the fool multitude who choose by show" more important. And from the standpoint of medicine as an art for the prevention and cure of disease, the man who translates the hieroglyphics of science into the plain language of healing is certainly the more useful. He is more favoured inasmuch as the laboratory in which he works, the hospital, is a necessity in every centre of population. The same obligation rests on him to know and to teach the best that is known and taught in the world—on the surgeon the obligation to know thoroughly the scientific principles on which his art is based, to be a master in the technique of his handicraft, ever studying, modifying, improving;—

on the physician, the obligation to study the natural history of diseases and the means for their prevention, to know the true value of regimen, diet and drugs in their treatment, ever testing, devising, thinking;—and upon both, to teach to their students habits of reliance, and to be to them examples of gentleness, forbearance and courtesy in dealing with their suffering brethren.

I would fain dwell upon many other points in the relation of the hospital to the medical school—on the necessity of ample, full and prolonged clinical instruction, and on the importance of bringing the student and the patient into close contact, not through the cloudy knowledge of the amphitheatre, but by means of the accurate, critical knowledge of the wards; on the propriety of encouraging the younger men as instructors and helpers in ward work; and on the duty of hospital physicians and surgeons to contribute to the advance of their art—but I pass on with an allusion to a very delicate matter in college faculties.

From one who, like themselves, has passed *la crise de quarante ans*, the seniors present will pardon a few plain remarks upon the disadvantages to a school of having too many men of mature, not to say riper, years. Insensibly, in the fifth and sixth decades, there begins to creep over most of us a change, noted physically among other ways in the silvering of the hair and that lessening of elasticity, which impels a man to open rather than to vault a five-barred gate. It comes to all sooner or later; to some it is only too painfully evident, to others it comes unconsciously, with no pace perceived. And with most of us this physical change has its mental equivalent, not necessarily accompanied by loss of the powers of application or of judgment; on the contrary, often the mind grows clearer and the memory more retentive, but the change is seen in a weakened receptivity and in an inability to adapt oneself to an altered intellectual environment. It is this loss of mental elasticity which makes men over forty so slow to receive new truths. Harvey complained in his day that few men above this critical age seemed able to accept the doctrine of the circulation of the blood, and in our own time it is interesting to note how the theory of the bacterial origin of certain diseases has had, as other truths, to grow to acceptance with the generation in which it was announced. The only safeguard in the teacher against this lamentable condition is to live in, and with the third decade, in company with the younger, more receptive and progressive minds.

There is no sadder picture than the Professor who has outgrown his usefulness, and, the only one unconscious of the fact, insists, with a praiseworthy zeal, upon the performance of duties for which the circumstances of the time have rendered him unfit. When a man nor wax nor honey can bring home, he should, in the interests of an institution, be dissolved from the hive to give more labourers room; though it is not every teacher who will echo the sentiment—

> Let me not live . . .
> After my flame lacks oil, to be the snuff
> Of younger spirits whose apprehensive senses
> All but new things disdain.

As we travel farther from the East, our salvation lies in keeping our faces toward the rising sun, and in letting the fates drag us, like Cacus his oxen, backward into the cave of oblivion.

III

Students of Medicine, Apprentices of the Guild, with whom are the promises, and in whom centre our hopes—let me congratulate you on the choice of calling which offers a combination of intellectual and moral interests found in no other profession, and not met with at all in the common pursuits of life—a combination which, in the words of Sir James Paget, "offers the most complete and constant union of those three qualities which have the greatest charm for pure and active minds—novelty, utility, and charity." But I am not here to laud our profession; your presence here on these benches is a guarantee that such praise is superfluous. Rather allow me, in the time remaining at my disposal, to talk of the influences which may make you good students— now in the days of your pupilage, and hereafter when you enter upon the more serious duties of life.

In the first place, acquire early the *Art of Detachment*, by which I mean the faculty of isolating yourselves from the pursuits and pleasures incident to youth. By nature man is the incarnation of idleness, which quality alone, amid the ruined remnants of Edenic characters, remains in all its primitive intensity. Occasionally we do find an individual who takes to toil as others to pleasure, but the majority of us have to wrestle hard with the original Adam, and find it no easy matter to scorn delights and live laborious days. Of special importance is this gift to those of you who reside for the first time in a large city, the many attractions of which offer a serious obstacle to its acquisition. The discipline necessary to secure this art brings in its train habits of self-control and forms a valuable introduction to the sterner realities of life.

I need scarcely warn you against too close attention to your studies. I have yet to meet a medical student, the hey-day in whose blood had been quite tamed in his college days; but if you think I have placed too much stress upon isolation in putting the Art of Detachment first in order amongst the *desiderata* let me temper the hard saying by telling you how with "labors assiduous due pleasures to mix." Ask of any active business man or a leader in a profession the secret which enables him to accomplish much work, and he will reply in one word, *system;* or as I shall term it, the *Virtue of Method*, the harness without which only the horses of genius travel. There are two aspects of this subject; the first relates to the orderly arrangement of your work, which is to some extent enforced by the roster of demonstrations and lectures, but this you would do well to supplement in private study by a schedule in which each hour finds its allotted duty. Thus faithfully followed day by day system may become at last engrained in the most shiftless nature, and at the end of a semester a youth of moderate ability may find himself far in advance of the student who works spasmodically, and trusts to *cramming.* Priceless as this virtue is now in the time of your probation, it becomes in the practising physician an incalculable blessing. The incessant and irregular demands upon a busy doctor make it very difficult to retain, but the public in this matter can be educated, and the men who practise with system, allotting a definite time of the day to certain work, accomplish much more and have at any rate a little leisure; while those who are unmethodical never catch up with the day's duties and worry themselves, their *confrères,* and their patients.

The other aspect of method has a deeper significance, hard for you to reach, not consoling when attained, since it lays bare our weaknesses. The practice of medicine is an art, based on science. Working with science, in science, for science, it has not reached, perhaps never will, the dignity of a complete science, with exact laws, like astronomy or engineering. Is there then no science of medicine? Yes, but in parts only, such as anatomy and physiology,

and the extraordinary development of these branches during
the present century has been due to the cultivation of
method, by which we have reached some degree of exactness, some certainty of truth.   Thus we can weigh the
secretions in the balance and measure the work of the heart
in foot-pounds.   The deep secrets of generation have been
revealed and the sesame of evolution has given us fairy
tales of science more enchanting than the Arabian Nights'
entertainment.   With this great increase in our knowledge
of the laws governing the processes of life, has been a corresponding, not less remarkable, advance in all that relates to
life in disorder, that is, disease.   The mysteries of heredity
are less mysterious, the operating room has been twice over
robbed of its terrors; the laws of epidemics are known, and
the miracle of the threshing floor of Araunah the Jebusite,
may be repeated in any town out of Bumbledom.   All this
change has come about by the observation of facts, by their
classification, and by the founding upon them of general
laws.   Emulating the persistence and care of Darwin, we
must collect facts with open-minded watchfulness, unbiased
by crotchets or notions; fact on fact, instance on instance,
experiment on experiment, facts which fitly joined together
by some master who grasps the idea of their relationship
may establish a general principle.   But in the practice of
medicine, where our strength should be lies our great weakness.   Our study is man, as the subject of accidents or
diseases.   Were he always, inside and outside, cast in the
same mould, instead of differing from his fellow man as
much in constitution and in his reaction to stimulus as in
feature, we should ere this have reached some settled principles in our art.   And not only are the reactions themselves
variable, but we, the doctors, are so fallible, ever beset with
the common and fatal facility of reaching conclusions from

superficial observations, and constantly misled by the ease with which our minds fall into the ruts of one or two experiences.

And thirdly add to the Virtue of Method, the *Quality of Thoroughness*, an element of such importance that I had thought of making it the only subject of my remarks. Unfortunately, in the present arrangement of the curriculum, few of you as students can hope to obtain more than a measure of it, but all can learn its value now, and ultimately with patience become living examples of its benefit.   Let me tell you briefly what it means.   A knowledge of the fundamental sciences upon which our art is based—chemistry, anatomy, and physiology—not a smattering, but a full and deep acquaintance, not with all the facts, that is impossible, but with the great principles based upon them.   You should, as students, become familiar with the methods by which advances in knowledge are made, and in the laboratory see clearly the paths the great masters have trodden, though you yourselves cannot walk therein.   With a good preliminary training and a due apportioning of time you can reach in these three essential studies a degree of accuracy which is the true preparation for your life duties.   It means such a knowledge of diseases and of the emergencies of life and of the means for their alleviation, that you are safe and trustworthy guides for your fellowmen.   You cannot of course in the brief years of pupilage so grasp the details of the various branches that you can surely recognize and successfully treat all cases.   But here if you have mastered certain principles is at any rate one benefit of thoroughness —you will avoid the sloughs of charlatanism.   Napoleon, according to Sainte Beuve, one day said when somebody was spoken of in his presence as a charlatan, "Charlatan as much as you please, but where is there not charlatanism?"

Now, thoroughness is the sole preventive of this widespread malady, which in medicine is not met with only outside of the profession. Matthew Arnold, who quotes the above from Sainte Beuve, defines charlatanism as the "confusing or obliterating the distinctions between excellent and inferior, sound and unsound, or only half sound, true and untrue or half true." The higher the standard of education in a profession the less marked will be the charlatanism, whereas no greater incentive to its development can be found than in sending out from our colleges men who have not had mental training sufficient to enable them to judge between the excellent and the inferior, the sound and the unsound, the true and the half true. And if we of the household are not free from the seductions of this vice, what of the people among whom we work? From the days of the sage of Endor, even the rulers have loved to dabble in it, while the public of all ages have ever revelled in its methods—today, as in the time of the Father of Medicine, one of whose contemporaries (Plato) thus sketches the world old trait: "And what a delightful life they lead! they are always doctoring and increasing and complicating their disorders and always fancying they will be cured by any nostrum which anybody advises them to try."

The Art of Detachment, the Virtue of Method, and the Quality of Thoroughness may make you students, in the true sense of the word, successful practitioners, or even great investigators; but your characters may still lack that which can alone give permanence to powers—the *Grace of Humility*. As the divine Italian at the very entrance to Purgatory was led by his gentle Master to the banks of the island and girt with a rush, indicating thereby that he had cast off all pride and self-conceit, and was prepared for his perilous ascent to the realms above, so should you, now at the outset of your journey take the reed of humility in your hands, in token that you appreciate the length of the way, the difficulties to be overcome, and the fallibility of the faculties upon which you depend.

In these days of aggressive self-assertion, when the stress of competition is so keen and the desire to make the most of oneself so universal, it may seem a little old-fashioned to preach the necessity of this virtue, but I insist for its own sake, and for the sake of what it brings, that a due humility should take the place of honour on the list. For its own sake, since with it comes not only a reverence for truth, but also a proper estimation of the difficulties encountered in our search for it. More perhaps than any other professional man, the doctor has a curious—shall I say morbid?—sensitiveness to (what he regards) personal error. In a way this is right; but it is too often accompanied by a *cocksureness* of opinion which, if encouraged, leads him to so lively a conceit that the mere suggestion of mistake under any circumstances is regarded as a reflection on his honour, a reflection equally resented whether of lay or of professional origin. Start out with the conviction that absolute truth is hard to reach in matters relating to our fellow creatures, healthy or diseased, that slips in observation are inevitable even with the best trained faculties, that errors in judgment must occur in the practice of an art which consists largely of balancing probabilities;—start, I say, with this attitude in mind, and mistakes will be acknowledged and regretted; but instead of a slow process of self-deception, with ever increasing inability to recognize truth, you will draw from your errors the very lessons which may enable you to avoid their repetition.

And, for the sake of what it brings, this grace of humility is a precious gift. When to the sessions of sweet silent thought you summon up the remembrance of your own imperfections, the faults of your brothers will seem less grievous, and, in the quaint language of Sir Thomas Browne, you will "allow one eye for what is laudable in them." The wrangling and unseemly disputes which have too often disgraced our profession arise, in a great majority of cases, on the one hand, from this morbid sensitiveness to the confession of error, and, on the other, from a lack of brotherly consideration, and a convenient forgetfulness of our own failings. Take to heart the words of the son of Sirach, winged words to the sensitive souls of the sons of Esculapius: "Admonish a friend, it may be he has not done it; and if he have done it, that he do it no more. Admonish thy friend, it may be he hath not said it; and if he have, that he speak it not again. Admonish a friend, for many times it is a slander, and believe not every tale." Yes, many times it is a slander, and believe not every tale.

The truth that lowliness is young ambition's ladder is hard to grasp, and when accepted harder to maintain. It is so difficult to be still amidst bustle, to be quiet amidst noise; yet, "*es bildet ein Talent sich in der Stille*" alone, in the calm life necessary to continuous work for a high purpose. The spirit abroad at present in this country is not favourable to this Teutonic view, which galls the quick apprehension and dampens the enthusiasm of the young American. All the same, it is true, and irksome at first though the discipline may be, there will come a time when the very fetters in which you chafed shall be a strong defence, and your chains a robe of glory.

Sitting in Lincoln Cathedral and gazing at one of the loveliest of human works—for such the angel Choir has been said to be—there arose within me, obliterating for the moment the thousand heraldries and twilight saints and dim emblazonings, a strong sense of reverence for the minds which had conceived and the hands which had executed such things of beauty. What manner of men were they who could, in those (to us) dark days, build such transcendent monuments? What was the secret of their art? By what spirit were they moved? Absorbed in thought, I did not hear the beginning of the music, and then, as a response to my reverie and arousing me from it, rang out the clear voice of the boy leading the antiphon, "That thy power, thy glory and the mightiness of thy kingdom might be known unto men." Here was the answer. Moving in a world not realized, these men sought, however feebly, to express in glorious structures their conceptions of the beauty of holiness, and these works, our wonder, are but the outward and visible signs of the ideals which animated them.

To us in very different days life offers nearly the same problems, but the conditions have changed, and, as has happened before in the world's history, great material prosperity has weakened the influence of ideals, and blurred the eternal difference between means and end. Still, the ideal State, the ideal Life, the ideal Church—what they are and how best to realize them—such dreams continue to haunt the minds of men, and who can doubt that their contemplation greatly assists the upward progress of our race? We, too, as a profession, have cherished standards, some of which, in words sadly disproportionate to my subject, I have attempted to portray.

My message is chiefly to you, Students of Medicine, since with the ideals entertained now your future is indissolubly bound. The choice lies open, the paths are plain before you. Always seek your own interests, make of a high and sacred calling a sordid business, regard your fellow creatures as so many tools of trade, and, if your heart's desire is for riches, they may be yours; but you will have bartered away the birthright of a noble heritage, traduced the physician's well-deserved title of the Friend of Man, and falsified the best traditions of an ancient and honourable Guild. On the other hand, I have tried to indicate some of the ideals which you may reasonably cherish. No matter though they are paradoxical in comparison with the ordinary conditions in which you work, they will have, if encouraged, an ennobling influence, even if it be for you only to say with Rabbi Ben Ezra, "what I aspired to be and was not, comforts me." And though this course does not necessarily bring position or renown, consistently followed it will at any rate give to your youth an exhilarating zeal and a cheerfulness which will enable you to surmount all obstacles—to your maturity a serene judgment of men and things, and that broad charity without which all else is nought—to your old age that greatest of blessings, peace of mind, a realization, maybe, of the prayer of Socrates for the beauty in the inward soul and for unity of the outer and the inner man; perhaps, of the promise of St. Bernard, *"pax sine crimine, pax sine turbine, pax sine rixa."*

IV
PHYSIC AND PHYSICIANS AS
DEPICTED IN PLATO

To one small people . . . it was given to create the principle of Progress. That people was the Greek. Except the blind forces of Nature, nothing moves in this world which is not Greek in its origin.

SIR HENRY MAINE, *Village Communities*, p. 238.

From the lifeless background of an unprogressive world—Egypt Syria, frozen Scythia—a world in which the unconscious social aggregate had been everything, the conscious individual, his capacity and rights, almost nothing, the Greek had stepped forth, like the young prince in the fable, to set things going.

WALTER PATER, *Plato and Platonism.*

These (years of vague, restless speculation) had now lasted long enough, and it was time for the *Meisterjahre* of quiet, methodical research to succeed if science was to acquire steady and sedentary habits instead of losing itself in a maze of phantasies, revolving in idle circles. It is the undying glory of the medical school of Cos that it introduced this innovation in the domain of its art, and thus exercised the most beneficial influence on the whole intellectual life of mankind. "Fiction to the right! Reality to the left!" was the battle-cry of this school in the war they were the first to wage against the excesses and defects of the nature-philosophy. Nor could it have found any more suitable champions, for the serious and noble calling of the physician, which brings him every day and every hour in close communion with nature, in the exercise of which mistakes in theory engender the most fatal practical consequences, has served in all ages as a nursery of the most genuine and incorruptible sense of truth. The best physicians must be the best observers, but the man who sees keenly, who hears clearly, and whose senses, powerful at the start, are sharpened and refined by constant exercise, will only in exceptional instances be a visionary or a dreamer.

GOMPERZ, *Greek Thinkers*, vol i.

IV

PHYSIC AND PHYSICIANS AS DEPICTED IN PLATO[1]

OUR Historical Club had under consideration last winter the subject of Greek Medicine. After introductory remarks and a description of the Æsculapian temples and worship by Dr. Welch, we proceeded to a systematic study of the Hippocratic writings, taking up in order, as found in them, medicine, hygiene, surgery, and gynæcology. Among much of interest which we gleaned, not the least important was the knowledge that as an art, medicine had made, even before Hippocrates, great progress, as much almost as was possible without a basis in the sciences of anatomy and physiology. Minds inquisitive, acute, and independent had been studying the problems of nature and of man; and several among the pre-Socratic philsophers had been distinguished physicians, notably, Pythagoras, Empedocles, and Democritus. Unfortunately we know but little of their views, or even of the subjects in medicine on which they wrote. In the case of Democritus, however, Diogenes Laërtius has preserved a list of his medical writings, which intensifies the regret at the loss of the works of this great man, the title of one of whose essays, "On Those who are Attacked with Cough after Illness," indicates a critical observation of disease, which Daremberg seems unwilling to allow to the pre-Hippocratic philosopher-physicians.

[1] Johns Hopkins Hospital Historical Club, 1893.

We gathered also that in the golden age of Greece, medicine had, as to-day, a triple relationship, with science, with gymnastics, and with theology. We can imagine an Athenian father of the early fourth century worried about the enfeebled health of one of his growing lads, asking the advice of Hippocrates about a suspicious cough, or sending him to the palæstra of Taureas for a systematic course in gymnastics; or, as Socrates advised, "when human skill was exhausted," asking the assistance of the divine Apollo, through his son, the "hero-physician," Æsculapius, at his temple in Epidaurus or at Athens itself. Could the Greek live over his parental troubles at the end of the nineteenth century, he would get a more exact diagnosis and a more rational treatment; but he might travel far to find so eminent a "professor" of gymnastic as Miccus for his boy, and in Christian science or faith-healing he would find our bastard substitute for the stately and gracious worship of the Æsculapian temple.[1]

From the Hippocratic writings alone we have a very imperfect knowledge of the state of medicine in the most brilliant period of Grecian history; and many details relating to the character and to the life of physicians are gleaned only from secular authors. So much of the daily life of a civilized community relates to problems of health and disease that the great writers of every age of necessity throw an important side-light, not only on the opinions of the people on these questions, but often on the condition of special knowledge in various branches. Thus a consider-

[1] For an account of "Æsculapius at Epidaurus and Athens," see chap. vi of Dyer's *Gods of Greece* (Macmillan, 1891), a chapter which contains also an excellent discussion on the relation of secular to priestly medicine. In chapter III of Pater's delightful story *Marius the Epicurean*, is a description of one of the Roman Æsculapia, and an account of the method of procedure in the "cure," the ridiculous aspects of which are so graphically described in the "Plutus" of Aristophanes.

able literature already illustrates the medical knowledge of Shakespeare, from whose doctors, apothecaries, and mad-folk much may be gathered as to the state of the profession in the latter part of the sixteenth century. So also the satire of Molière, malicious though it be, has preserved for us phases of medical life in the seventeenth century, for which we scan in vain the strictly medical writings of that period; and writers of our times, like George Eliot, have told for future generations in a character such as Lydgate, the little every-day details of the struggles and aspirations of the profession of the nineteenth century, of which we find no account whatever in the files of the *Lancet*.

We are fortunate in having had preserved the writings of the two most famous of the Greek philosophers—the great idealist, Plato, whose "contemplation of all time and all existence" was more searching than that of his predecessors, fuller than that of any of his disciples, and the great realist, Aristotle, to whose memory every department of knowledge still pays homage, and who has swayed the master-minds of twenty-two centuries. From the writings of both much may be gathered about Greek physic and physicians; but I propose in this essay to restrict myself to what I have culled from the *Dialogues of Plato*. I shall first speak of his physiological and pathological speculations; then I shall refer to the many interesting allusions to, and analogies drawn from, medicine and physicians; and, lastly, I shall try to estimate from the *Dialogues* the social standing of the Greek doctor, and shall speak on other points which bear upon the general condition of the profession. The quotations are made in every instance from Professor Jowett's translation, the third edition, 1892.[1]

[1] *The Dialogues of Plato*, translated into English by B. Jowett, M.A., Master of Balliol College, Oxford. At the Clarendon Press; first edition, 1871; third edition, 1892.

I

To our enlightened minds the anatomy and physiology
of Plato are crude and imperfect; as much or even more so
than those of Hippocrates.   In the *Timæus* he conceived
the elements to be made up of bodies in the form of triangles,
the different varieties and combinations of which accounted
for the existence of the four elementary bodies of Empedocles—fire, earth, water, and air.   The differences in the
elementary bodies are due to differences in the size and
arrangement of the elementary triangles, which, like the
atoms of the atomist, are too small to be visible.   Marrow
had the most perfect of the elementary triangles, and from
it bone, flesh, and the other structures of the body were
made.   "God took such of the primary triangles as were
straight and smooth, and were adapted by their perfection
to produce fire and water, and air and earth; these, I say, he
separated from their kinds, and mingling them in due proportions with one another, made the marrow out of them
to be a universal seed of the whole race of mankind; and in
this seed he then planted and enclosed the souls, and in the
original distribution gave to the marrow as many and
various forms as the different kinds of souls were hereafter
to receive.   That which, like a field, was to receive the
divine seed, he made round every way, and called that portion of the marrow brain, intending that, when an animal
was perfected, the vessel containing this substance should
be the head; but that which was intended to contain the
remaining and mortal part of the soul he distributed into
figures at once round and elongated, and he called them all
Jy the name 'marrow'; and to these, as to anchors, fasten-
ing the bonds of the whole soul, he proceeded to fashion
around them the entire framework of our body, constructing

for the marrow, first of all, a complete covering of bone."[1]

The account of the structure of bone and flesh, and of functions of respiration, digestion, and circulation is unintelligible to our modern notions. Plato knew that the blood was in constant motion; in speaking of inspiration and expiration, and the network of fire which interpenetrates the body, he says: "For when the respiration is going in and out, and the fire, which is fast bound within, follows it, and ever and anon moving to and fro, enters the belly and reaches the meat and drink, it dissolves them, and dividing them into small portions, and guiding them through the passages where it goes, pumps them as from a fountain into the channels of the veins, *and makes the stream of the veins flow through the body as through a conduit.*"[2] A complete circulation was unknown; but Plato understood fully that the blood was the source of nourishment,—"the liquid itself we call blood, which nourishes the flesh and the whole body, whence all parts are watered and empty spaces filled."[3] In the young, the triangles, or in modern parlance we would say the atoms, are new, and are compared to the keel of a vessel just off the stocks. They are locked firmly together, but form a soft and delicate mass freshly made of marrow and nourished on milk. The process of digestion is described as a struggle between the triangles out of which the meats and drinks are composed, and those of the bodily frame; and as the former are older and weaker the newer triangles of the body cut them up, and in this way the animal grows great, being nourished by a multitude of similar particles. The triangles are in constant fluctuation and change, and in the "Symposium" Socrates makes Diotima say, "A man is called the same, and yet in the short

[1] *Dialogues*, iii. 493   [2] Ibid. iii. 501.   [3] Ibid. iii. 503.

interval which elapses between youth and age, and in which every animal is said to have life and identity, he is undergoing a perpetual process of loss and reparation—hair, flesh, bones, and the whole body are always changing."[1]

The description of senility, euthanasia, and death is worth quoting: "But when the roots of the triangles are loosened by having undergone many conflicts with many things in the course of time, they are no longer able to cut or assimilate the food which enters, but are themselves easily divided by the bodies which come in from without. In this way every animal is overcome and decays, and this affection is called old age. And at last, when the bonds by which the triangles of the marrow are united no longer hold, and are parted by the strain of existence, they in turn loosen the bonds of the soul, and she, obtaining a natural release, flies away with joy. For that which takes place according to nature is pleasant, but that which is contrary to nature is painful. And thus death, if caused by disease or produced by wounds, is painful and violent; but that sort of death which comes with old age and fulfils the debt of nature is the easiest of deaths, and is accompanied with pleasure rather than with pain."[2]

The mode of origin and the nature of disease, as described in the *Timæus*, are in keeping with this primitive and imperfect science. The diseases of the body arise when any one of the four elements is out of place, or when the blood, sinews and flesh are produced in a wrong order. Much influence is attributed to the various kinds of bile. The worst of all diseases, he thinks, are those of the spinal marrow, in which the whole course of the body is reversed. Other diseases are produced by disorders of respiration; as by phlegm "when detained within by reason of the air

[1] *Dialogues*, i. 578.   [2] Ibid. iii. 503–4.

bubbles." This, if mingled with black bile and dispersed about the courses of the head produces epilepsy, attacks of which during sleep, he says, are not so severe, but when it assails those who are awake it is hard to be got rid of, and "being an affection of a sacred part, is most justly called sacred" *morbus sacer.* Of other disorders, excess of fire causes a continuous fever; of air, quotidian fever; of water, which is a more sluggish element than either fire or air, tertian fever; of earth, the most sluggish element of the four, is only purged away in a four-fold period, that is in a quartan fever.[1]

The psychology of Plato, in contrast to his anatomy and physiology, has a strangely modern savour, and the three-fold divisions of the mind into reason, spirit and appetite, represents very much the mental types recognized by students of the present day. The rational, immortal principle of the soul "the golden cord of reason" dwells in the brain "and inasmuch as we are a plant not of earthly but of heavenly growth, raises us from earth to our kindred who are in heaven." The mortal soul consists of two parts; the one with which man "loves and hungers and thirsts, and feels the flutterings of any other desire," is placed between the midriff and the boundary of the navel; the other, passion or spirit, is situated in the breast between the midriff and the neck, "in order that it might be under the rule of reason and might join with it in controlling and restraining the desires when they are no longer willing of their own accord to obey the word of command issuing from the citadel."[2]

No more graphic picture of the struggle between the rational and appetitive parts of the soul has ever been given than in the comparison of man in the *Phædrus* to a charioteer

[1] *Dialogues,* iii. 507–8.   [2] Ibid. iii. 491–2.

driving a pair of winged horses, one of which is noble and of noble breed; the other ignoble and of ignoble breed, so that "the driving of them of necessity gives a great deal of trouble to him."[1]

The comparison of the mind of man in the *Theœtetus* to a block of wax, "which is of different sizes in different men; harder, moister, and having more or less of purity in one than another, and in some of an intermediate quality," is one of the happiest of Plato's conceptions. This wax tablet is a gift of Memory, the mother of the Muses; "and when we wish to remember anything which we have seen, or heard or thought in our own minds, we hold the wax to the perceptions and thoughts, and in that material receive the impression of them as from the seal of a ring; and we remember and know what is imprinted as long as the image lasts; but when the image is effaced, or cannot be taken, then we forget and do not know."[2]

Another especially fortunate comparison is that of the mind to an aviary which is gradually occupied by different kinds of birds, which correspond to the varieties of knowledge. When we were children the aviary was empty, and as we grow up we go about "catching" the various kinds of knowledge.[3]

Plato recognized, in the *Timœus*, two kinds of mental disease, to wit, madness and ignorance. He has the notion advocated by advanced psychologists to-day, that much of the prevalent vice is due to an ill disposition of the body, and is involuntary; "for no man is voluntarily bad; but the bad become bad by reason of ill disposition of the body and bad education, things which are hateful to every man and happen to him against his will."[4]   A fuller discussion

---

[1] *Dialogues*, i. 452.   [2] Ibid. iv. 254–5.   [3] Ibid. iv. 262.
[4] Ibid. iii. 509.

of the theorem that madness and the want of sense are the same is found in the *Alcibiades* (II.); which is not, however, one of the genuine *Dialogues*. The different kinds of want of sense are very graphically described:

Socrates. In like manner men differ in regard to want of sense. Those who are most out of their wits we call "madmen," while we term those who are less far gone "stupid," or "idiotic," or if we prefer gentle language, describe them as "romantic" or "simple-minded," or again as "innocent," or "inexperienced," or "foolish." You may even find other names if you seek for them, but by all of them lack of sense is intended. They only differ as one art appears to us to differ from another, or one disease from another.

There is a shrewd remark in the *Republic* "that the most gifted minds, when they are ill-educated, become pre-eminently bad. Do not great crimes and the spirit of pure evil spring out of a fulness of nature ruined by education rather than from any inferiority, whereas weak natures are scarcely capable of any very great good or very great evil."[1]

In the *Phædrus* there is recognized a form of madness "which is a divine gift and a source of the chiefest blessings granted to man." Of this there are four kinds—prophecy, inspiration, poetry and love. That indefinable something which makes the poet as contrasted with the rhymster and which is above and beyond all art, is well characterized in the following sentence: "But he who, having no touch of the Muse's madness in his soul, comes to the door and thinks that he will get into the temple by the help of art—he, I say, and his poetry are not admitted. The sane man disappears and is nowhere when he enters into rivalry with a madman."[2] Certain crimes, too, are definitely recognized as manifestations of insanity; in the *Laws* the incurable

[1] *Dialogues*, iii. 189.
[2] Ibid. i. 450–1, "Not by wisdom do poets write poetry, but by a sort of inspiration and genius."—*Apology*.

criminal is thus addressed: "Oh, sir, the impulse which moves you to rob temples is not an ordinary human malady, nor yet a visitation of heaven, but a madness which is begotten in man from ancient and unexpiated crimes of his race." In the *Laws*, too, it is stated that there are many sorts of madness, some arising out of disease, and others originating in an evil and passionate temperament, and increased by bad education. Respecting the care of the insane, it is stated that a madman shall not be at large in the city, but his relations shall keep him at home in any way they can, or if not, certain fines are mentioned.[1]

The greatest aid in the prevention of disease is to preserve the due proportion of mind and body, "for there is no proportion or disproportion more productive of health and disease, and virtue and vice, than that between soul and body." In the double nature of the living being if there is in this compound an impassioned soul more powerful than the body, "that soul, I say, convulses and fills with disorders the whole inner nature of man; and when eager in the pursuit of some sort of learning or study, causes wasting; or again, when teaching or disputing in private or in public, and considerations and controversies arise, inflames and dissolves the composite form of man and introduces rheums; and the nature of this phenomenon is not understood by most professors of medicine, who ascribe it to the opposite of the real cause." . . . Body and mind should both be equally exercised to protect against this disproportion, and "we should not move the body without the soul or the soul without the body. In this way they will be on their guard against each other, and be healthy and well balanced." He urges the mathematician to practise gymnastic, and the gymnast to cultivate music and philosophy.[2]

[1] *Dialogues*, v. 236, 323, 324.   [2] *Dialogues*, iii. 510–1.

The modes of treatment advised are simple, and it is evident that Plato had not much faith in medicines. Professor Jowett's commentary is here worth quoting: "Plato is still the enemy of the purgative treatment of physicians, which, except in extreme cases, no man of sense will ever adopt. For, as he adds, with an insight into the truth, 'every disease is akin to the nature of the living being and is only irritated by stimulants.' He is of opinion that nature should be left to herself, and is inclined to think that physicians are in vain (cf. *Laws*, VI. 761 C., where he says that warm baths would be more beneficial to the limbs of the aged rustic than the prescriptions of a not overwise doctor). If he seems to be extreme in his condemnation of medicine and to rely too much on diet and exercise, he might appeal to nearly all the best physicians of our own age in support of his opinions, who often speak to their patients of the worthlessness of drugs. For we ourselves are sceptical about medicine, and very unwilling to submit to the purgative treatment of physicians. May we not claim for Plato an anticipation of modern ideas as about some questions of astronomy and physics, so also about medicine? As in the *Charmides* (156, 7) he tells us that the body cannot be cured without the soul, so in the *Timæus* he strongly asserts the sympathy of soul and body; any defect of either is the occasion of the greatest discord and disproportion in the other. Here too may be a presentiment that in the medicine of the future the interdependence of mind and body will be more fully recognized, and that the influence of the one over the other may be exerted in a manner which is not now thought possible."[1]

The effect of the purgative method to which Plato was so opposed is probably referred to in the following passage.

[1] *Dialogues,* iii. 413

"When a man goes of his own accord to a doctor's shop and takes medicine, is he not quite aware that soon and for many days afterwards, he will be in a state of body which he would rather die than accept as a permanent condition of his life?"

It is somewhat remarkable that nowhere in the *Dialogues* is any reference made to the method of healing at the Æsculapian temples. The comments upon physic and physicians are made without allusion to these institutions. Hippocrates and other practitioners at Athens were probably secular Asclepiads, but as Dyer remarks, "in spite of the severance the doctors kept in touch with the worship of Æsculapius, and the priests in his temples did not scorn such secular knowledge as they could gain from lay practitioners."[1]

II

So much for the general conception of the structure and functions of the body, in order and disorder, as conceived by Plato. Were nothing more to be gleaned, the thoughts on these questions of one of the greatest minds of what was intellectually the most brilliant period of the race, would be of interest, but scattered throughout his writings are innumerably little *obiter dicta*, which indicate a profound knowledge of that side of human nature which turns uppermost when the machinery is out of gear. There are, in addition, many charming analogies drawn from medicine, and many acute suggestions, some of which have a modern flavour. The noble pilot and the wise physician who, as Nestor remarks, "is worth many another man," furnish some of the most striking illustrations of the *Dialogues*.

[1] *The Gods of Greece*

One of the most admirable definitions of the Art of Medicine I selected as a rubric with which to grace my text-book, "And I said of medicine, that this is an Art which considers the constitution of the patient, and has principles of action and reasons in each case." Or, again, the comprehensive view taken in the statement, "There is one science of medicine which is concerned with the inspection of health equally in all times, present, past and future."

Plato gives a delicious account of the origin of the modern medicine, as contrasted with the art of the guild of Asclepius.[1]

Well, I said, and to require the help of medicine, not when a wound has to be cured, or on occasion of an epidemic, but just because by indolence and a habit of life such as we have been describing, men fill themselves with waters and winds, as if their bodies were a marsh, compelling the ingenious sons of Asclepius to find more names for diseases, such as flatulence and catarrh; is not this, too, a disgrace?

Yes, he said, they do certainly give very strange and new-fangled names to diseases.

Yes, I said, and I do not believe there were any such diseases in the days of Asclepius; and this I infer from the circumstance that the hero Eurypylus, after he has been wounded in Homer, drinks a posset of Pramnian wine well besprinkled with barley-meal and grated cheese, which are certainly inflammatory, and yet the sons of Asclepius who were at the Trojan war do not blame the damsel who gives him the drink, or rebuke Patroclus, who is treating his case.

Well, he said, that was surely an extraordinary drink to be given to a person in his condition.

Not so extraordinary, I replied, if you bear in mind that in former days, as is commonly said, before the time of Herodicus, the guild of Asclepius did not practise our present system of medicine, which may be said to educate diseases. But Herodicus, being a trainer, and himself of a sickly constitution, by a combination of training and doctoring found out a way of torturing first and chiefly himself, and secondly the rest of the world.

How was that? he said.

By the invention of lingering death; for he had a mortal disease which he perpetually tended, and as recovery was out of the question, he passed

---

[1] *Dialogues*, iii. 93.

his entire life as a valetudinarian; he could do nothing but attend upon himself, and he was in constant torment whenever he departed in anything from his usual regimen, and so dying hard, by the help of science he struggled on to old age.

A rare reward of his skill!

He goes on to say that Asclepius did not instruct his descendants in valetudinarian arts because he knew that in well-ordered states individuals with occupations had no time to be ill.   If a carpenter falls sick, he asks the doctor for a "rough and ready cure—an emetic, or a purge, or a cautery, or the knife—these are his remedies."   Should any one prescribe for him a course of dietetics and tell him to swathe and swaddle his head, and all that sort of thing, he says, "he sees no good in a life spent in nursing his disease to the neglect of his customary employment; and therefore bidding good-bye to this sort of physician, he resumes his ordinary habits, and either gets well and lives and does his business, or, if his constitution fails, he dies and has no more trouble."[1]

He is more in earnest in another place (*Gorgias*) in an account of the relations of the arts of medicine and gymnastics: "The soul and the body being two, have two arts corresponding to them: there is the art of politics attending on the soul; and another art attending on the body, of which I know no specific name, but which may be described as having two divisions, one of them gymnastic, and the other medicine.   And in politics there is a legislative part, which answers to gymnastic, as justice does to medicine; and the two parts run into one another, justice having to do with the same subject as legislation, and medicine with the same subject as gymnastic, but with a difference. . . . Cookery simulates the disguise of medicine, and pretends to

[1] *Dialogues*, iii. 93–4.

know what food is the best for the body; and if the physician
and the cook had to enter into a competition in which
children were the judges, or men who had no more sense
than children, as to which of them best understands the
goodness or badness of food, the physician would be starved
to death."[1]

And later in the same dialogue Socrates claims to be the
only true politician of his time who speaks, not with any
view of pleasing, but for the good of the State, and is
unwilling to practise the graces of rhetoric—and so would
make a bad figure in a court of justice. He says: "I shall
be tried just as a physician would be tried in a court of
little boys at the indictment of the cook. What would he
reply under such circumstances, if some one were to accuse
him, saying, 'O my boys, many evil things has this man
done to you; he is the death of you, especially of the younger
ones among you, cutting and burning and starving and
suffocating you, until you know not what to do; he gives
you the bitterest potions, and compels you to hunger and
fast? How unlike the variety of meats and sweets on
which I feasted for you.' What do you suppose that the
physician would be able to reply when he found himself in
such a predicament? If he told the truth he could only
say: 'All these evil things, my boys I did for your health,'
and then would there not just be a clamour among a jury
like that? How they would cry out!"[2]

The principle of continuity, of uniformity, so striking in
ancient physics was transferred to the body, which, like
the world, was conceived as a whole. Several striking
passages illustrative of this are to be found. Thus to the
question of Socrates, "Do you think that you can know the
nature of the soul intelligently without knowing the nature

[1] *Dialogues,* ii. 345–6.   [2] Ibid. ii. 415.

of the whole?" Phædrus replies, "Hippocrates, the Asclepiad, says that the nature even of the body can only be understood as a whole."[1] The importance of treating the whole and not the part is insisted upon. In the case of a patient who comes to them with bad eyes the saying is "that they cannot cure his eyes by themselves, but that if his eyes are to be cured his head must be treated": and then again they say "that to think of curing the head alone and not the rest of the body also is the height of folly."

Charmides had been complaining of a headache, and Critias had asked Socrates to make believe that he could cure him of it. He said that he had a charm, which he had learnt, when serving with the army, of one of the physicians of the Thracian king, Zamolxis. This physician had told Socrates that the cure of the part should not be attempted without treatment of the whole, and also that no attempt should be made to cure the body without the soul, "and, therefore, if the head and body are to be well you must begin by curing the soul; that is the first thing. . . . And he who taught me the cure and the charm added a special direction, 'Let no one,' he said, 'persuade you to cure the head until he has first given you his soul to be cured. For this,' he said, 'is the great error of our day in the treatment of the human body, that physicians separate the soul from the body.' " The charms to which he referred were fair words by which temperance was implanted in the soul.[2]

Though a contemporary, Hippocrates is only once again referred to in the *Dialogues*—where the young Hippocrates, son of Apollodorus, who has come to Protagoras, "that almighty wise man," as Socrates terms him in another place, to learn the science and knowledge of human life, is asked by Socrates, "If you were going to Hippocrates of Cos, the

[1] *Dialogues*, i. 479.   [2] Ibid. i. 11–13.

Asclepiad, and were about to give him your money, and
some one had said to you, 'You are paying money to your
namesake, Hippocrates, O Hippocrates; tell me, what is he
that you give him money?' how would you have answered?"
"I should say," he replied, "that I gave money to him as a
physician." "And what will he make of you?" "A
physician,' he said[1]—a paragraph which would indicate that
Hippocrates was in the habit of taking pupils and teaching
them the art of medicine; and in the *Euthydemus*, with
reference to the education of physicians, Socrates says,
"that he would send such to those who profess the art, and
to those who demand payment for teaching the art, and
profess to teach it to any one who will come and learn."

We get a glimpse of the method of diagnosis, derived
doubtless from personal observation, possibly of the great
Hippocrates himself, whose critical knowledge of pulmonary
complaints we daily recognize in the use of his name in
association with the clubbed fingers of phthisis, and with
the succussion splash of pneumo-thorax. "Suppose some
one, who is inquiring into the health or some other bodily
quality of another: he looks at his face and at the tips of
his fingers, and then he says, 'Uncover your chest and back
to me that I may have a better view.' " And then Socrates
says to Protagoras, "Uncover your mind to me; reveal your
opinion, etc."[2]

One of the most celebrated medical passages is that in
which Socrates professes the art of a midwife practising
on the souls of men when they are in labour, and diagnos-
ing their condition, whether pregnant with the truth or
with some "darling folly." The entire section, though
long, must be quoted. Socrates is in one of his "little
difficulties" and wishes to know of the young Theætetus,

[1] *Dialogues*, i. 131–2.   [2] Ibid. i. 176.

who has been presented to him as a paragon of learning, and whose progress in the path of knowledge has been sure and smooth—"flowing on silently like a river of oil"— what is knowledge?   Theætetus is soon entangled and cannot shake off a feeling of anxiety.

Theæt.   I can assure you, Socrates, that I have tried very often, when the report of questions asked by you was brought to me; but I can neither persuade myself that I have any answer to give, nor hear of any one who answers as you would have him; and I cannot shake off a feeling of anxiety.

Soc.   These are the pangs of labour, my dear Theætetus; you have something within you which you are bringing to the birth.

Theæt.   I do not know, Socrates; I only say what I feel.

Soc.   And did you never hear, simpleton, that I am the son of a midwife, brave and burly, whose name was Phænarete?

Theæt.   Yes, I have.

Soc.   And that I myself practise midwifery?

Theæt.   No, never.

Soc.   Let me tell you that I do though, my friend; but you must not reveal the secret, as the world in general have not found me out; and therefore they only say of me, that I am the strangest of mortals, and drive men to their wits' end.   Did you ever hear that too?

Theæt.   Yes.

Soc.   Shall I tell you the reason?

Theæt.   By all means.

Soc.   Bear in mind the whole business of the midwives, and then you will see my meaning better.   No woman, as you are probably aware, who is still able to conceive and bear, attends other women, but only those who are past bearing.

Theæt.   Yes, I know.

Soc.   The reason of this is said to be that Artemis—the goddess of childbirth—is not a mother, and she honours those who are like herself; but she could not allow the barren to be midwives, because human nature cannot know the mystery of an art without experience; and therefore she assigned this office to those who are too old to bear.

Theæt.   I dare say.

Soc.   And I dare say, too, or rather I am absolutely certain, that the midwives know better than others who is pregnant and who is not?

Theæt.   Very true.

Soc.   And by the use of potions and incantations they are able to arouse the pangs and to soothe them at will; they can make those bear who have a difficulty in bearing, and if they think fit, they can smother the embryo in the womb.

Theæt. They can.

Soc. Did you ever remark that they are also most cunning match-makers, and have a thorough knowledge of what unions are likely to produce a brave brood?

Theæt. No, never.

Soc. Then let me tell you that this is their greatest pride, more than cutting the umbilical cord. And if you reflect, you will see that the same art which cultivates and gathers in the fruits of the earth, will be most likely to know in what soils the several plants or seeds should be deposited.

Theæt. Yes, the same art.

Soc. And do you suppose that with women the case is otherwise?

Theæt. I should think not.

Soc. Certainly not; but midwives are respectable women and have a character to lose, and they avoid this department of their profession, because they are afraid of being called procuresses, which is a name given to those who join together man and woman in an unlawful and unscientific way; and yet the true midwife is also the true and only matchmaker.

Theæt. Clearly.

Soc. Such are the midwives, whose task is a very important one, but not so important as mine; for women do not bring into the world at one time real children, and at another time counterfeits which are with difficulty distinguished from them; if they did, then the discernment of the true and false birth would be the crowning achievement of the art of midwifery—you would think so?

Theæt. Indeed I should.

Soc. Well, my art of midwifery is in most respects like theirs; but differs in that I attend men and not women, and I look after their souls when they are in labour, and not after their bodies; and the triumph of my art is in thoroughly examining whether the thought which the mind of the young man is bringing to the birth, is a false idol or a noble and true birth. And like the midwives, I am barren, and the reproach which is often made against me, that I ask questions of others and have not the wit to answer them myself, is very just; the reason is, that the god compels me to be a midwife, but forbids me to bring forth. And therefore I am not myself at all wise, nor have I anything to show which is the invention or birth of my own soul, but those who converse with me profit. Some of them appear dull enough at first, but afterwards, as our acquaintance ripens, if the god is gracious to them, they all make astonishing progress; and this in the opinion of others as well as their own. It is quite clear that they had never learned anything from me; the many fine discoveries to which they cling are of their own making. But to me and the god they owe their delivery. And the proof of my words is, that many of them in their ignorance, either in their self-conceit despising me, or falling under the influence of others, have gone away too soon; and have not only lost the children of whom I had previously delivered them by an ill bringing up, but have stifled whatever else they had in them by evil communications, being fonder of lies and shams than of the truth; and they have at last ended by seeing themselves, as others see them, to be great fools. Aristeides, the son of Lysimachus, is one of them, and there are many others. The truants often return to me, and beg that I would consort with them again—they are ready to go to me on their knees—and then, if my familiar allows, which is not always the case, I receive them and they begin to grow again. Dire are the pangs which my art is able to arouse and to allay in those who consort with me, just like the pangs of women in childbirth; night and day they are full of perplexity and travail which is even worse than that of the women. So much for them. And there are others, Theætetus, who come to me apparently having nothing in them; and as I know that they have no need of my art, I coax them into marrying some one, and by the grace of God I can generally tell who is likely to do them good. Many of them I have given away to Prodicus, and many to other inspired sages. I tell you this long story, friend Theætetus, because I suspect, as indeed you seem to think yourself, that you are in labour— great with some conception. Come then to me, who am a midwife's son and myself a midwife, and try to answer the questions which I will ask you. And if I abstract and expose your first-born, because I discover upon inspection that the conception which you have formed is a vain shadow, do not quarrel with me on that account, as the manner of women is when their first children are taken from them. For I have actually known some who were ready to bite me when I deprived them of a darling folly; they did not perceive that I acted from good will, not knowing that no god is the enemy of man—that was not within the range of their ideas; neither am I their enemy in all this, but it would be wrong in me to admit falsehood, or to stifle the truth. Once more, then, Theætetus, I repeat my old question, "What is knowledge?" and do not say that you cannot tell; but quit yourself like a man, and by the help of God you will be able to tell.[1]

Socrates proceeds to determine whether the intellectual babe brought forth by Theætetus is a wind-egg or a real and genuine birth. "This then is the child, however he may turn out, which you and I have with difficulty brought

[1] *Dialogues*, iv. 201–4.

into the world, and now that he is born we must run round
the hearth with him and see whether he is worth rearing or
only a wind-egg and a sham.   Is he to be reared in any case
and not exposed? or will you bear to see him rejected and not
get into a passion if I take away your first-born?" The
conclusion is "that you have brought forth wind, and that
the offspring of your brain are not worth bringing up." And
the dialogue ends as it began with a reference to the midwife:
"The office of a midwife I, like my mother, have received
from God; she delivered women, and I deliver men; but
they must be young and noble and fair."

III

From the writings of Plato we may gather many details
about the status of physicians in his time. It is very
evident that the profession was far advanced and had been
progressively developing for a long period before Hippocrates, whom we erroneously, yet with a certain propriety,
call the *Father of Medicine*. The little by-play between
Socrates and Euthydemus suggests an advanced condition
of medical literature: "Of course, you who have so many
books are going in for being a doctor," says Socrates, and
then he adds, "there are so many books on medicine, you
know." As Dyer remarks, whatever the quality of these
books may have been, their number must have been great
to give point to this chaff.

It may be clearly gathered from the writings of Plato that
two sorts of physicians (apart altogether from quacks and
the Æsculapian guild) existed in Athens, the private practitioner, and the State-physician. The latter, though the
smaller numerically, representing apparently the most
distinguished class. From a reference in one of the dia-

logues (*Gorgias*) they evidently were elected by public assembly,—"when the assembly meets to elect a physician."[1] The office was apparently yearly, for in the *Statesman* is the remark, "when the year of office has expired, the pilot or physician has to come before a court of review" to answer any charges that may be made against him. In the same dialogue occurs the remark, "and if anyone who is in a private station has the art to advise one of the public physicians, must he not be called a physician?"[2] Apparently a physician must have been in practice for some time and attained great eminence before he was deemed worthy of the post of State-physician. "If you and I were physicians, and were advising one another that we were competent to practise as state-physicians, should I not ask you, and would you not ask me, Well, but how about Socrates himself, has he good health? And was any one else ever known to be cured by him whether slave or freeman?"[3]

A reference to the two sorts of doctors is also found in the *Republic:* "Now you know that when patients do not require medicine, but have only to be put under a regimen, the inferior sort of practitioner is deemed to be good enough; but when medicine has to be given, then the doctor should be more of a man."[4]

The office of State-physician was in existence fully two generations before this time, for Democedes held this post at Athens in the second half of the sixth century at a salary of £406, and, very much as a modern professor might be, he was seduced away by the offer of a great increase in salary by Polycrates, the tyrant of Samos. It is evident, too, from the *Laws*, that the doctors had assistants, often among the slaves.

[1] *Dialogues*, ii. 335. [2] Ibid. iv. 453, 502. [3] Ibid. ii. 407.
[4] Ibid. iii. 153.

For of doctors, as I may remind you, some have a gentler, others a ruder method of cure; and as children ask the doctor to be gentle with them, so we will ask the legislator to cure our disorders with the gentlest remedies. What I mean to say is, that besides doctors there are doctors' servants, who are also styled doctors.

Cle. Very true.

Œth. And whether they are slaves or freemen makes no difference; they acquire their knowledge of medicine by obeying and observing their masters; empirically and not according to the natural way of learning, as the manner of freemen is, who have learned scientifically themselves the art which they impart scientifically to their pupils. You are aware that there are these two classes of doctors?

Cle. To be sure.

Œth. And did you ever observe that there are two classes of patients in states, slaves and freemen; and the slave doctors run about and cure the slaves, or wait for them in the dispensaries—practitioners of this sort never talk to their patients individually, or let them talk about their own individual complaints? The slave-doctor prescribes what mere experience suggests, as if he had exact knowledge; and when he has given his orders, like a tyrant, he rushes off with equal assurance to some other servant who is ill; and so he relieves the master of the house of the care of his invalid slaves. But the other doctor, who is a freeman, attends and practises upon freemen; and he carries his inquiries far back, and goes into the nature of the disorder; he enters into discourse with the patient and with his friends, and is at once getting information from the sick man, and also instructing him as far as he is able, and he will not prescribe for him until he has first convinced him; at last, when he has brought the patient more and more under his persuasive influences and set him on the road to health, he attempts to effect a cure. Now which is the better way of proceeding in a physician and in a trainer? Is he the better who accomplishes his ends in a double way, or he who works in one way, and that the ruder and inferior?[1]

This idea of first convincing a patient by argument is also mentioned in the *Gorgias*, and would appear indeed to have furnished occupation for some of the numerous sophists of that period. Gorgias, lauding the virtues of rhetoric and claiming that she holds under her sway all the inferior arts, says: "Let me offer you a striking example of this. On several occasions I have been with my brother Herodicus,

[1] *Dialogues*, v. 103–4.

or some other physician, to see one of his patients, who
would not allow the physician to give him medicine or apply
the knife or hot iron to him; and I have persuaded him to do
for me what he would not do for the physician just by the
use of rhetoric. And I say that if a rhetorician and a
physician were to go to any city, and had there to argue in
the Ecclesia or any other assembly as to which of them
should be elected state-physician, the physician would have
no chance; but he who could speak would be chosen if he
wished."[1] In another place (*Laws*) Plato satirizes this
custom: "For of this you may be very sure, that if one of
those empirical physicians, who practise medicine without
science, were to come upon the gentleman physician talking
to his gentleman patient, and using the language almost of
philosophy—beginning at the beginning of the disease, and
discoursing about the whole nature of the body, he would
burst into a hearty laugh—he would say what most of those
who are called doctors always have at their tongue's end:
foolish fellow, he would say, you are not healing the sick
man, but you are educating him; and he does not want to be
made a doctor, but to get well."[2]

Of the personal qualifications of the physician not much
is said; but in the *Republic* (III. 408) there is an original,
and to us not very agreeable, idea: "Now the most skilful
physicians are those who, from their youth upwards, have
combined with a knowledge of their art, the greatest experience of disease; they had better not be in robust health, and
should have had all manner of diseases in their own person.
For the body, as I conceive, is not the instrument with
which they cure the body; in that case we could not allow
them ever to be or to have been sickly; but they cure the

<hr>

[1] *Dialogues*, ii. 336.   [2] Ibid. v. 240.

body with the mind, and the mind which has become and is sick can cure nothing."[1]

Some idea of the estimate which Plato put on the physician may be gathered from the mystical account in the *Phædrus* of the nature of the soul and of life in the upper world. We are but animated failures—the residua of the souls above, which have attained a vision of truth, but have fallen "hence beneath the double load of forgetfulness and vice." There are nine grades of human existence into which these souls may pass, from that of a philosopher or artist to that of a tyrant. The physician or lover of gymnastic toils comes in the fourth class.[2]

But if Plato assigns the physician a place in the middle tier in his mystery, he welcomes him socially into the most select and aristocratic circle of Athens. In that most festive of all festal occasions, at the house of Agathon; described in the *Symposium*, Eryximachus, a physician and the son of one, is a chief speaker, and in his praise of love says, "from medicine I will begin that I may do honour to my art." We find him, too, on the side of temperance and sobriety: "The weak heads like myself, Aristodemus, Phædrus, and others who never can drink, are fortunate in finding that the stronger ones are not in a drinking mood. (I do not include Socrates, who is able either to drink or to abstain, and will not mind, whichever we do.) Well, as none of the company seem disposed to drink much, I may be forgiven for saying, as a physician, that drinking deep is a bad practice, which I never follow, if I can help, and certainly do not recommend to another, least of all to any one who still feels the effect of yesterday's carouse." The prescriptions for hiccough, given by Eryximachus, give verisimilitude to the dialogue. When the turn of Aristo-

---

[1] *Dialogues*, iii. 96.   [2] Ibid. i. 454.

phanes came he had eaten too much and had the hiccough, and he said to Eryximachus, "You ought either to stop my hiccough or speak in my turn." Eryximachus recommended him to hold his breath, or if that failed to gargle with a little water, and if the hiccough still continued, to tickle his nose with something and sneeze, adding, "if you sneeze once or twice even the most violent hiccough is sure to go."[1]

Upon the medical symptoms narrated in that memorable scene, unparalleled in literature, after Socrates had drunk the poison in prison, it is unnecessary to dwell; but I may refer to one aspect as indicating the reverence felt for the representative of the great Healer. Denied his wish (by the warning of the jailor, who says that there is only sufficient poison) to offer a libation to a god, Socrates' dying words were, "Crito, we owe a cock to Æsculapius." "The meaning of this solemnly smiling farewell of Socrates would seem to be," according to Dyer, "that to Æsculapius, a god who always is prescribing potions and whose power is manifest in their effects, was due that most welcome and sovereign remedy which cured all the pains and ended all the woes of Socrates—the hemlock, which cured him of life which is death, and gave him the glorious realities of hereafter. For this great boon of awakening into real life Socrates owed Æsculapius a thankoffering. This offering of a cock to Æsculapius was plainly intended for him as the awakener of the dead to life everlasting."

And permit me to conclude this already too long account with the eulogium of Professor Jowett—words worthy of the master, worthy of his great interpreter to this generation:

"More than two thousand two hundred years have passed away since he returned to the place of Apollo and the Muses.

[1] *Dialogues,* i. 546, 555, 556.

Yet the echo of his words continues to be heard among men, because of all philosophers he has the most melodious voice. He is the inspired prophet or teacher who can never die, the only one in whom the outward form adequately represents the fair soul within; in whom the thoughts of all who went before him are reflected and of all who come after him are partly anticipated. Other teachers of philosophy are dried up and withered—after a few centuries they have become dust; but he is fresh and blooming, and is always begetting new ideas in the minds of men. They are one-sided and abstract; but he has many sides of wisdom. Nor is he always consistent with himself, because he is always moving onward, and knows that there are many more things in philosophy than can be expressed in words, and that truth is greater than consistency. He who approaches him in the most reverent spirit shall reap most of the fruits of his wisdom; he who reads him by the light of ancient commentators will have the least understanding of him.

"We may see him with the eye of the mind in the groves of the Academy, or on the banks of the Ilissus, or in the streets of Athens, alone or walking with Socrates, full of these thoughts which have since become the common possession of mankind. Or we may compare him to a statue hid away in some temple of Zeus or Apollo, no longer existing on earth, a statue which has a look as of the God himself. Or we may once more imagine him following in another state of being the great company of heaven which he beheld of old in a vision (*Phædrus*, 248). So, 'partly trifling but with a degree of seriousness' (*Symposium*, 197, E), we linger around the memory of a world which has passed away (*Phædrus*, 250, C)."

V
THE LEAVEN OF SCIENCE

Knowledge comes, but wisdom lingers.

Locksley Hall, TENNYSON.

Who loves not knowledge?   Who shall rail
  Against her beauty?   May she mix
  With men and prosper!   Who shall fix
Her pillars?   Let her work prevail.

In Memoriam, CXIV, TENNYSON

V

THE LEAVEN OF SCIENCE[1]

I

IN the continual remembrance of a glorious past individuals and nations find their noblest inspiration, and if to-day this inspiration, so valuable for its own sake, so important in its associations, is weakened, is it not because in the strong dominance of the individual, so characteristic of a democracy, we have lost the sense of continuity? As we read in Roman history of the ceremonies commemorative of the departed, and of the scrupulous care with which, even at such private festivals as the Ambarvalia, the dead were invoked and remembered, we appreciate, though feebly, the part which this sense of continuity played in the lives of their successors—an ennobling, influence, through which the cold routine of the present received a glow of energy from "the touch divine of noble natures gone." In our modern lives no equivalent to this feeling exists, and the sweet and gracious sense of an ever-present immortality, recognized so keenly and so closely in the religion of Numa, has lost all value to us. We are even impatient of those who would recall the past, and who would insist upon the importance of its recognition as a factor in our lives, impatient as we are of everything save the present with its prospects, the future with its possibilities. Year by year the memory of the men who made this institution fades from out the circle of the hills, and the shadow of oblivion

[1] An address delivered at the opening of The Wistar Institute of Anatomy and Biology, May 21, 1894.

falls deeper and deeper over their forms, until a portrait, or perhaps a name alone, remains to link the dead with the quick. To be forgotten seems inevitable, but not without a sense of melancholy do we recognize that the daily life of three thousand students and teachers is passed heedless of the fame, careless of the renown of these men; and in the second state sublime it must sadden the "circle of the wise," as they cast their eyes below, to look down on festivals in which they play no part, on gatherings in which their names are neither invoked nor blessed. But ours the loss, since to us, distant in humanity, the need is ever present to cherish the memories of the men who in days of trial and hardship laid on broad lines the foundations of the old colonial colleges.

To-day, through the liberality of General Wistar, we dedicate a fitting monument to one of the mighty dead of the University—Caspar Wistar. The tribute of deeds has already been paid to him in this splendid structure, to all in the stately group of academic buildings which you now see adorning the campus—the tribute of words remains, to be able to offer which I regard a very special honour.

But as this is an Institute of Anatomy, our tribute to-day may be justly restricted, in its details at least, to a eulogy upon the men who have taught the subject in this University. About the professorship of anatomy cluster memories which give it precedence of all others, and in the septemviri of the old school the chairs were arranged, with that of anatomy in the centre, with those of physiology, chemistry, and materia medica on the left, and with those of practice, surgery, and obstetrics on the right. With the revival of learning anatomy brought life and liberty to the healing art, and throughout the sixteenth, seventeenth, and eighteenth centuries the great names of the profession, with but one or two exceptions, are those of the great anatomists. The University of Pennsylvania has had an extraordinary experience in the occupancy of this important chair. In the century and a quarter which ended with the death of Leidy, six names appear on the faculty roll as professors of this branch. Dorsey, however, only delivered the introductory lecture to the course, and was seized the same evening with his fatal illness; and in the next year Physick was transferred from the chair of surgery, with Horner as his adjunct. In reality, therefore, only four men have taught anatomy in this school since its foundation. Physick's name must ever be associated with the chair of surgery. We do not know the faculty exigencies which led to the transfer, but we can readily surmise that the youthfulness of Horner, who was only twenty-six, and the opportunity of filching for surgery so strong a man as Gibson from the Faculty of the University of Maryland, then a stout rival, must have been among the most weighty considerations.

If in the average length of the period of each incumbency the chair of anatomy in the University is remarkable, much more so is it for the quality of the men who followed each other at such long intervals. It is easy to praise the Athenians among the Athenians, but where is the school in this country which can show such a succession of names in this branch: Shippen, the first teacher of anatomy; Wistar, the author of the first text-book of anatomy; Horner, the first contributor to human anatomy in this country; and Leidy, one of the greatest comparative anatomists of his generation? Of European schools, Edinburgh alone presents a parallel picture, as during the same period only four men have held the chair. The longevity and tenacity of the three Monros have become proverbial; in succession they held the chair of anatomy for 126 years.

Shortly before the foundation of this school Monro *secundus* had succeeded his father, and taught uninterruptedly for fifty years. His son, Monro *tertius*, held the chair for nearly the same length of time, and the remainder of the period has been covered by the occupancy of John Goodsir, and his successor, Sir William Turner, the present incumbent.

To one feature in the history of anatomy in this school I must refer in passing. Shippen was a warm personal friend and house-pupil of John Hunter. Physick not only had the same advantages, but became in addition his house-surgeon at St. George's Hospital. Both had enjoyed the intimate companionship of the most remarkable observer of nature since Aristotle, of a man with wider and more scientific conceptions and sympathies than had ever before been united in a member of our profession, and whose fundamental notions of disease are only now becoming prevalent. Can we doubt that from this source was derived the powerful inspiration which sustained these young men. One of them, on his return from England, at once began the first anatomical classes which were held in the colonies; the other entered upon that career so notable and so honourable, which led to the just title of the Father of American Surgery. It is pleasant to think that direct from John Hunter came the influence which made anatomy so strong in this school, and that zeal in the acquisition of specimens which ultimately led to the splendid collections of the Wistar-Horner Museum.

William Shippen the younger shares with John Morgan the honour of establishing medical instruction in this city. When students in England they had discussed plans, but it was Morgan who seems to have had the ear of the trustees, and who broached a definite scheme in his celebrated "Discourse," delivered in May, 1765. It was not until the autumn of the year that Shippen signified to the board his willingness to accept a professorship of anatomy and surgery.   He had enjoyed, as I have mentioned, the friendship of John Hunter, and had studied also with his celebrated brother, William.   Associated with him as fellow-pupil was William Hewson, who subsequently became so famous as an anatomist and physiologist, and as the discoverer of the leucocytes of the blood, and whose descendants have been so prominent in the profession of this city.   No wonder, then, with such an education, that Shippen, on his return in 1762, in his twenty-sixth year, should have begun a course of lectures in anatomy, the introductory to which was delivered in the State House on November 16.   To him belongs the great merit of having made a beginning, and of having brought from the Hunters methods and traditions which long held sway in this school.   Wistar in his eulogium pays a warm tribute to his skill as a lecturer and as a demonstrator, and to the faithfulness with which he taught the subject for more than forty years.   Apart from his connection with this institution he served as Director-General of the Military Hospitals from 1777 to 1781, and was the second president of the College of Physicians.

In the history of the profession of this country Caspar Wistar holds an unique position.   He is its Avicenna, its Mead, its Fothergill, the very embodiment of the physician who, to paraphrase the words of Armstrong, used by Wistar in his Edinburgh Graduation Thesis, "Sought the cheerful haunts of men, and mingled with the bustling crowd."   He taught anatomy in this school as adjunct and professor for twenty-six years.   From the records of his contemporaries we learn that he was a brilliant teacher, "the idol of his class," as one of his eulogists says.   As an anatomist he will be remembered as the author of the first American Text-

Book on Anatomy, a work which was exceedingly popular, and ran through several editions. His interest in the subject was not, however, of the "knife and fork" kind, for he was an early student of mammalian palæontology, in the development of which one of his successors was to be a chief promotor. But Wistar's claim to remembrance rests less upon his writings than upon the impress which remains to this day of his methods of teaching anatomy. Speaking of these, Horner, who was his adjunct and intimate associate, in a letter dated February 1, 1818, says, "In reviewing the several particulars of his course of instruction, it is difficult to say in what part his chief merit consisted; he undertook everything with so much zeal, and such a conscientious desire to benefit those who came to be instructed by him, that he seldom failed of giving the most complete satisfaction. There were, however, some parts of his course peculiar to himself. These were the addition of models on a very large scale to illustrate small parts of the human structure; and the division of the general class into a number of sub-classes, each of which he supplied with a box of bones, in order that they might become thoroughly acquainted with the human skeleton, a subject which is acknowledged by all to be at the very foundation of anatomical knowledge. The idea of the former mode of instruction was acted on for the first time about fifteen years ago." We have no knowledge of a collection of specimens by Shippen, though it is hard to believe that he could have dwelt in John Hunter's house and remained free from the insatiable hunger for specimens which characterized his master. But the establishment of a museum as an important adjunct to the medical school was due to Wistar, whose collections formed the nucleus of the splendid array which you will inspect to-day. The trustees, in accepting the gift on the death of

Dr. Wistar, agreed that it should be styled the Wistar Museum, and now, after the lapse of seventy-six years, the collection has found an appropriate home in an Institute of Anatomy which bears his honoured name.

But Wistar has established a wider claim to remembrance. Genial and hospitable, he reigned supreme in society by virtue of exceptional qualities of heart and head, and became, in the language of Charles Caldwell, "the *sensorium commune* of a large circle of friends." About no other name in our ranks cluster such memories of good fellowship and good cheer, and it stands to-day in this city a synonym for *esprit* and social intercourse. Year by year his face, printed on the invitations to the "Wistar Parties" (still an important function of winter life in Philadelphia) perpetuates the message of his life, "Go seek the cheerful haunts of men."

How different was the young prosector and adjunct who next taught the subject! Horner was naturally reserved and diffident, and throughout his life those obstinate questionings which in doubt and suffering have so often wrung the heart of man were ever present. Fightings within and fears without harassed his gentle and sensitive soul, on which mortality weighed heavily, and to which the four last things were more real than the materials in which he worked. He has left us a *journal intime*, in which he found, as did Amiel of whom he was a sort of medical prototype, "a safe shelter wherein his questionings of fate and the future, the voice of grief, of self-examination and confession, the soul's cry for inward peace, might make themselves freely heard." Listen to him: "I have risen early in the morning, ere yet the watchman had cried the last hour of his vigil, and in undisturbed solitude giving my whole heart and understanding to my Maker, prayed fervently that I might be enlightened on this momentous subject, that I might be freed from the errors of an excited imagination, from the allurements of personal friendship, from the prejudices of education, and that I might, under the influence of Divine grace, be permitted to settle this question in its true merits." How familiar is the cry, the great and exceeding bitter cry of the strong soul in the toils and doubtful of the victory! Horner however, was one of those on whom both blessings rested. Facing the spectres of the mind, he laid them, and reached the desired haven. In spite of feeble bodily health and fits of depression, he carried on his anatomical studies with zeal, and as an original worker and author brought much reputation to the University. Particularly he enriched the museum with many valuable preparations, and his name will ever be associated with that of Wistar in the anatomical collection which bears their names.

But what shall I say of Leidy, the man in whom the leaven of science wrought with labour and travail for so many years? The written record survives, scarcely equalled in variety and extent by any naturalist, but how meagre is the picture of the man as known to his friends. The traits which made his life of such value—the patient spirit, the kindly disposition, the sustained zeal—we shall not see again incarnate. The memory of them alone remains. As the echoes of the eulogies upon his life have scarcely died away, I need not recount to this audience his ways and work, but upon one aspect of his character I may dwell for a moment, as illustrating an influence of science which has attracted much attention and aroused discussion. So far as the facts of sense were concerned, there was not a trace of Pyrrhonism in his composition, but in all that relates to the ultra-rational no more consistent disciple of the great sceptic ever lived. There was in him, too, that delightful "ataraxia," that imperturbability which is the distinguishing feature of the Pyrrhonist, in the truest sense of the word. A striking parallel exists between Leidy and Darwin in this respect, and it is an interesting fact that the two men of this century who have lived in closest intercourse with nature should have found full satisfaction in their studies and in their domestic affections. In the autobiographical section of the life of Charles Darwin, edited by his son Francis, in which are laid bare with such charming frankness the inner thoughts of the great naturalist, we find that he, too, had reached in suprasensuous affairs that state of mental imperturbability in which, to borrow the quaint expression of Sir Thomas Browne, they stretched not his *pia mater*. But while acknowledging that in science scepticism is advisable, Darwin says that he was not himself very sceptical. Of these two men, alike in this point, and with minds distinctly of the Aristotelian type, Darwin yet retained amid an overwhelming accumulation of facts—and here was his great superiority—an extraordinary power of generalizing principles from them. Deficient as was this quality in Leidy, he did not, on the other hand, experience "the curious and lamentable loss of the higher æsthetic taste" which Darwin mourned, and which may have been due in part to protracted ill health, and to an absolute necessity of devoting all his powers to collecting facts in support of his great theory.

When I think of Leidy's simple life, of his devotion to the study of nature, of the closeness of his communion with her for so many years, there recur to my mind time and again the lines,—

> He is made one with nature: there is heard
> His voice in all her music, from the moan
> Of thunder, to the song of night's sweet bird;

He is a presence to be felt and known
In darkness and in light, from herb and stone,
  Spreading itself where'er that Power may move
Which has withdrawn his being to its own.

II

Turning from the men to the subject in which they
worked, from the past to the present, let us take a hasty
glance at some of the developments of human anatomy and
biology. Truth has been well called the daughter of Time,
and even in anatomy, which is a science in a state of fact,
the point of view changes with successive generations. The
following story, told by Sir Robert Christison, of Barclay,
one of the leading anatomists of the early part of this
century, illustrates the old attitude of mind still met with
among "bread and butter" teachers of the subject. Barclay spoke to his class as follows: "Gentlemen, while
carrying on your work in the dissecting-room, beware of
making anatomical discoveries; and above all beware of
rushing with them into print. Our precursors have left us
little to discover. You may, perhaps, fall in with a super-
numerary muscle or tendon, a slight deviation or extra
branchlet of an artery, or, perhaps, a minute stray twig of
a nerve—that will be all. But beware! Publish the fact,
and ten chances to one you will have it shown that you
have been forestalled long ago. Anatomy may be likened
to a harvest-field. First come the reapers, who, entering
upon untrodden ground, cut down great store of corn from
all sides of them. These are the early anatomists of modern
Europe, such as Vesalius, Fallopius, Malpighi, and Harvey.
Then come the gleaners, who gather up ears enough from
the bare ridges to make a few loaves of bread. Such were
the anatomists of last century—Valsalva, Cotunnius,

Haller, Winslow, Vicq d'Azyr, Camper, Hunter, and the two Monros. Last of all come the geese, who still contrive to pick up a few grains scattered here and there among the stubble, and waddle home in the evening, poor things, cackling with joy because of their success. Gentlemen, we are the geese." Yes, geese they were, gleaning amid the stubble of a restricted field, when the broad acres of biology were open before them. Those were the days when anatomy meant a knowledge of the human frame alone; and yet the way had been opened to the larger view by the work of John Hunter, whose comprehensive mind grasped as proper subjects of study for the anatomist all the manifestations of life in order and disorder.

The determination of structure with a view to the discovery of function has been the foundation of progress. The meaning may not always have been for "him who runs to read;" often, indeed, it has been at the time far from clear; and yet a knowledge in full detail of the form and relations must precede a correct physiology. The extraordinary development of all the physical sciences, and the corresponding refinement of means of research, have contributed most largely to the enlightenment of the "geese" of Barclay's witticism. Take the progress in any one department which has a practical aspect, such as, in the anatomy and physiology of the nervous system. Read, for example, in the third edition of Wistar's *Anatomy*, edited by Horner in 1825, the description of the convolutions of the brain, on which to-day a whole army of special students are at work, medical, surgical, and anthropological, and the functions of which are the objective point of physiological and psychological research—the whole subject is thus disposed of: "The surface of the brain resembles that of the mass of the small intestine, or of a convoluted. cylindrical tube; it is, therefore, said to be convoluted. The fissures between these convolutions do not extend very deep into the substance of the brain." The knowledge of function correlated with this meagre picture of structure is best expressed, perhaps, in Shakesperian diction, "that when the brains were out, the man would die." The laborious, careful establishment of structure by the first two generations in this century led to those brilliant discoveries in the functions of the nervous system which have not only revolutionized medicine, but have almost enabled psychologists to dispense with metaphysics altogether. It is particularly interesting to note the widespread dependence of many departments on accurate anatomical knowledge. The new cerebral anatomy, particularly the study of the surface of the brain, so summarily dismissed in a few lines by Wistar, made plain the path for Hitzig and Fritsch, the careful dissection of cases of disease of the brain prepared the way for Hughlings Jackson; and gradually a new phrenology on a scientific basis has replaced the crude notions of Gall and Spurzheim; so that with the present generation, little by little, there has been established on a solid structure of anatomy, the localization of many of the functions of the brain. Excite with a rough touch, from within or from without, a small region of that mysterious surface, and my lips may move, but not in the articulate expression of thought, and I may see, but I cannot read the page before me; touch here and sight is gone, and there again and hearing fails. One by one the centres may be touched which preside over the muscles, and they may, singly or together, lose their power. All these functions may go without the loss of consciousness. Touch with the slow finger of Time the nutrition of that thin layer, and backward by slow degrees creep the intellectual faculties, back to childish simplicity, back to infantile silliness, back to the oblivion of the womb.

To this new cerebral physiology, which has thus gradually developed with increasing knowledge of structure, the study of cases of disease has contributed enormously, and to-day the diagnosis of affections of the nervous system has reached an astonishing degree of accuracy. The interdependence and sequence of knowledge in various branches of science is nowhere better shown than in this very subject. The facts obtained by precise anatomical investigation, from experiments on animals in the laboratory, from the study of nature's experiments upon us in disease, slowly and painfully acquired by many minds in many lands, have brought order out of the chaos of fifty years ago. In a practical age this vast change has wrought a corresponding alteration in our ideas of what may or may not be done in the condition of perverted health which we call disease, and we not only know better what to do, but also what to leave undone. The localization of centres in the surface of the brain has rendered it possible to make, with a considerable degree of certainty, the diagnosis of focal disease, and Macewen and Horsley have supplemented the new cerebral physiology and pathology by a new cerebro-spinal surgery, the achievements of which are scarcely credible.

But this is not all; in addition to the determination of the centres of sight, hearing, speech, and motor activities, we are gradually reaching a knowledge of the physical basis of mental phenomena. The correlation of intelligence and brain weight, of mental endowment and increased convolution of the brain surface, was recognized even by the *gleaners* of Barclay's story; but within the past twenty-five years the minute anatomy of the organ has been subjected to extensive study by methods of ever-increasing delicacy, which have laid bare its complex mechanism. The pyramidal cells of the cerebral grey matter constitute the anatomical basis of thought, and with the development, association, and complex connection of these psychical cells, as they have been termed, the psychical functions are correlated. How far these mechanical conceptions have been carried, may be gathered from the recent Croonian Lecture before the Royal Society, in which Ramón y Cajal based the action and the degree, and the development of intelligence upon the complexity of the cell mechanism and its associations. Even the physical basis of a moody madness has not evaded demonstration. Researches upon the finer structure of the cerebral cortex lead to the conclusion that imbecility, mental derangement, and the various forms of insanity are but symptoms of diseased conditions of the pyramidal cells, and not separate affections of an indefinable entity, the mind. Still further; there is a school of anthropologists which strives to associate moral derangement with physical abnormalities, particularly of the brain, and urges a belief in a criminal psychosis, in which men are "villains by necessity, fools by heavenly compulsion, knaves, thieves, and treachers by spherical predominance." This remarkable revolution in our knowledge of brain functions has resulted directly from the careful and accurate study by Barclay's "geese," of the anatomy of the nervous system. Truly the gleaning of the grapes of Ephraim has been better than the vintage of Abi-ezer.

The study of structure, however, as the basis of vital phenomena, the strict province of anatomy, forms but a small part of the wide subject of biology, which deals with the multiform manifestations of life, and seeks to know the laws governing the growth, development, and actions of living things. John Hunter, the master of Shippen and Physick, was the first great biologist of the moderns, not alone because of his extraordinary powers of observation and the comprehensive sweep of his intellect, but chiefly because he first looked at life as a whole, and studied all of its manifestations, in order and disorder, in health and in disease. He first, in the words of Buckle, "determined to contemplate nature as a vast and united whole, exhibiting, indeed, at different times, different appearances, but preserving amidst every change, a principle of uniform, and uninterrupted order, admitting of no division, undergoing no disturbance, and presenting no real irregularity albeit to the common eye irregularities abound on every side." We of the medical profession may take no little pride in the thought that there have never been wanting men in our ranks who have trodden in the footsteps of this great man; not only such giants as Owen, Huxley, and Leidy, but in a more humble way many of the most diligent students of biology have been physicians. From John Hunter to Charles Darwin enormous progress was made in every department of zoology and botany, and not only in the accumulation of facts relating to structure, but in the knowledge of function, so that the conception of the phenomena of living matter was progressively widened. Then with the *Origin of Species* came the awakening, and the theory of evolution has not only changed the entire aspect of biology, but has revolutionized every department of human thought.

Even the theory itself has come within the law; and to those of us whose biology is ten years old, the new conceptions are, perhaps, a little bewildering. The recent literature shows, however, a remarkable fertility and strength. Around the nature of cell-organization the battle wages most fiercely, and here again the knowledge of structure is sought eagerly as the basis of explanation of the vital phenomena. So radical have been the changes in this direction that a new and complicated terminology has sprung up, and the simple, undifferentiated bit of proto-plasm has now its cytosome, cytolymph, caryosome, chromosome, with their somacules and biophores. These accurate studies in the vital units have led to material modifications in the theory of descent. Weismann's views, particularly on the immortality of the unicellular organisms, and of the reproductive cells of the higher forms, and on the transmission or non-transmission of acquired characters, have been based directly upon studies of cell-structure and cell-fission.

In no way has biological science so widened the thoughts of men as in its application to social problems. That throughout the ages, in the gradual evolution of life, one unceasing purpose runs; that progress comes through unceasing competition, through unceasing selection and rejection; in a word, that evolution is the one great law controlling all living things, "the one divine event to which the whole creation moves," this conception has been the great gift of biology to the nineteenth century. In his work on *Social Evolution*, Kidd thus states the problem in clear terms: "Nothing tends to exhibit more strikingly the extent to which the study of our social phenomena must in future be based on the biological sciences, than the fact that the technical controversy now being waged by biologists as to the transmission or non-transmission to offspring of qualities acquired during the lifetime of the parent, is one which, if decided in the latter sense, must produce the most revolutionary effect throughout the whole domain of social and political philosophy. If the old view is correct, and the effects of use and education *are* transmitted by inheritance, then the Utopian dreams of philosophy in the past are undoubtedly possible of realization. If we tend to inherit in our own persons the result of the education and mental and moral culture of past generations, then we may venture to anticipate a future society which will not deteriorate, but which may continue to make progress, even though the struggle for existence be suspended, the population regulated exactly to the means of subsistence, and the antagonism between the individual and the social organism extinguished. But if the views of the Weismann party are in the main correct; if there can be no progress except by the accumulation of congenital variations above the average to the exclusion of others below; if, without the constant stress of selection which this involves, the tendency of every higher form of life *is actually retrograde;* then is the whole human race caught in the toils of that struggle and rivalry of life which has been in progress from the beginning. Then must the rivalry of existence continue, humanized as to conditions it may be, but immutable and inevitable to the end. Then also must all the phenomena of human life, individual, political, social, and religious, be considered as aspects of this cosmic process, capable of being studied and understood by science only in their relations thereto."[1]

Biology touches the problems of life at every point, and may claim, as no other science, completeness of view and a comprehensiveness which pertains to it alone. To all whose daily work lies in her manifestations the value of a deep insight into her relations cannot be overestimated. The study of biology trains the mind in accurate methods of observation and correct methods of reasoning, and gives

[1] *Social Evolution.* By Benjamin Kidd. London. 1894.

to a man clearer points of view, and an attitude of mind more serviceable in the working-day-world than that given by other sciences, or even by the humanities. Year by year it is to be hoped that young men will obtain in this Institute a fundamental knowledge of the laws of life.

To the physician particularly a scientific discipline is an incalculable gift, which leavens his whole life, giving exactness to habits of thought and tempering the mind with that judicious faculty of distrust which can alone, amid the uncertainties of practice, make him wise unto salvation. For perdition inevitably awaits the mind of the practitioner who has never had the full inoculation with the leaven, who has never grasped clearly the relations of science to his art, and who knows nothing, and perhaps cares less, for the limitations of either.

And I may be permitted on higher grounds to congratulate the University of Pennsylvania on the acquisition of this Institute. There is great need in the colleges of this country of men who are thinkers as well as workers—men with ideas, men who have drunk deep of the Astral wine, and whose energies are not sapped in the tread-mill of the class-room. In these laboratories will be given opportunities for this higher sort of university work. The conditions about us are changing rapidly: in the older states utility is no longer regarded as the test of fitness, and the value of the intellectual life has risen enormously in every department. Germany must be our model in this respect. She is great because she has a large group of men pursuing pure science with unflagging industry, with self-denying zeal, and with high ideals. No secondary motives sway their minds, no cry reaches them in the recesses of their laboratories, "of what practical utility is your work?" but, unhampered by social or theological prejudices, they have been enabled to cherish "the truth which has never been deceived—that complete truth which carries with it the antidote against the bane and danger which follow in the train of half-knowledge." (Helmholtz.)

The leaven of science gives to men habits of mental accuracy, modes of thought which enlarge the mental vision, and strengthens—to use an expression of Epicharmus—"the sinews of the understanding." But is there nothing further? Has science, the last gift of the gods, no message of hope for the race as a whole; can it do no more than impart to the individual imperturbability amid the storms of life, judgment in times of perplexity? Where are the bright promises of the days when "the kindly earth should slumber rapt in universal law"? Are these, then, futile hopes, vain imaginings of the dreamers, who from Plato to Comte have sought for law, for order, for the *civitas Dei* in the *regnum hominis?*

Science has done much, and will do more, to alleviate the unhappy condition in which so many millions of our fellow-creatures live, and in no way more than in mitigating some of the horrors of disease; but we are too apt to forget that apart from and beyond her domain lie those irresistible forces which alone sway the hearts of men. With reason science never parts company, but with feeling, emotion, passion, what has she to do? They are not of her; they owe her no allegiance. She may study, analyze, and define, she can never control them, and by no possibility can their ways be justified to her. The great philosopher who took such a deep interest in the foundation of this University, chained the lightnings, but who has chained the wayward spirit of man? Strange compound, now wrapt in the ecstasy of the beatific vision, now wallowing in the sloughs of iniquity, no leaven, earthly or divine, has worked any permanent change in him. Listen to the words of a student of the heart of man, a depictor of his emotions: "In all ages the reason of the world has been at the mercy of brute force. The reign of law has never had more than a passing reality, and never can have more than that so long as man is human. The individual intellect, and the aggregate intelligence of nations and races, have alike perished in the struggle of mankind, to revive again, indeed, but as surely to be again put to the edge of the sword. Look where you will throughout the length and breadth of all that was the world, 5000 or 500 years ago; everywhere passion has swept thought before it, and belief, reason. Passion rules the world, and rules alone. And passion is neither of the head nor of the hand, but of the heart. Love, hate, ambition, anger, avarice, either make a slave of intelligence to serve their impulses, or break down its impotent opposition with the unanswerable argument of brute force, and tear it to pieces with iron hands." (Marion Crawford.)

Who runs may read the scroll which reason has placed as a warning over the human menageries: "chained, not tamed." And yet who can doubt that the leaven of science, working in the individual, leavens in some slight degree the whole social fabric. Reason is at least free, or nearly so; the shackles of dogma have been removed, and faith herself, freed from a morganatic alliance, finds in the release great gain.

One of the many fertile fancies of the "laughing philosopher," a happy anticipation again of an idea peculiarly modern, was that of the influence upon us for weal or woe of Externals, of the idola, images, and effluences which encompass us—of Externals upon which so much of our happiness, yes, so much of our every character depends.

The trend of scientific thought in this, as in the atomic theory, has reverted to the Sage of Abdera; and if environment really means so much, how all-important a feature in education must be the nature of these encompassing effluences. This magnificent structure, so admirably adapted to the prosecution of that science from which modern thought has drawn its most fruitful inspirations, gives completeness to the already exhilarating *milieu* of this University. Here at last, and largely owing to your indomitable energy, Mr. Provost, are gathered all the externals which make up a *Schola major* worthy of this great Commonwealth. What, after all, is education but a subtle, slowly-affected change, due to the action upon us of the Externals; of the written record of the great minds of all ages, of the beautiful and harmonious surroundings of nature and of art, and of the lives, good or ill, of our fellows—these alone educate us, these alone mould the developing minds. Within the bounds of this campus these influences will lead successive generations of youth from matriculation in the college to graduation in the special school, the complex, varied influences of Art, of Science, and of Charity; of Art, the highest development of which can only come with that sustaining love for ideals which, "burns bright or dim as each are mirrors of the fire for which all thirst;" of Science, the cold logic of which keeps the mind independent and free from toils of self-deception and half-knowledge; of Charity, in which we of the medical profession, to walk worthily, must live and move and have our being.

VI
THE ARMY SURGEON

Nor Mars his sword nor war's quick fire shall burn
The living record of your memory.
'Gainst death and all-oblivious enmity
Shall you pace forth; your praise shall still find room
Even in the eyes of all posterity.

SHAKESPEARE, Sonnets, LV

VI

THE ARMY SURGEON[1]

AT the outset I am sure you will permit me, on behalf
of the profession, to offer to the Army Medical
Department hearty congratulations on the completion
of the arrangements which have made possible this gathering. With capacities strained to the utmost in furnishing
to students an ordinary medical education, the schools at
large cannot be expected to equip army surgeons with
the full details of special training. A glance at the curriculum just completed brings into sharp relief the dis-
abilities under which previous classes must have proceeded
to their labours, the members of which have had to pick up
at random—in many cases have probably never acquired—
the valuable knowledge traversed in the lectures and
laboratory exercises of the session. But greatest of all the
advantages of an army medical school must be counted
the contact of the young officers with their seniors, with
the men under whose directions they subsequently have
to work. In comparison with their predecessors, with
what different feelings and ideas will the men before us
enter upon their duties in the various posts to which they
have been assigned. Instead of hazy notions—perhaps to
one fresh from the Examining Board not pleasant ones—of
a central authority at Washington, of a Yama enthroned
as Secretary of War, and of an exacting Surgeon-General,
the young officer who has enjoyed the delightful opportunities of four months' study amid these inspiring sur-

[1] Army Medical School, Washington, February 28, 1894.

roundings, which teem with reminders of the glories of the corps and of the greatness of his profession, the young officer, I say, must be indeed a muddy-mettled fellow who does not carry away, not alone rich stores of information, but, most precious of all educational gifts, a true ideal of what his life-work should be.

Members of the Graduating Class: Though to you it may not, to me it seems peculiarly appropriate that the Surgeon-General should have asked a civilian to make an address on this occasion. With the strictly military aspects of your future life you have made yourselves familiar; of the merits and demerits of the army as a career for a physician you have in the past four months heard very much; but about all subjects there are some questions which are more freely handled by one who is unhampered by too particular knowledge, and this is my position, I may say my advantage, to-day. For me the Army Medical Department, so far as particulars are concerned, means a library with unsurpassed facilities, the worth of which is doubled by the liberality of its management; a museum in which I have spent some delightful hours; an index-catalogue, which is at my elbow like a dictionary; and the medical history of the late war, particularly the volumes by Woodward and Smart. Further, in my general reading in the history of the profession of this country, I have here and there gleaned facts about the corps and its members. I have read the spirited vindication of John Morgan, who may be called the first Surgeon-General, and I am familiar with the names and works of many of your distinguished predecessors who have left their mark in our literature.

But as I write an aspiration of the past occurs, bringing me, it seems, closer to you than any of the points just mentioned, a recollection of the days when the desire of my life was to enter the India Medical Service, a dream of youth, dim now and almost forgotten—a dream of "Vishnu land, what Avatar!"

Speaking, then, from the vantage ground of my ignorance, let me tell you briefly of the opportunities of the life you have chosen. First among your privileges I shall place a feature often spoken of as a hardship, viz., the frequent change from station to station. Permanence of residence. good undoubtedly for the pocket, is not always best for wide mental vision in the physician. You are modern representatives of a professional age long past, of a day when physicians of distinction had no settled homes. You are Cyprid larvæ, unattached, free-swimming, seeing much in many places; not fixed, as we barnacles of civil life, head downward, degenerate descendants of the old professional Cirripeds, who laid under contribution not one, but a score of cities.

Without local ties, independent of the public, in, while not exactly of, our ranks, you will escape many of the anxieties which fret the young physician—the pangs of disprized worth, the years of weary waiting, the uncertainty of the effort; and perhaps those sorer trials inevitable in an art engaging equally heart and head, in which, from the very nature of the occupation, the former is apt—in finer spirits—to be touched with a grievous sensibility. In change, that leaven of life denied to so many, you will find a strong corrective to some of the most unpleasant of the foibles which beset us. Self-satisfaction, a frame of mind widely diffused, is manifest often in greatest intensity where it should be least encouraged, and in individuals and communities is sometimes so active on such slender grounds that the condition is comparable to the delusions of grandeur in the insane. In a nomad life this common infirmity, to the entertainment of which the twin sisters, Use and Wont, lend their ever-ready aid, will scarcely touch you, and for this mercy give thanks; and while you must, as men, entertain many idols of the tribe, you may at least escape this idol of the cave. Enjoying the privilege of wide acquaintance with men of very varied capabilities and training, you can, as spectators of their many crotchets and of their little weaknesses, avoid placing an undue estimate on your own individual powers and position. As Sir Thomas Browne says, it is the "nimbler and conceited heads that never looked a degree beyond their nests that tower and plume themselves on light attainments," but "heads of capacity and such as are not full with a handful or easy measure of knowledge think they know nothing till they know all!"

Per contra, in thus attaining a broader mental platform, you may miss one of the great prizes of the profession —a position in a community reached in length of days by one or two, who, having added to learning, culture, to wisdom, charity, pass the evening of their lives in the hearts of their colleagues and of their kind. No gift of Apollo, not the Surgeon-Generalship, not distinguished position in science, no professorship, however honoured, can equal this, this which, as wandering Army Surgeons, you must forego. Fortunate is it for you that the service in one place is never long enough to let the roots strike so deeply as to make the process of transplantation too painful. Myself a peripatetic, I know what it is to bear the scars of partings from comrades and friends, scars which sometimes ache as the memories recur of the days which have flown and of the old familiar faces which have gone.

Another aspect of the life of the Army Surgeon, isolation in some degree from professional colleagues, will influence you in different ways—hurtfully in the more dependent natures, helpfully in those who may have learned that "not from without us, only from within comes, or can ever come, upon us light"—and to such the early years of separation from medical societies and gatherings will prove a useful seed-time for habits of study, and for the cultivation of the self-reliance that forms so important an element in the outfit of the practitioner. And, after all, the isolation is neither so enduring nor so corroding as might have fallen to your lot in the routine of country practice. In it may be retained, too, some measure of individuality, lost with astonishing rapidity in the city mills that rub our angles down and soon stamp us all alike. In the history of the profession there are grounds for the statement that isolation promotes originality. Some of the most brilliant work has been done by men in extremely limited spheres of action, and during the past hundred years it is surprising how many of the notable achievements have been made by physicans dwelling far from educational centres—Jenner worked out his discovery in a village; McDowell, Long, and Sims were country doctors; Koch was a district physician.

So much depends upon the sort of start that a man makes in his profession that I cannot refrain from congratulating you again on the opportunities enjoyed during the past four months, which have not only added enormously to your capabilities for work, but have familiarized you with life at the heart of the organization of which hereafter you will form part, and doubtless have given you fruitful ideas on the possibilities of your individual development. Naturally each one of you will desire to

make the best use of his talents and education, and let me
sketch briefly what I think should be your plan of action.

Throw away, in the first place, all ambition beyond
that of doing the day's work well. The travellers on
the road to success live in the present, heedless of taking
thought for the morrow, having been able at some time,
and in some form or other, to receive into their heart of
hearts this maxim of the Sage of Chelsea: Your business
is "not to *see* what lies dimly at a distance, but to *do*
what lies clearly at hand." Fevered haste is not
encouraged in military circles, and if you can adapt your
intellectual progress to army rules, making each step in
your mental promotion the lawful successor of some
other, you will acquire little by little those staying powers
without which no man is of much value in the ranks.
Your opportunities for study will cover at first a wide
field in medicine and surgery, and this diffuseness in your
work may be your salvation. In the next five or ten years
note with accuracy and care everything that comes within
your professional ken. There are, in truth, no specialties
in medicine, since to know fully many of the most important diseases a man must be familiar with their manifestations in many organs. Let nothing slip by you; the
ordinary humdrum cases of the morning routine may have
been accurately described and pictured, but study each
one separately as though it were new— so it is so far as
your special experience goes; and if the spirit of the student
is in you the lesson will be there. Look at the cases not
from the standpoint of text-books and monographs, but as
so many stepping-stones in the progress of your individual
development in the art. This will save you from the
pitiable mental attitude of the men who travel the road of
practice from Dan to Beersheba, and at every step cry out

upon its desolation, its dreariness, and its monotony.   With
Laurence Sterne, we can afford to pity such, since they
know not that the barrenness of which they complain is
within themselves, a result of a lack of appreciation of the
meaning and method of work.

In the early years of service your advantages will be
fully as great as if you had remained in civil life.   Faithfulness in the day of small things will insensibly widen
your powers, correct your faculties, and, in moments of
despondency, comfort may be derived from a knowledge
that some of the best work of the profession has come from
men whose clinical field was limited but well-tilled.   The
important thing is to make the lesson of each case tell
on your education.   The value of experience is not in
seeing much, but in seeing wisely.   Experience in the
true sense of the term does not come to all with years,
or with increasing opportunities.   Growth in the acquisition
of facts is not necessarily associated with development.
Many grow through life mentally as the crystal, by simple
accretion, and at fifty possess, to vary the figure, the
unicellular mental blastoderm with which they started.
The growth which is organic and enduring, is totally
different, marked by changes of an unmistakable character.
The observations are made with accuracy and care, no
pains are spared, nothing is thought a trouble in the
investigation of a problem.   The facts are looked at in
connexion with similar ones, their relation to others is
studied, and the experience of the recorder is compared
with that of others who have worked upon the question.
Insensibly, year by year, a man finds that there has been
in his mental protoplasm not only growth by assimilation
but an actual development, bringing fuller powers of
observation, additional capabilities of mental nutrition,

and that increased breadth of view which is of the very essence of wisdom.

As clinical observers, we study the experiments which Nature makes upon our fellow-creatures. These experiments, however, in striking contrast to those of the laboratory, lack exactness, possessing as they do a variability at once a despair and a delight—the despair of those who look for nothing but fixed laws in an art which is still deep in the sloughs of Empiricism; the delight of those who find in it an expression of a universal law transcending, even scorning, the petty accuracy of test-tube and balance, the law that in man "the measure of all things," mutability, variability, mobility, are the very marrow of his being. The *clientèle* in which you work has, however, more stability, a less extended range of variation than that with which we deal in civil life. In a body of carefully selected active young men, you have a material for study in which the oscillations are less striking, and in which the results of the experiments, i.e., the diseases, have a greater uniformity than in infancy and old age, in the enfeebled and debauched. This adds a value to the studies of army medical officers, who often have made investigations in hygiene, dietetics, and medicine, so trustworthy and thorough that they serve us as a standard of comparison, as a sort of *abscissa* or base-line. Thus you have demonstrated to us, and to the community at large, the possibilities of stamping out small-pox by systematic revaccination; in civil practice we strive to reach the low rate of mortality of army hospitals in the treatment of typhoid fever and of pneumonia. Many of the most important facts relating to etiology and symptomatology have come from camp or barrack. I often think that army surgeons scarcely appreciate that in their work they may follow the natural history of a disease under the

most favourable circumstances; the experiments are more
ideal, the conditions less disturbing than those which
prevail either in family practice or in the routine of the
general hospital. Many of the common disorders can be
tracked from inception to close, as can be done in no other
line of medical work, and the facilities for the continuous
study of certain affections are unequalled. This, which
is a point to be appreciated in the intrinsic education of
which I spoke, gives you a decided advantage over your
less favoured brethren.

Your extraordinary range of observation, from the
Florida Keys to Montana, from Maine to Southern Cali-
fornia, affords unequalled facilities for the study of many
of the vexed problems in medicine—facilities, indeed,
which in the diversity of morbid conditions to be studied
are equalled in no position in civil life. Let me here
mention a few of the subjects that may profitably engage
your attention. No question is of more importance at
present than the settlement, definitely, of the varieties of
fever in the West and South. The studies of Baumgarten
in St. Louis, and of Guitéras and others in the Southern
States, suggest the possibility that in addition to typhoid
fever and malaria—the common affections—there are other
fevers the symptomatology and morbid anatomy of which
still require careful elucidation. In this you will be walking
in the footsteps of notable predecessors in the corps, and
in the exhaustive works of Woodward and Smart, to which
I have already alluded, and which are always available,
you will find a basis from which you may start your personal
observations. More particularly in this direction do we
need careful anatomical investigation, since the symptomatology of certain of the affections in question has much in
common with that of the ordinary continued fevers of the

North. I may call your attention to the satisfactory settlement of the nature of mountain fever by army surgeons, and need hardly add that the specimens contributed by Hoff and by Girard to this museum demonstrate conclusively that it is in reality typhoid fever.

In the Southern posts malaria with its protean manifestations presents still many interesting problems for solution, and you will leave this school better equipped than any of your predecessors for the study and differentiation of its less known varieties. With positive knowledge as to the etiology, and a practical familiarity with methods of blood-examination, you can do much in many localities to give to malaria a more definite position than it at present occupies in the profession, and can offer in doubtful cases the positive and satisfactory test of the microscope. The hæmaturia of the South requires to be studied anew—the filarial cases separated from the malarial, and, most important of all, the relation of quinine to hæmaturia positively settled.

In the more distant posts, where, so far as the soldier is concerned, your opportunities for study may be limited, you may add greatly to our knowledge of the disorders prevalent among the Indians. More particularly do we need additional information as to the frequency of tuberculosis among them, and its clinical history. One of your number, Dr. Edwards, has already furnished admirable statistics upon this point, but the field is still open, and much remains to be done. In this connexion, too, you may be able to carry saving knowledge upon the etiology of the disease, and enforce regulations for its prevention. You have only to turn to the Index-catalogue to see how scanty in reality are the facts in the nosology of the North American Indian.

At many posts there will be presented to you the interesting effects of altitude, with problems of the greatest
physiological importance. An excellent piece of work
may be done upon its influences upon the red blood-corpuscles, in determining whether, as has been maintained,
there is an increase numerically per cubic millimetre, so
long as the individual remains in the more rarefied atmosphere. Points remain to be settled also upon the effects of
altitude upon the chest-capacity, the chest-measurement,
and the heart, and our knowledge is still lacking on questions
relating to the influence of high altitudes upon many of
the ordinary diseases.

To one of you, perhaps, another peculiarly American
disease—milk-sickness—may reveal its secret. Our knowledge of its etiology has not been materially increased
since the early papers on the subject, which so well described
its symptomatology.

These are but a few of the questions suggesting themselves to my mind, to which, as chance affords, you could
direct your attention. In a ten or fifteen years' service,
travelling with seeing eyes and hearing ears, and carefully-
kept note-books, just think what a store-house of clinical
material may be at the command of any one of you—
material not only valuable in itself to the profession, but
of infinite value to you personally in its acquisition, render-
ing you painstaking and accurate, and giving you, year by
year, an increasing experience of the sort to which I have
already more than once referred.

In what I have said hitherto I have dwelt chiefly on
your personal development, and on the direction in which
your activities might be engaged, but while you are thus
laying the foundation of an education in all that relates
to the technical side of the profession, there are other

duties which call for a word or two. In the communities to which you may be sent do not forget that, though army officers, you owe allegiance to an honourable profession, to the members of which you are linked by ties of a most binding character. In situations in which the advantages of a more critical training give you a measure of superiority over your *confrères* in civil life, let it not be apparent in your demeanour, but so order yourselves that in all things you may appear to receive, not to grant favours. There are regions, *in partibus infidelium*, to which you will go as missionaries, carrying the gospel of loyalty to truth in the science and in the art of medicine, and your lives of devotion may prove to many a stimulating example. You cannot afford to stand aloof from your professional colleagues in any place. Join their associations, mingle in their meetings, giving of the best of your talents, gathering here, scattering there; but everywhere showing that you are at all times faithful students, as willing to teach as to be taught. Shun as most pernicious that frame of mind, too often, I fear, seen in physicians, which assumes an air of superiority and limits as worthy of your communion only those with satisfactory collegiate or sartorial credentials. The passports of your fellowship should be honesty of purpose, and a devotion to the highest interests of our profession, and these you will find widely diffused, sometimes apparent only when you get beneath the crust of a rough exterior.

If I have laid stress upon the more strictly professional aspects of your career it has been with a purpose. I believe the arrangements in the department are such that, with habits of ordinary diligence, each one of you may attain not only a high grade of personal development, but may become an important contributor in the advancement of our art. I have said nothing of the pursuit of the sciences cognate to medicine, of botany, zoology, geology, ethnology and archæology. In every one of these, so fascinating in themselves, it is true that army medical officers have risen to distinction, but I claim that your first duty is to medicine, which should have your best services and your loyal devotion. Not, too, in the perfunctory discharge of the daily routine, but in zealous endeavour to keep pace with, and to aid in, the progress of knowledge. In this way you will best serve the department, the profession, and the public.

Generalities, of the kind in which I have been indulging, though appropriate to the occasion, are close kin, I fear, to the fancies fond, that vanish like the gay motes which float for a moment in the sunbeams of our mind. But I would fain leave with you, in closing, something of a more enduring kind—a picture that for me has always had a singular attraction, the picture of a man who, amid circumstances the most unfavourable, saw his opportunity and was quick to "grasp the skirts of happy chance." Far away in the northern wilds, where the waters of Lake Michigan and Lake Huron unite, stands the fort of Michili-mackinac, rich in memories of Indian and *voyageur*, one of the four important posts on the upper lakes in the days when the Rose and the Fleur-de-lis strove for the mastery of the Western world. Here was the scene of Marquette's mission, and here beneath the chapel of St. Ignace they laid his bones to rest. Here the intrepid La Salle, the brave Tonty, and the resolute Du Lhut had halted in their wild wanderings. Its palisades and bastions had echoed the war-whoops of Ojibwas and Ottawas, of Hurons and Iroquois, and had been the scene of bloody massacres and of hard-fought fights. At the conclusion of the war of 1812, after two centuries of struggle, peace settled at last upon the old fort, and early in her reign celebrated one of the most famous of her minor victories, one which carried the high-sounding name of Michilimackinac far and wide, and into circles where Marquette, Du Lhut and La Salle were unknown.   Here, in 1820, was assigned to duty at the fort, which had been continued in use to keep the Indians in check, Surgeon William Beaumont, then a young man in the prime of life.   On June 22, 1822, the accidental discharge of a musket made St. Martin, a *voyageur*, one of the most famous subjects in the history of physiology, for the wound laid open his stomach, and he recovered with a permanent gastric fistula of an exceptionally favourable kind.   Beaumont was not slow to see the extraordinary possibilities that were before him.   Early in the second decade of the century the process of gastric digestion was believed to be due to direct mechanical maceration or to the action of a vital principle, and though the idea of a solvent juice had long been entertained, the whole question was *sub judice*.   The series of studies made by Beaumont on St. Martin settled for ever the existence of a solvent fluid capable of acting on food outside as well as within the body, and in addition enriched our knowledge of the processes of digestion by new observations on the movements of the stomach, the temperature of the interior of the body, and the digestibility of the various articles of food.   The results of his work were published in 1833, in an octavo volume of less than 300 pages.[1]   In looking through it one cannot but recognize that it is the source of a very large part of the current statements about digestion; but apart altogether from the value of the facts, there are qualities about the

[1] *Experiments and Observations on the Gastric Juice and the Physiology of Digestion.*   By William Beaumont, M.D., Surgeon in the United States Army.   Plattsburg.   1833.

work which make it a model of its kind, and on every page is revealed the character of the man. From the first experiment, dated August 1, 1825, to the last, dated November 1, 1833, the observations are made with accuracy and care, and noted in plain, terse language. A remarkable feature was the persistence with which for eight years Beaumont pursued the subject, except during two intervals when St. Martin escaped to his relatives in Lower Canada. On one occasion Beaumont brought him a distance of two thousand miles to Fort Crawford, on the upper Mississippi, where, in 1829, the second series of experiments was made. The third series was conducted in Washington, in 1832; and the fourth at Plattsburg in 1833. The determination to sift the question thoroughly, to keep at it persistently until the truth was reached, is shown in every one of the 238 experiments which he has recorded.

The opportunity presented itself, the observer had the necessary mental equipment and the needed store of endurance to carry to a successful termination a long and laborious research. William Beaumont is indeed a bright example in the annals of the Army Medical Department, and there is no name on its roll more deserving to live in the memory of the profession of this country.

And in closing let me express the wish that each one of you, in all your works begun, continued and ended, may be able to say with him: "Truth, like beauty, 'when unadorned is adorned the most,' and in prosecuting experiments and inquiries I believe I have been guided by its light."

VII
TEACHING AND THINKING

Let us then blush, in this so ample and so wonderful field of nature (where performance still exceeds what is promised), to credit other men's traditions only, and thence come uncertain problems to spin out thorny and captious questions. *Nature* her selfe must be our adviser; the path she chalks must be our walk: for so while we confer with our own eies, and take our rise from meaner things to higher, we shall at length be received into her Closet-secrets.

Preface to *Anatomical Exercitations concerning the Generation of Living Creatures*, 1653.

WILLIAM HARVEY.

VII

TEACHING AND THINKING[1]

The Two Functions of a Medical School

I

MANY things have been urged against our nineteenth century civilization—that political enfranchisement only ends in anarchy, that the widespread unrest in spiritual matters leads only to unbelief, and that the best commentary on our boasted enlightenment is the picture of Europe in arms and the nations everywhere gnarring at each other's heels. Of practical progress in one direction, however, there can be no doubt; no one can dispute the enormous increase in the comfort of each individual life. Collectively the human race, or portions of it at any rate, may in the past have enjoyed periods of greater repose, and longer intervals of freedom from strife and anxiety; but the day has never been when the unit has been of such value, when the man, and the man alone, has been so much the measure, when the individual as a living organism has seemed so sacred, when the obligations to regard his rights have seemed so imperative. But even these changes are as nothing in comparison with the remarkable increase in his physical well-being. The bitter cry of Isaiah that with the multiplication of the nations their joys have not been increased, still echoes in our ears. The sorrows and troubles of men, it is true, may not have been materially

[1] McGill Medical School, January 8, 1895.

diminished, but bodily pain and suffering, though not abolished, have been assuaged as never before, and the share of each in the *Weltschmerz* has been enormously lessened.

Sorrows and griefs are companions sure sooner or later to join us on our pilgrimage, and we have become perhaps more sensitive to them, and perhaps less amenable to the old time remedies of the physicians of the soul; but the pains and woes of the body, to which we doctors minister, are decreasing at an extraordinary rate, and in a way that makes one fairly gasp in hopeful anticipation.

In his *Grammar of Assent*, in a notable passage on suffering, John Henry Newman asks, "Who can weigh and measure the aggregate of pain which this one generation has endured, and will endure, from birth to death? Then add to this all the pain which has fallen and will fall upon our race through centuries past and to come." But take the other view of it—think of the Nemesis which has overtaken pain during the past fifty years! Anæsthetics and antiseptic surgery have almost manacled the demon, and since their introduction the aggregate of pain which has been prevented far outweighs in civilized communities that which has been suffered. Even the curse of travail has been lifted from the soul of women.

The greatest art is in the concealment of art, and I may say that we of the medical profession excel in this respect. You of the public who hear me, go about the duties of the day profoundly indifferent to the facts I have just mentioned. You do not know, many of you do not care, that for the cross-legged Juno who presided over the arrival of your grandparents, there now sits a benign and straight-legged goddess. You take it for granted that if a shoulder is dislocated there is chloroform and a delicious Nepenthe

instead of the agony of the pulleys and paraphernalia of
fifty years ago.   You accept with a selfish complacency, as
if you were yourselves to be thanked for it, that the arrows
of destruction fly not so thickly, and that the pestilence now
rarely walketh in the darkness; still less do you realize that
you may now pray the prayer of Hezekiah with a reasonable
prospect of its fulfilment, since modern science has made
to almost everyone of you the present of a few years.

I say you do not know these things.   You hear of them,
and the more intelligent among you perhaps ponder them
in your hearts, but they are among the things which you
take for granted, like the sunshine, and the flowers and the
glorious heavens.

'Tis no idle challenge which we physicians throw out to
the world when we claim that our mission is of the highest
and of the noblest kind, not alone in curing disease but in
educating the people in the laws of health, and in preventing
the spread of plagues and pestilences; nor can it be gainsaid
that of late years our record as a body has been more encouraging in its practical results than those of the other learned
professions.   Not that we all live up to the highest ideals,
far from it—we are only men.   But we have ideals, which
mean much, and they are realizable, which means more.
Of course there are Gehazis among us who serve for shekels,
whose ears hear only the lowing of the oxen and the jingling
of the guineas, but these are exceptions.   The rank and file
labour earnestly for your good, and self-sacrificing devotion
to your interests animates our best work.

The exercises in which we are to-day engaged form an
incident in this beneficent work which is in progress everywhere; an incident which will enable me to dwell upon
certain aspects of the university as a factor in the promotion
of the physical well-being of the race.

II

A great university has a dual function, to teach and to think. The educational aspects at first absorb all its energies, and in equipping various departments and providing salaries, it finds itself hard pressed to fulfil even the first of the duties. The story of the progress of the medical school of this institution illustrates the struggles and difficulties, the worries and vexations attendant upon the effort to place it in the first rank as a teaching body. I know them well, since I was in the thick of them for ten years, and see to-day the realization of many of my daydreams. Indeed in my wildest flights I never thought to see such a splendid group of buildings as I have just inspected. We were modest in those days, and I remember when Dr. Howard showed me in great confidence the letter of the Chancellor, in which he conveyed his first generous bequest to the Faculty, it seemed so great that in my joy I was almost ready to sing my *Nunc dimittis*. The great advances here, at the Montreal General Hospital, and at the Royal Victoria (both of which institutions form most essential parts of the medical schools of this city) mean increased teaching facilities, and of necessity better equipped graduates, better equipped doctors! Here is the kernel of the whole matter, and it is for this that we ask the aid necessary to build large laboratories and large hospitals in which the student may learn the science and art of medicine. Chemistry, anatomy and physiology give that perspective which enables him to place man and his diseases in their proper position in the scheme of life, and afford at the same time that essential basis upon which alone a trustworthy experience may be built. Each one of these is a science in itself, complicated and difficult, demanding much time and labour for its acquisition, so that in the few years which are given to their study the student can only master the principles and certain of the facts upon which they are founded.   Only so far as they bear upon a due understanding of the phenomena of disease do these subjects form part of the medical curriculum, and for us they are but means— essential means it is true—to this end.   A man cannot become a competent surgeon without a full knowledge of human anatomy and physiology, and the physician without physiology and chemistry flounders along in an aimless fashion, never able to gain any accurate conception of disease, practising a sort of popgun pharmacy, hitting now the malady and again the patient, he himself not knowing which.

The primary function of this department of the university is to instruct men about disease, what it is, what are its manifestations, how it may be prevented, and how it may be cured; and to learn these things the four hundred young men who sit on these benches have come from all parts of the land.   But it is no light responsibility which a faculty assumes in this matter.   The task is beset with difficulties, some inherent in the subject and others in the men themselves, while not a few are caused by the lack of common sense in medical matters of the people among whom we doctors work.

The processes of disease are so complex that it is excessively difficult to search out the laws which control them, and, although we have seen a complete revolution in our ideas, what has been accomplished by the new school of medicine is only an earnest of what the future has in store. The three great advances of the century have been a knowledge of the mode of controlling epidemic diseases, the introduction of anæsthetics, and the adoption of antiseptic methods in surgery. Beside them all others sink into insignificance, as these three contribute so enormously to the personal comfort of the individual. The study of the causes of so-called infectious disorders has led directly to the discovery of the methods for their control, for example, such a scourge as typhoid fever becomes almost unknown in the presence of perfect drainage and an uncontaminated water supply. The outlook, too, for specific methods of treatment in these affections is most hopeful. The public must not be discouraged by a few, or even by many failures. The thinkers who are doing the work for you are on the right path, and it is no vain fancy that before the twentieth century is very old there may be effective vaccines against many of the contagious diseases.

But a shrewd old fellow remarked to me the other day, "Yes, many diseases are less frequent, others have disappeared, but new ones are always cropping up, and I notice that with it all there is not only no decrease, but a very great increase in the number of doctors."

The total abolition of the infectious group we cannot expect, and for many years to come there will remain hosts of bodily ills, even among preventable maladies, to occupy our labours; but there are two reasons which explain the relative numerical increase in the profession in spite of the great decrease in the number of certain diseases. The development of specialties has given employment to many extra men who now do much of the work of the old family practitioner, and again people employ doctors more frequently and so give occupation to many more than formerly.

It cannot be denied that we have learned more rapidly how to prevent than how to cure diseases, but with a definite outline of our ignorance we no longer live now in a fool's Paradise, and fondly imagine that in all cases we control the

issues of life and death with our pills and potions.   It took
the profession many generations to learn that fevers ran
their course, influenced very little, if at all, by drugs, and
the £60 which old Dover complained were spent in drugs
in a case of ordinary fever about the middle of the last
century is now better expended on a trained nurse, with
infinitely less risk, and with infinitely greater comfort to
the patient.   Of the difficulties inherent in the art not one
is so serious as this which relates to the cure of disease by
drugs.   There is so much uncertainty and discord even
among the best authorities (upon non-essentials it is true)
that I always feel the force of a well-known stanza in *Rabbi
Ben Ezra*—

> Now, who shall arbitrate?
> Ten men love what I hate,
> Shun what I follow, slight what I receive;
> Ten, who in ears and eyes
> Match me: we all surmise,
> They this thing, and I that: whom shall my soul believe?

One of the chief reasons for this uncertainty is the
increasing variability in the manifestations of any one disease.   As no two faces, so no two cases are alike in all
respects, and unfortunately it is not only the disease itself
which is so varied, but the subjects themselves have peculiarities which modify its action.

With the diminished reliance upon drugs, there has been
a return with profit to the older measures of diet, exercise,
baths, and frictions, the remedies with which the Bithynian
Asclepiades doctored the Romans so successfully in the
first century.   Though used less frequently, medicines are
now given with infinitely greater skill; we know better their
indications and contradictions, and we may safely say

(reversing the proportion of fifty years ago) that for one damaged by dosing, one hundred are saved.

Many of the difficulties which surround the subject relate to the men who practise the art. The commonest as well as the saddest mistake is to mistake one's profession, and this we doctors do often enough, some of us, without knowing it. There are men who have never had the preliminary education which would enable them to grasp the fundamental truths of the science on which medicine is based. Others have poor teachers, and never receive that bent of mind which is the all important factor in education; others again fall early into the error of thinking that they know it all, and benefiting neither by their mistakes or their successes, miss the very essence of all experience, and die bigger fools, if possible, than when they started. There are only two sorts of doctors; those who practise with their brains, and those who practise with their tongues. The studious, hardworking man who wishes to know his profession thoroughly, who lives in the hospitals and dispensaries, and who strives to obtain a wide and philosophical conception of disease and its processes, often has a hard struggle, and it may take years of waiting before he becomes successful; but such form the bulwarks of our ranks, and outweigh scores of the voluble Cassios who talk themselves into, and often out of, practice.

Now of the difficulties bound up with the public in which we doctors work, I hesitate to speak in a mixed audience. Common sense in matters medical is rare, and is usually in inverse ratio to the degree of education. I suppose as a body, clergymen are better educated than any other, yet they are notorious supporters of all the nostrums and humbuggery with which the daily and religious papers abound, and I find that the further away they have wandered from the decrees of the Council of Trent, the more apt are they to be steeped in thaumaturgic and Galenical superstition. But know also, man has an inborn craving for medicine. Heroic dosing for several generations has given his tissues a thirst for drugs. As I once before remarked, the desire to take medicine is one feature which distinguishes man, the animal, from his fellow creatures. It is really one of the most serious difficulties with which we have to contend. Even in minor ailments, which would yield to dieting or to simple home remedies, the doctor's visit is not thought to be complete without the prescription. And now that the pharmacists have cloaked even the most nauseous remedies, the temptation is to use medicine on every occasion, and I fear we may return to that state of polypharmacy, the emancipation from which has been the sole gift of Hahnemann and his followers to the race. As the public becomes more enlightened, and as we get more sense, dosing will be recognized as a very minor function in the practice of medicine in comparison with the old measures of Asclepiades.

After all, these difficulties—in the subject itself, in us, and in you—are lessening gradually, and we have the consolation of knowing that year by year the total amount of unnecessary suffering is decreasing at a rapid rate.

In teaching men what disease is, how it may be prevented, and how it may be cured, a University is fulfilling one of its very noblest functions. The wise instruction and the splendid example of such men as Holmes, Sutherland, Campbell, Howard, Ross, Macdonnell, and others have carried comfort into thousands of homes throughout this land. The benefits derived from the increased facilities for the teaching of medicine which have come with the great changes made here and at the hospitals during the past few years, will not be confined to the citizens of this town, but will be widely diffused and felt in every locality to which the graduates of this school may go; and every gift which promotes higher medical education, and which enables the medical faculties throughout the country to turn out better doctors, means fewer mistakes in diagnosis, greater skill in dealing with emergencies, and the saving of pain and anxiety to countless sufferers and their friends.

The physician needs a clear head and a kind heart; his work is arduous and complex, requiring the exercise of the very highest faculties of the mind, while constantly appealing to the emotions and finer feelings. At no time has his influence been more potent than at present, at no time has he been so powerful a factor for good, and as it is one of the highest possible duties of a great University to fit men for this calling, so it will be your highest mission, students of medicine, to carry on the never-ending warfare against disease and death, better equipped, abler men than your predecessors, but animated with their spirit and sustained by their hopes, "for the hope of every creature is the banner that we bear."

III

The other function of a University is to think. Teaching current knowledge in all departments, teaching the steps by which the *status præsens* has been reached, and teaching how to teach, form the routine work of the various college faculties. All this may be done in a perfunctory manner by men who have never gone deeply enough into the subjects to know that really thinking about them is in any way necessary or important. What I mean by the thinking function of a University, is that duty which the professional corps owes to enlarge the boundaries of human knowledge.

Work of this sort makes a University great, and alone enables it to exercise a wide influence on the minds of men.

We stand to-day at a critical point in the history of this faculty. The equipment for teaching, to supply which has taken years of hard struggle, is approaching completion, and with the co-operation of the General and the Royal Victoria Hospitals students can obtain in all branches a thorough training. We have now reached a position in which the higher university work may at any rate be discussed, and towards it progress in the future must trend. It may seem to be discouraging, after so much has been done and so much has been so generously given, to say that there remains a most important function to foster and sustain, but this aspect of the question must be considered when a school has reached a certain stage of development. In a progressive institution the changes come slowly, the pace may not be perceived by those most concerned, except on such occasions as the present, which serve as land-marks in its evolution. The men and methods of the old Coté street school were better than those with which the faculty started; we and our ways at the new building on University street were better than those of Coté street; and now you of the present faculty teach and work much better than we did ten years ago. Everywhere the old order changeth, and happy those who can change with it. Like the defeated gods in Keats's "Hyperion," too many unable to receive the balm of the truth, resent the wise words of Oceanus (which I quoted here with very different feelings some eighteeen years ago in an introductory lecture).

> So on our heels a fresh perfection treads,
> *   *   *   *   *   born of us
> And fated to excel us.

Now the fresh perfection which will tread on our heels will come with the opportunities for higher university work. Let me indicate in a few words its scope and aims.   Teachers who teach current knowledge are not necessarily investigators; many have not had the needful training; others have not the needful time.   The very best instructor for students may have no conception of the higher lines of work in his branch, and contrariwise, how many brilliant investigators have been wretched teachers?   In a school which has reached this stage and wishes to do thinking as well as teaching, men must be selected who are not only thoroughly *au courant* with the best work in their department the world over, but who also have ideas, with ambition and energy to put them into force—men who can add each one in his sphere, to the store of the world's knowledge.   Men of this stamp alone confer greatness upon a university.   They should be sought for far and wide; an institution which wraps itself in Strabo's cloak and does not look beyond the college gates in selecting professors may get good teachers, but rarely good thinkers.

One of the chief difficulties in the way of advanced work is the stress of routine class and laboratory duties, which often sap the energies of men capable of higher things.   To meet this difficulty it is essential, first, to give the professors plenty of assistance, so that they will not be worn out with teaching; and, secondly, to give encouragement to graduates and others to carry on researches under their direction. With a system of fellowships and research scholarships a university may have a body of able young men, who on the outposts of knowledge are exploring, surveying, defining and correcting.   Their work is the outward and visible sign that a university is thinking.   Surrounded by a group of bright young minds, well trained in advanced methods, not only is the professor himself stimulated to do his best work, but he has to keep far afield and to know what is stirring in every part of his own domain.

With the wise co-operation of the university and the hospital authorities Montreal may become the Edinburgh of America, a great medical centre to which men will flock for sound learning, whose laboratories will attract the ablest students, and whose teaching will go out into all lands, universally recognized as of the highest and of the best type.

Nowhere is the outlook more encouraging than at McGill. What a guarantee for the future does the progress of the past decade afford! No city on this continent has endowed higher education so liberally. There remains now to foster that undefinable something which, for want of a better term, we call the university spirit, a something which a rich institution may not have, and with which a poor one may be saturated, a something which is associated with men and not with money, which cannot be purchased in the market or grown to order, but which comes insensibly with loyal devotion to duty and to high ideals, and without which *Nehushtan* is written on the portals of any school of Medicine, however famous.

VIII
INTERNAL MEDICINE AS A VOCATION

A physician in a great city seems to be the mere plaything of fortune; his degree of reputation is for the most part totally casual; they that employ him know not his excellence; they that reject him know not his deficience.

SAMUEL JOHNSON.

It happens to us, as it happeneth to wayfaring men: sometimes our way is clean, sometimes oul; sometimes up hill, sometimes down hill; we are seldom at a certainty; the wind is not always at our backs, nor is every one a friend that we meet in the way.

BUNYAN'S *Pilgrim's Progress*, Part II.

In the mind, as in the body, there is the necessity of getting rid of waste, and a man of active literary habits will write for the *fire* as well as for the *press*.

JEROME CARDAN.

VIII

INTERNAL MEDICINE AS A VOCATION[1]

I

IT was with the greatest pleasure that I accepted an invitation to address this section of the Academy on the importance of internal medicine as a vocation. I wish there were another term to designate the wide field of medical practice which remains after the separation of surgery, midwifery, and gynæcology. Not itself a specialty (though it embraces at least half a dozen), its cultivators cannot be called specialists, but bear without reproach the good old name physician, in contradistinction to general practitioners, surgeons, obstetricians, and gynæcologists. I have heard the fear expressed that in this country the sphere of the physician proper is becoming more and more restricted, and perhaps this is true; but I maintain (and I hope to convince you) that the opportunities are still great, that the harvest truly is plenteous, and the labourers scarcely sufficient to meet the demand.

At the outset I would like to emphasize the fact that the student of internal medicine cannot be a specialist. The manifestations of almost any one of the important diseases in the course of a few years will "box the compass" of the specialties. Typhoid fever, for example, will not only go the rounds of those embraced in medicine proper, but will carry its student far afield in morbid psychology, and some-

[1] New York Academy of Medicine, 1897

138

times teach him, perhaps at the cost of the patient, a little surgery. So, too, with syphilis, which after the first few weeks I claim as a medical affection. I often tell my students that it is the only disease which they require to study thoroughly. Know syphilis in all its manifestations and relations, and all other things clinical will be added unto you.

Each generation has to grow its own consultants. Hossack, Samuel Mitchill, Swett, Alonzo Clark, Austin Flint, Fordyce Barker, and Alfred Loomis, served their day in this city, and then passed on into silence. Their works remain; but enough of a great physician's experience dies with him to justify the saying "there is no wisdom in the grave." The author of *Rab and His Friends* has a couple of paragraphs on this point which are worth quoting: "Much that made such a man what the community, to their highest profit, found him to be, dies with him. His inborn gifts, and much of what was most valuable in his experience, were necessarily incommunicable to others; this depending much on his forgetting the process by which, in particular cases, he made up his mind, and its minute successive steps, . . . but mainly, we believe, because no man can explain directly to another man *how* he does any one practical thing, the doing of which he himself has accomplished not at once or by imitation, or by teaching, but by repeated personal trials, by missing much before ultimately hitting."

Wherewithal shall a young man prepare himself, should the ambition arise in him to follow in the footsteps of such a teacher as, let us say, the late Austin Flint—the young man just starting, and who will from 1915 to 1940 stand in relation to the profession of this city and this country as did Dr. Flint between 1861 and the time of his death. We will assume that he starts with equivalent advantages, though this is taking a great deal for granted, since Austin Flint had a strong hereditary bias toward medicine, and early in life fell under the influence of remarkable men whose teachings moulded his thought to the very end. We must not forget that Dr. Flint was a New Englander, and of the same type of mind as his great teachers—James Jackson and Jacob Bigelow.

Our future consultant has just left the hospital, where, for the first time realizing the possibilities of his profession, he has had his ambition fired. Shall he go abroad? It is not necessary. The man whom we have chosen as his exemplar did not, but found his opportunities in country-practice, in Buffalo and Louisville, then frontier towns, and in New Orleans, and had a national reputation before he reached New York. But would it be useful to him? Undoubtedly. He will have a broader foundation on which to build, and a year or two in the laboratories and clinics of the great European cities will be most helpful. To walk the wards of Guy's or St. Bartholomew's, to see the work at the St. Louis and at the Salpêtrière, to spend a few quiet months of study at one of the German university towns will store the young man's mind with priceless treasures. I assume that he has a mind. I am not heedless of the truth of the sharp taunt—

> How much the fool that hath been sent to Rome,
> Exceeds the fool that hath been kept at home.

At any rate, whether he goes abroad or not, let him early escape from the besetting sin of the young physician, *Chauvinism*, that intolerant attitude of mind, which brooks no regard for anything outside his own circle and his own school. If he cannot go abroad let him spend part of his short vacations in seeing how it fares with the brethern in his own country. Even a New Yorker could learn some-thing in the Massachusetts General and the Boston City Hospitals. A trip to Philadelphia would be most helpful; there is much to stimulate the mind at the old Pennsylvania Hospital and at the University, and he would be none the worse for a few weeks spent still farther south on the banks of the Chesapeake. The all-important matter is to get breadth of view as early as possible, and this is difficult without travel.

Poll the successful consulting physicians of this country to-day, and you will find they have been evolved either from general practice or from laboratory and clinical work; many of the most prominent having risen from the ranks of general practitioners. I once heard an eminent consultant rise in wrath because some one had made a remark reflecting upon this class. He declared that no single part of his profes-sional experience had been of such value. But I wish to speak here of the training of men who start with the object of becoming pure physicians. From the vantage ground of more than forty years of hard work, Sir Andrew Clark told me that he had striven ten years for bread, ten years for bread and butter, and twenty years for cakes and ale; and this is really a very good partition of the life of the student of internal medicine, of some at least, since all do not reach the last stage.

It is high time we had our young Lydgate started.[1] If he has shown any signs of *nous* during his student and hospital days a dispensary assistantship should be available; anything should be acceptable which brings him into con-

---

[1] This well-drawn character in George Eliot's *Middlemarch* may be studied with advantage by the physician; one of the most important lessons to be gathered from it is—marry the right woman!

tact with patients. By all means, if possible, let him be a pluralist, and—as he values his future life—let him not get early entangled in the meshes of specialism. Once established as a clinical assistant he can begin his education, and nowadays this is a very complicated matter. There are three lines of work which he may follow, all of the most intense interest, all of the greatest value to him—chemistry, physiology, and morbid anatomy. Professional chemists look askance at physiological chemistry, and physiological chemists criticize pretty sharply the work of some clinical chemists, but there can be no doubt of the value to the physician of a very thorough training in methods and ways of organic chemistry. We sorely want, in this country, men of this line of training, and the outlook for them has never before been so bright. If at the start he has not had a good chemical training, the other lines should be more closely followed.

Physiology, which for him will mean very largely experimental therapeutics and experimental pathology, will open a wider view and render possible a deeper grasp of the problems of disease. To Traube and men of his stamp, the physiological clinicians, this generation owes much more than to the chemical or *post-mortem*-room group. The training is more difficult to get, and nowadays, when physiology is cultivated as a specialty, few physicians will graduate into clinical medicine directly from the laboratory. On the other hand, the opportunities for work are now more numerous, and the training which a young fellow gets in a laboratory controlled by a pure physiologist will help to give that scientific impress, which is only enduring when early received. A thorough chemical training and a complete equipment in methods of experimental research are less often met with in the clinical physician than a good practical knowledge of morbid anatomy; and, if our prospective consultant has to limit his work, chemistry and physiology should yield to the claims of the dead-house. In this dry-bread period he should see autopsies daily, if possible. Successful knowledge of the infinite variations of disease can only be obtained by a prolonged study of morbid anatomy. While of special value in training the physician in diagnosis, it also enables him to correct his mistakes, and, if he reads its lessons aright, it may serve to keep him humble.

This is, of course, a very full programme, but in ten years a bright man, with what Sydenham calls "the ancient and serious diligence of Hippocrates," will pick up a very fair education, and will be fit to pass from the dispensary to the wards. If he cannot go abroad after his hospital term, let it be an incentive to save money, and with the first $600 let him take a summer semester in Germany, working quietly at one of the smaller places. Another year let him spend three months or longer in Paris. When schemes are laid in advance, it is surprising how often the circumstances fit in with them. How shall he live meanwhile? On crumbs—on pickings obtained from men in the cakes-and-ale stage (who always can put paying work into the hands of young men), and on fees from classes, journal work, private instruction, and from work in the schools. Any sort of medical practice should be taken, but with caution— too much of it early may prove a good man's ruin. He cannot expect to do more than just eke out a living. He must put his emotions on ice; there must be no "Amaryllis in the shade," and he must beware the tangles of "Neæra's hair." Success during the first ten years means endurance and perseverance; all things come to him who has learned to labour and wait, who bides his time "ohne Hast, aber ohne Rast," whose talent develops "in der Stille," in the quiet fruitful years of unselfish devoted work. A few words in addition about this dry-bread decade. He should stick closely to the dispensaries. A first-class reputation may be built up in them. Byrom Bramwell's *Atlas of Medicine* largely represents his work while an assistant physician to the Royal Infirmary, Edinburgh. Many of the best-known men in London serve ten, fifteen, or even twenty years in the out-patient departments before getting wards. Lauder Brunton only obtained his full physician-ship at St. Bartholomew's after a service of more than twenty years in the out-patient department. During this period let him not lose the substance of ultimate success in grasping at the shadow of present opportunity. Time is now his money, and he must not barter away too much of it in profitless work—profitless so far as his education is con-cerned, though it may mean ready cash. Too many "quiz" classes or too much journal work has ruined many a promising clinical physician. While the Pythagorean silence of nearly seven years, which the great Louis followed (and broke to burst into a full-blown reputation) cannot be enjoined, the young physician should be careful what and how he writes. Let him take heed to his education, and his reputation will take care of itself, and in a development under the guidance of seniors he will find plenty of material for papers before medical societies and for publication in scientific journals.

I would like to add here a few words on the question of clinical instruction, as with the great prospective increase of it in our schools there will be many chances of employ-ment for young physicians who wish to follow medicine proper as a vocation. To-day this serious problem con-fronts the professors in many of our schools—how to teach practical medicine to the large classes; how to give them protracted and systematic ward instruction? I know of no teacher in the country who controls enough clinical material for the instruction of classes say of 200 men during the third and fourth years. It seems to me that there are two plans open to the schools: The first is to utilize dispensaries for clinical instruction much more than is at present the rule. For this purpose a teaching-room for a class of twenty-five or thirty students immediately adjoining the dispensary is essential. For instruction in physical diagnosis, for the objective teaching of disease, and for the instruction of students in the use of their senses, such an arrangement is invaluable. There are hundreds of dispensaries in which this plan is feasible, and in which the material now is not properly worked up because of the lack of this very stimulus. In the second place, I feel sure that ultimately we shall develop a system of extra-mural teaching similar to that which has been so successful in Edinburgh; and this will give employment to a large number of the younger men. At any large university school of medicine there might be four or five extra-mural teachers of medicine, selected from men who could show that they were fully qualified to teach and that they had a sufficient number of beds at their command, with proper equipment for clinical work. At Edinburgh there are eight extra-mural teachers of internal medicine whose courses qualify the student to present himself for examination either before the Royal Colleges or the University. If we ever are to give our third and fourth year students protracted and complete courses in physical diagnosis and clinical medicine, extending throughout the session, and not in classes of a brief period of six weeks' duration, I am confident that the number of men engaged in teaching must be greatly increased.

II

Ten years' hard work tells with colleagues and friends in the profession, and with enlarged clinical facilities the physician enters upon the second, or bread-and-butter period. This, to most men, is the great trial, since the risks are greater, and many now drop out of the race, wearied at the length of the way and drift into specialism or general practice. The physician develops more slowly than the surgeon, and success comes later. There are surgeons at forty years in full practice and at the very top of the wave, a time at which the physician is only preparing to reap the harvest of years of patient toil. The surgeon must have hands, and better, young hands. He should have a head, too, but this does not seem so essential to success, and he cannot have an old head with young hands. At the end of twenty years, when about forty-five, our Lydgate should have a first-class reputation in the profession, and a large circle of friends and students. He will probably have precious little capital in the bank, but a very large accumulation of interest-bearing funds in his brain-pan. He has gathered a stock of special knowledge which his friends in the profession appreciate, and they begin to seek his counsel in doubtful cases, and gradually learn to lean upon him in times of trial. He may awake some day, perhaps, quite suddenly, to find that twenty years of quiet work, done for the love of it, has a very solid value.

The environment of a large city is not essential to the growth of a good clinical physician. Even in small towns a man can, if he has it in him, become well versed in methods of work, and with the assistance of an occasional visit to some medical centre he can become an expert diagnostician and reach a position of dignity and worth in the community in which he lives. I wish to plead particularly for the wasted opportunities in the smaller hospitals of our large cities, and in those of more moderate size. There are in this State a score or more of hospitals with from thirty to fifty medical beds, offering splendid material for good men on which to build reputations. Take, for example, the town of Thelema, which I know well, to which young Rondibilis, a recent interne at the Hôtel Dieu, has just gone. He wrote asking me for a letter of advice, from which I take the liberty of extracting one or two paragraphs:—

"Your training warrants a high aim. To those who ask, say that you intend to practise medicine only, and will not take surgical or midwifery cases. X. has promised that you may help in the dispensary, and as you can count blood and percuss a chest you will be useful to him in the wards, which, by the way, he now rarely visits. Be careful with the house physicians, and if you teach them anything do it gently, and never crow when you are right. The crow of the young rooster before his spurs are on always jars and antagonizes. Get your own little clinical laboratory in order. Old Dr. Rolando will be sure to visit you, and bear with him as he tells you how he can tell casts from the ascending limb of the loop of Henle. Once he was as you are now, a modern, twenty years ago; but he crawled up the bank, and the stream has left him there, but he does not know it. He means to impress you; be civil and show him the new Nissl-stain preparations, and you will have him as a warm friend. His good heart has kept him with a large general practice, and he can put *post-mortems* in your way, and may send for you to sit up o' nights with his rich patients. If Y. asks you to help in the teaching, jump at the chance. The school is not what you might wish, but the men are in earnest, and a clinical microscopy-class or a voluntary ward-class, with Y.'s cases, will put you on the first rung of the ladder. Yes, join both the city and the county society, and never miss a meeting. Keep your mouth shut too, for a few years, particularly in discussions.

Let the old men read new books; you read the journals and the old books. Study Laënnec this winter; Forbes's *Translation* can be cheaply obtained, but it will help to keep up your French to read it in the original. The old Sydenham Society editions of the Greek writers and of Sydenham are easily got and are really very helpful. As a teacher you can never get *orientiert* without a knowledge of the Fathers, ancient and modern. And do not forget, above all things, the famous advice to Blackmore, to whom, when he first began the study of physic, and asked what books he should read, Sydenham replied, *Don Quixote*, meaning thereby, as I take it, that the only book of physic suitable for permanent reading is the book of Nature."

A young fellow with staying powers who avoids entanglements, may look forward in twenty years to a good consultation practice in any town of 40,000 to 50,000 inhabitants. Some such man, perhaps, in a town far distant, taking care of his education, and not of his bank book, may be the Austin Flint of New York in 1930.

"Many are called, but few are chosen," and of the many who start out with high aims, few see the goal. Even when reached the final period of "cakes and ale" has serious drawbacks. There are two groups of consultants, the intra- and the extra-professional; the one gets work through his colleagues, the other, having outgrown the narrow limits of professional reputation, is at the mercy of the *profanum vulgus*. Then for him "farewell the tranquil mind, farewell content." His life becomes an incessant struggle, and between the attempt to carry on an exhausting and irksome practice, and to keep abreast with young fellows still in the bread-and-butter stage, the consultant at this period is worthy of our sincerest sympathy.

One thing may save him. It was the wish of Walter Savage Landor always to walk with Epicurus on the right hand and Epictetus on the left, and I would urge the clinical physician, as he travels farther from the East, to look well to his companions—to see that they are not of his own age and generation. He must walk with the "boys," else he is lost, irrevocably lost; not all at once, but by easy grades, and every one perceives his ruin before he, "good, easy man," is aware of it. I would not have him a basil plant, to feed on the brains of the bright young fellows who follow the great wheel uphill, but to keep his mind receptive, plastic, and impressionable he must travel with the men who are doing the work of the world, the men between the ages of twenty-five and forty.

In the life of every successful physician there comes the temptation to toy with the Delilah of the press—daily and otherwise. There are times when she may be courted with satisfaction, but beware! sooner or later she is sure to play the harlot, and has left many a man shorn of his strength, viz., the confidence of his professional brethren. Not altogether with justice have some notable members of our profession laboured under the accusation of pandering too much to the public. When a man reaches the climacteric, and has long passed beyond the professional stage of his reputation, we who are still "in the ring" must exercise a good deal of charity, and discount largely the *on dits* which indiscreet friends circulate. It cannot be denied that in dealings with the public just a little touch of humbug is immensely effective, but it is not necessary. In a large city there were three eminent consultants of world-wide reputation; one was said to be a good physician but no humbug, the second was no physician but a great humbug, the third was a great physician and a great humbug. The first achieved the greatest success, professional and social, possibly not financial.

While living laborious days, happy in his work, happy in the growing recognition which he is receiving from his colleagues, no shadow of doubt haunts the mind of the young physician, other than the fear of failure; but I warn him to cherish the days of his freedom, the days when he can follow his bent, untrammeled, undisturbed, and not as yet in the coils of the octopus. In a play of Oscar Wilde's one of the characters remarks, "there are only two great tragedies in life, not getting what you want—and getting it!" and I have known consultants whose treadmill life illustrated the bitterness of this *mot*, and whose great success at sixty did not bring the comfort they had anticipated at forty. The mournful echo of the words of the preacher rings in their ears, words which I not long ago heard quoted with deep feeling by a distinguished physician, "Better is an handful with quietness, than both the hands full with travail and vexation of spirit."

NURSE AND PATIENT

I said, I will take heed to my ways, that I offend not in my tongue.
I will keep my mouth as it were with a bridle.

PSALM xxxix. 1, 2.

If thou hast heard a word, let it die with thee; and be bold, it will not
burst thee.

ECCLESIASTICUS xix. 10.

Lo, in the vale of years beneath
A grisly troop are seen,
The painful family of death,
More hideous than their queen:
This racks the joints, this fires the veins,
That every labouring sinew strains,
Those in the deeper vitals rage:

THOMAS GRAY

IX

NURSE AND PATIENT[1]

THE trained nurse as a factor in life may be regarded from many points of view—philanthropic, social, personal, professional and domestic. To her virtues we have been exceeding kind—tongues have dropped manna in their description. To her faults—well let us be blind, since this is neither the place nor the time to expose them. I would rather call your attention to a few problems connected with her of interest to us collectively,—and individually, too, since who can tell the day of her coming.

Is she an added blessing or an added horror in our beginning civilization? Speaking from the point of view of a sick man, I take my stand firmly on the latter view, for several reasons. No man with any self-respect cares to be taken off guard, in *mufti*, so to speak. Sickness dims the eye, pales the cheek, roughens the chin, and makes a man a scarecrow, not fit to be seen by his wife, to say nothing of a strange woman all in white or blue or gray. Moreover she will take such unwarrantable liberties with a fellow, particularly if she catches him with fever; *then* her special virtues could be depicted by King Lemuel alone. So far as she is concerned you are again in swathing bands, and in her hands you are, as of yore, a helpless lump of human clay. She will stop at nothing, and between baths and spongings and feeding and temperature-taking you are ready to cry with Job the cry of every sick man—"*Cease then, and let me alone.*" For generations has not this been his immemorial

[1] Johns Hopkins Hospital, 1897.

privilege, a privilege with vested rights as a deep-seated animal instinct—to turn his face toward the wall, to sicken in peace, and, if he so wishes, to die undisturbed? All this the trained nurse has, alas! made impossible. And more, too. The tender mother, the loving wife, the devoted sister, the faithful friend, and the old servant who ministered to his wants and carried out the doctor's instructions so far as were consistent with the sick man's wishes—all, all are gone, these old familiar faces; and now you reign supreme, and have added to every illness a domestic complication of which our fathers knew nothing. You have upturned an inalienable right in displacing those whom I have just mentioned. You are intruders, innovators, and usurpers, dislocating, as you do, from their tenderest and most loving duties these mothers, wives and sisters. Seriously, you but lightly reck the pangs which your advent may cause. The handing over to a stranger the care of a life precious beyond all computation may be one of the greatest earthly trials. Not a little of all that is most sacred is sacrificed to your greater skill and methodical ways. In the complicated fabric of modern society both our nursing and our charity appear to be better done second-hand, though at the cost in the one case as in the other of many Beatitudes, links of that golden chain, of which the poet sings, let down from heaven to earth.

Except in the warped judgment of the sick man, for which I have the warmest sympathy, but no respect, you are regarded as an added blessing, with, of course, certain limitations. Certainly you have made the practice of medicine easier to the physician; you are more than the equivalent of the old two hourly doses to a fever patient; and as the public grows in intelligence you should save in many instances the entire apothecary's bill. In his chapter on Instinct, in the

Origin of the Species, Darwin gives a graphic account of the marvellous care-taking capacity of the little Formica fusca—a slave ant. One of these "introduced into a company of her masters who were helpless and actually dying for lack of assistance, instantly set to work, fed and saved the survivors, made some cells, and tended the larvae and put all to rights." *Put all to rights!* How often have I thought of this expression and of this incident when at your word I have seen order and quiet replace chaos and confusion, not alone in the sick-room, but in the household.

As a rule, a messenger of joy and happiness, the trained nurse may become an incarnate tragedy. A protracted illness, an attractive and weak Mrs. Ebb-Smith as nurse, and a weak husband—and all husbands are weak—make fit elements for a domestic tragedy which would be far more common were your principles less fixed.

While thus a source of real terror to a wife, you may become a more enduring misery to a husband. In our hurried progress the weak-nerved sisters have suffered sorely, and that deep mysterious undercurrent of the emotions, which flows along silently in each one of us, is apt to break out in the rapids, eddies and whirls of hysteria or neurasthenia. By a finely measured sympathy and a wise combination of affection with firmness, you gain the full confidence of one of these unfortunates, and become to her a rock of defence, to which she clings, and without which she feels again adrift. You become essential in her life, a fixture in the family, and at times a dark shadow between husband and wife. As one poor victim expressed it, "She owns my wife body and soul, and, so far as I am concerned, she has become the equivalent of her disease." Sometimes there develops that occult attraction between women, only to be explained by the theory of Aristophanes as to the origin of the race; but usually it grows out of the natural leaning of the weak upon the strong, and in the nurse the wife may find that "stern strength and promise of control" for which in the husband she looked in vain.

To measure finely and nicely your sympathy in these cases is a very delicate operation. The individual temperament controls the situation, and the more mobile of you will have a hard lesson to learn in subduing your emotions. It is essential, however, and never let your outward action demonstrate the native act and figure of your heart. You are lost irrevocably, should you so far give the reins to your feelings as to "ope the sacred source of sympathetic tears." Do enter upon your duties with a becoming sense of your frailties. Women can fool men always, women only sometimes, and it may be the lot of any one of you to be such a castaway as the nurse of whom I was told a few weeks ago. The patient was one of those Alphonsine Plessis-like creatures whom everybody had to love, and for whom the primrose path of dalliance had ended in a rigid rest cure. After three weary months she was sent to a quiet place in the mountains with the more sedate of the two nurses who had been with her. Miss Blank had had a good training and a large experience, and was a New England women of the very best type. Alas! hers the greater fall! An accomplishment of this siren, which had produced serious symptoms, was excessive cigarette smoking, and Dr. —— had strictly forbidden tobacco. Three weeks later, my informant paid a visit to the secluded resort, and to his dismay found patient and nurse on the verandah enjoying the choicest brand of Egyptian cigarette!

While not the recipient of all the wretched secrets of life, as are the parson and the doctor, you will frequently be in households the miseries of which cannot be hid, all the cupboards of which are open to you, and you become the involuntary possessor of the most sacred confidences, known perhaps to no other soul. Nowadays that part of the Hippocratic oath which enjoins secrecy as to the things seen and heard among the sick, should be administered to you at graduation.

Printed in your remembrance, written as headlines on the tablets of your chatelaines, I would have two maxims: "I will keep my mouth as it were with a bridle," and "If thou hast heard a word let it die with thee." Taciturnity, a discreet silence, is a virtue little cultivated in these garrulous days when the chatter of the bander-log is everywhere about us, when, as some one has remarked, speech has taken the place of thought. As an inherited trait it is perhaps an infirmity, but the kind to which I refer is an acquired faculty of infinite value. Sir Thomas Browne drew the distinction nicely when he said, "Think not silence the wisdom of fools, but, if rightly timed, the honour of wise men, who had not the infirmity but the virtue of taciturnity," the talent for silence Carlyle calls it.

Things medical and gruesome have a singular attraction for many people, and in the easy days of convalescence a facile-tongued nurse may be led on to tell of "moving incidents" in ward or theatre, and once untied, that unruly member is not apt to cease wagging with the simple narration of events. To talk of diseases is a sort of Arabian Nights' entertainment to which no discreet nurse will lend her talents.

With the growth of one abominable practice in recent days I am not certain you have anything to do, though I have heard your name mentioned in connexion with it. I refer to the habit of openly discussing ailments which should never be mentioned. Doubtless it is in a measure the result

of the disgusting publicity in which we live, and to the
pernicious habit of allowing the filth of the gutters as
purveyed in the newspapers to pollute the stream of our
daily lives. This open talk about personal maladies is an
atrocious breach of good manners. Not a month ago, I
heard two women, both tailor-made, who sat opposite to me
in a street-car, compare notes on their infirmities in Fulvian
accents audible to everyone. I have heard a young woman
at a dinner-table relate experiences which her mother would
have blushed to have told to the family physician. Everything nowadays is proclaimed from the house-tops, among
them our little bodily woes and worries. This is a sad lapse
from the good old practice of our grandfathers, of which
George Sand writes, "People knew how to live and die in
those days, and kept their infirmities out of sight. You
might have the gout, but you must walk about all the same
without making grimaces. It was a point of good breeding
to hide one's suffering." We doctors are great sinners in
this manner, and among ourselves and with the laity are
much too fond of "talking shop."

To another danger I may refer, now that I have waxed
bold. With the fullest kind of training you cannot escape
from the perils of half-knowledge, of pseudo-science, that
most fatal and common of mental states. In your daily
work you involuntarily catch the accents and learn the
language of science, often without a clear conception of its
meaning. I turned incidentally one day to a very fine
example of the nurse learned and asked in a humble tone
what the surgeon, whom I had failed to meet, had thought
of the case, and she promptly replied that "he thought there
were features suggestive of an intracanalicular myxoma;"
and when I looked anxious and queried, "had she happened
to hear if he thought it had an epiblastic or mesoblastic

origin?" this daughter of Eve never flinched; "mesoblastic, I believe," was her answer. She would have handed sponges—I mean gauze—with the same *sang froid* at a Waterloo.

It must be very difficult to resist the fascination of a desire to know more, much more, of the deeper depths of the things you see and hear, and often this ignorance must be very tantalizing, but it is more wholesome than an assurance which rests on a thin veneer of knowledge.

A friend, a distinguished surgeon, has written, in the Lady Priestley vein, an essay on "The Fall of the Trained Nurse," which, so far, he has very wisely refrained from publishing, but he has permitted me to make one extract for your delectation. "A fifth common declension is into the bonds of marriage. The facility with which these modern Vestals fall into this commonplace condition is a commentary, shall I not say rather an illustration, of the inconsistency so notorious in the sex. The Association of Superintendents has in hand, I believe, a Collective Investigation dealing with this question, and we shall shortly have accurate figures as to the percentage of lady superintendents, of head-nurses, of graduates and of pupils who have bartered away their heritage for a hoop of gold."

I am almost ashamed to quote this rude paragraph, but I am glad to do so to be able to enter a warm protest against such sentiments. Marriage is the natural end of the trained nurse. So truly as a young man married is a young man marred, is a woman unmarried, in a certain sense, a woman undone. Ideals, a career, ambition, touched though they be with the zeal of St. Theresa, all vanish before "the blind bow-boy's butt shaft." Are you to be blamed and scoffed at for so doing? Contrariwise, you are to be praised, with but this caution—which I insert at the special request of

Miss Nutting—that you abstain from philandering during your period of training, and, as much as in you lies, spare your fellow-workers, the physicians and surgeons of the staff. The trained nurse is a modern representative, not of the Roman Vestal, but of the female guardian in Plato's republic—a choice selection from the very best women of the community, who know the laws of health, and whose sympathies have been deepened by contact with the best and worst of men. The experiences of hospital and private work, while they may not make her a Martha, enhance her value in many ways as a life-companion, and it is a cause, not for reproach, but for congratulation, that she has not acquired immunity from that most ancient of all diseases— that malady of which the Rose of Sharon sang so plaintively, that sickness "to be stayed not with flagons nor comforted with apples."

A luxury, let us say, in her private capacity, in public the trained nurse has become one of the great blessings of humanity, taking a place beside the physician and the priest, and not inferior to either in her mission. Not that her calling here is in any way new. Time out of mind she has made one of a trinity. Kindly heads have always been ready to devise means for allaying suffering; tender hearts, surcharged with the miseries of this "battered caravan-serai," have ever been ready to speak to the sufferer of a way of peace, and loving hands have ever ministered to those in sorrow, need and sickness. Nursing as an art to be culti-vated, as a profession to be followed, is modern; nursing as a practice originated in the dim past, when some mother among the cave-dwellers cooled the forehead of her sick child with water from the brook, or first yielded to the prompting to leave a well-covered bone and a handful of meal by the side of a wounded man left in the hurried flight before an enemy.   As a profession, a vocation, nursing has already reached in this country a high development. Graduates are numerous, the directories are full, and in many places there is over-crowding, and a serious complaint that even very capable women find it hard to get employment.   This will correct itself in time, as the existing conditions adjust the supply and demand.

A majority of the applicants to our schools are women who seek in nursing a vocation in which they can gain a livelihood in a womanly way; but there is another aspect of the question which may now be seriously taken up in this country.   There is a gradually accumulating surplus of women who will not or who cannot fulfil the highest duties for which Nature has designed them.   I do not know at what age one dare call a woman a spinster.   I will put it, perhaps rashly, at twenty-five.   Now, at that critical period a woman who has not to work for her living, who is without urgent domestic ties, is very apt to become a dangerous element unless her energies and emotions are diverted in a proper channel.   One skilled in hearts can perhaps read in her face the old, old story; or she calls to mind that tender verse of Sappho—

> As the sweet-apple blushes on the end of the
> bough, the very end of the bough, which the
> gatherers overlooked, nay overlooked not but could
> not reach.

But left alone, with splendid capacities for good, she is apt to fritter away a precious life in an aimless round of social duties, or in spasmodic efforts at Church work.   Such a woman needs a vocation, a calling which will satisfy her heart, and she should be able to find it in nursing without entering a regular school or working in ecclesiastical harness.

An organized nursing guild, similar to the German

Deaconesses, could undertake the care of large or small institutions, without the establishment of training schools in the ordinary sense of the term. Such a guild might be entirely secular, with St. James, the Apostle of practical religion, as the patron. It would be of special advantage to smaller hospitals, particularly to those unattached to Medical Schools, and it would obviate the existing anomaly of scores of training schools, in which the pupils cannot get an education in any way commensurate with the importance of the profession. In the period of their training, the members of the Nursing Guild could be transferred from one institution to another until their education was complete. Such an organization would be of inestimable service in connexion with District Nursing. The noble work of Theodore Fliedner should be repeated at an early day in this country. The Kaiserswerth Deaconesses have shown the world the way. I doubt if we have progressed in secularism far enough successfully to establish such guilds apart from church organizations. The Religion of Humanity is thin stuff for women, whose souls ask for something more substantial upon which to feed.

There is no higher mission in this life than nursing God's poor. In so doing a woman may not reach the ideals of her soul; she may fall far short of the ideals of her head, but she will go far to satiate those longings of the heart from which no woman can escape. Romola, the student, helping her blind father, and full of the pride of learning, we admire; Romola, the devotee, carrying in her withered heart woman's heaviest disappointment, we pity; Romola, the nurse, doing noble deeds amid the pestilence, rescuing those who were ready to perish, we love.

On the stepping-stones of our dead selves we rise to higher things, and in the inner life the serene heights are reached only when we die unto those selfish habits and feelings which absorb so much of our lives. To each one of us at some time, I suppose, has come the blessed impulse to break away from all such ties and follow cherished ideals. Too often it is but a flash of youth, which darkens down with the growing years. Though the dream may never be realized, the impulse will not have been wholly in vain if it enables us to look with sympathy upon the more successful efforts of others. In Institutions the corroding effect of routine can be withstood only by maintaining high ideals of work; but these become the sounding brass and tinkling cymbals without corresponding sound practice. In some of us the ceaseless panorama of suffering tends to dull that fine edge of sympathy with which we started. A great corporation cannot have a very fervent charity; the very conditions of its existence limit the exercise. Against this benumbing influence, we physicians and nurses, the immediate agents of the Trust, have but one enduring corrective —the practice towards patients of the Golden Rule of Humanity as announced by Confucius: "What you do not like when done to yourself, do not do to others,"—so familiar to us in its positive form as the great Christian counsel of perfection, in which alone are embraced both the law and the prophets.

X
BRITISH MEDICINE IN GREATER BRITAIN

Cranmer. Nor shall this peace sleep with her; but as when
The bird of wonder dies, the maiden phœnix,
Her ashes new-create another heir
As great in admiration as herself.
So shall she leave her blessedness to one—
When heaven shall call her from this cloud of
    darkness—
Who from the sacred ashes of her honour
Shall star-like rise, as great in fame as she was,
And so stand fix'd. Peace, plenty, love, truth, terror,
That were the servants to this chosen infant,
Shall then be his, and like a vine grow to him:
Wherever the bright sun of heaven shall shine,
His honour and the greatness of his name
Shall be, and make new nations: he shall flourish,
And, like a mountain cedar, reach his branches
To all the plains about him. Our children's children
Shall see this, and bless heaven.

King. Thou speakest wonders.

SHAKESPEARE, *King Henry VIII*, Act *V*.

X

BRITISH MEDICINE IN GREATER BRITAIN[1]

I

TO trace successfully the evolution of any one of the learned professions would require the hand of a master —of one who, like Darwin, combined a capacity for patient observation with philosophic vision. In the case of medicine the difficulties are enormously increased by the extraordinary development which has taken place during the nineteenth century. The rate of progress has been too rapid for us to appreciate, and we stand bewildered and, as it were, in a state of intellectual giddiness, when we attempt to obtain a broad, comprehensive view of the subject. In a safer "middle flight" I propose to dwell on certain of the factors which have moulded the profession in English-speaking lands beyond the narrow seas—of British medicine in Greater Britain. Even for this lesser task (though my affiliations are wide and my sympathies deep) I recognize the limitations of my fitness, and am not unaware that in my ignorance I shall overlook much which might have rendered less sketchy a sketch necessarily imperfect.

Evolution advances by such slow and imperceptible degress that to those who are part of it the finger of time scarcely seems to move. Even the great epochs are seldom apparent to the participators. During the last century neither the colonists nor the mother country appreciated

---

[1] British Medical Association, Montreal, 1897.

the thrilling interest of the long-fought duel for the possession of this continent.   The acts and scenes of the drama,
to them detached, isolated and independent, now glide like
dissolving views into each other, and in the vitascope of
history we can see the true sequence of events.   That we
can meet here to-day, Britons on British soil, in a French
province, is one of the far-off results of that struggle.   This
was but a prelude to the other great event of the eighteenth
century: the revolt of the colonies and the founding of a
second great English-speaking nation—in the words of
Bishop Berkeley's prophecy, "Time's noblest offspring."

It is surely a unique spectacle that a century later
descendants of the actors of these two great dramas should
meet in an English city in New France.   Here, the American may forget Yorktown in Louisbourg, the Englishman
Bunker Hill in Quebec, and the Frenchman both Louisbourg and Quebec in Chateauguay; while we Canadians,
English and French, remembering former friendships and
forgetting past enmities can welcome you to our country—
the land in which and for which you have so often fought.

Once, and only once, before in the history of the world
could such a gathering as this have taken place.   Divided
though the Greeks were, a Hellenic sentiment of extraordinary strength united them in certain assemblies and
festivals.   No great flight of imagination is required to
picture a notable representation of our profession in the
fifth century B.C. meeting in such a colonial town as Agri-
gentum, under the presidency of Empedocles.   Delegates
from the mother cities, brilliant predecessors of Hippocrates
of the stamp of Democedes and Herodicus, delegates from
the sister colonies of Syracuse and other Sicilian towns,
from neighbouring Italy, from far distant Massilia, and
from still more distant Panticapæum and Istria.   And in

such an assemblage there would have been men capable of discussing problems of life and mind more brilliantly than in many subsequent periods, in the proportion as the pre-Hippocratic philosophers in things medical had thought more deeply than many of those who came after them.

We English are the modern Greeks, and we alone have colonised as they did, as free peoples. There have been other great colonial empires, Phœnician, Roman, Spanish, Dutch and French, but in civil liberty and intellectual freedom Magna Græcia and Greater Britain stand alone. The parallel so often drawn between them is of particular interest with reference to the similarity between the Greek settlements in Sicily and the English plantations on the Atlantic coast. Indeed, Freeman says: "I can never think of America without something suggesting Sicily, or of Sicily without something suggesting America." I wish to use the parallel only to emphasise two points, one of difference and one of resemblance. The Greek colonist took Greece with him. Hellas had no geographical bounds, "Massilia and Olbia were cities of Hellas in as full sense as Athens or Sparta." While the emigrant Britons changed their sky, not their character, in crossing the great sea, yet the home-stayers had never the same feeling toward the plantations as the Greeks had towards the colonial cities of Magna Græcia. If, as has been shrewdly surmised, Professor Seely was Herodotus reincarnate, how grieved the spirit of the father of history must have been to say of Englishmen, "nor have we even now ceased to think of ourselves as simply a race inhabiting an island off the northern coast of the Continent of Europe." The assumption of gracious superiority which, unless carefully cloaked, smacks just a little of our national arrogance, is apt to jar on sensitive colonial nerves. With the expansion of the Empire, and the supplanting of a national by an imperial spirit this will become impossible. That this sentiment never prevailed in Hellas, as it did later in the Roman Empire, was due largely to the fact that in literature, in science and in art, the colonial cities of Greece early overshadowed the mother cities. It may be because the settlements of greater Britain were of slower growth that it took several generations and several bitter trials to teach a lesson the Greeks never had to learn.

The Greek spirit was the leaven of the old world, the working of which no nationality could resist; thrice it saved western civilisation, for it had the magic power of leading captivity captive and making even captive conquerors the missionaries of her culture. What modern medicine owes to it will appear later. "The love of science, the love of art, the love of freedom—vitally correlated to each other, and brought into organic union," were the essential attributes of the Greek genius (Butcher). While we cannot claim for the Anglo-Saxon race all of these distinctions it has in a high degree that one which in practical life is the most valuable, and which has been the most precious gift of the race to the world—the love of freedom,

> Of freedom in her regal seat
> Of England.

It would carry me too far afield to discuss the differences between the native Briton and his children scattered so widely up and down the earth. In Canada, South Africa, Australia, and New Zealand, types of the Anglo-Saxon race are developing which will differ as much from each other, and from the English, as the American does to-day from the original stock; but amid these differences can everywhere be seen those race-qualities which have made us what we are—"courage, national integrity, steady good sense, and energy in work." At a future meeting of the Association, perhaps in Australia, a professional Sir Charles Dilke with a firm grasp of the subject may deal with the medical problems of Greater Britain in a manner worthy of the address in medicine. My task, as I mentioned at the outset, is much less ambitious.

Could some one with full knowledge patiently analyse the characteristics of British medicine, he would find certain national traits sufficiently distinct for recognition. Three centuries cannot accomplish very much (and that period has only just passed since the revival of medicine in England), but the local conditions of isolation, which have been singularly favourable to the development of special peculiarities in the national character, have not been without effect in the medical profession. I cannot do more than touch upon a few features, which may be useful as indicating the sources of influence upon Great Britain in the past, and which may perhaps be suggestive as to lines of progress in the future.

Above the fireplace in Sir Henry Acland's library are three panelled portraits of Linacre, Sydenham, and Harvey; the scroll upon them reads *Litteræ*, *Praxis*, *Scientia*. To this great triumvirate, as to the fountain heads, we may trace the streams of inspiration which have made British medicine what it is to-day.

Linacre, the type of the literary physician, must ever hold a unique place in the annals of our profession. To him was due in great measure the revival of Greek thought in the sixteenth century in England; and in the last Harveian oration Dr. Payne has pointed out his importance as a forerunner of Harvey. He made Greek methods available; through him the art of Hippocrates and the science of Galen became once more the subject of careful, first-hand study.

Linacre, as Dr. Payne remarks, "was possessed from his youth till his death by the enthusiasm of learning. He was an idealist devoted to objects which the world thought of little use." Painstaking, accurate, critical, hypercritical perhaps, he remains to-day the chief literary representative of British medicine. Neither in Britain nor in Greater Britain have we maintained the place in the world of letters created for us by Linacre's noble start. It is true that in no generation since has the profession lacked a man who might stand unabashed in the temple at Delos; but, judged by the fruits of learning, scholars of his type have been more common in France and Germany. Nor is it to our credit that so little provision is made for the encouragement of these studies. For years the reputation of Great Britain in this matter was sustained almost alone by the great Deeside scholar, the surgeon of Banchory, Francis Adams— the interpreter of Hippocrates to English students. In the nineteenth century he and Greenhill well maintained the traditions of Linacre. Their work, and that of a few of our contemporaries, among whom Ogle must be specially mentioned, has kept us in touch with the ancients. But by the neglect of the study of the humanities, which has been far too general, the profession loses a very precious quality.

While in critical scholarship and in accurate historical studies, British medicine must take a second place, the influence of Linacre exerted through the Royal College of Physicians and the old Universities, has given to the humanities an important part in education, so that they have moulded a larger section of the profession than in any other country. A physician may possess the science of Harvey and the art of Sydenham, and yet there may be lacking in him those finer qualities of heart and head which count for so much in life. Pasture is not everything and that indefin-

able, though well understood, something which we know as
breeding, is not always an accompaniment of great professional skill.   Medicine is seen at its best in men whose faculties have had the highest and most harmonious culture.
The Lathams, the Watsons, the Pagets, the Jenners, and the
Gairdners have influenced the profession less by their
special work than by exemplifying those graces of life and
refinements of heart which make up character.   And the
men of this stamp in Greater Britain have left the most
enduring mark,—Beaumont, Bovell and Hodder in Toronto;
Holmes, Campbell and Howard in this city; the Warrens,
the Jacksons, the Bigelows, the Bowditches, and the Shat-
tucks in Boston; Bard, Hosack, Francis, Clark, and Flint
of New York; Morgan, Shippen, Redman, Rush, Coxe, the
elder Wood, the elder Pepper, and the elder Mitchell of
Philadelphia—Brahmins all, in the language of the greatest
Brahmin among them, Oliver Wendell Holmes,—these and
men like unto them have been the leaven which has raised
our profession above the dead level of a business.

The *litteræ humaniores*, represented by Linacre, revived
Greek methods; but the Faculty during the sixteenth and
at the beginning of the seventeenth centuries was in a slough
of ignorance and self-conceit, and not to be aroused even
by Moses and the prophets in the form of Hippocrates
and the fathers of medicine.   In the pictures referred to,
Sydenham is placed between Linacre and Harvey; but
science preceded practice, and Harvey's great Lumleian
lectures were delivered before Sydenham was born.   Linacre
has been well called, by Payne, Harvey's intellectual grand-
father.   "The discovery of the circulation of the blood was
the climax of that movement which began a century and a
half before with the revival of Greek medical classics, and
especially of Galen."   (Payne.)   Harvey returned to Greek

methods and became the founder of modern experimental physiology and the great glory of British scientific medicine. The demonstration of the circulation of the blood remains in every detail a model research. I shall not repeat the oft-told tale of Harvey's great and enduring influence, but I must refer to one feature which, until lately, has been also a special characteristic of his direct successors in Great Britain. Harvey was a practitioner and a hospital physician. There are gossiping statements by Aubrey to the effect that "he fell mightily in his practice" after the publication of the *De motu cordis*, and that his "therapeutic way" was not admired; but to these his practical success is the best answer. It is remarkable that a large proportion of all the physiological work of Great Britain has been done by men who have become successful hospital physicians or surgeons. I was much impressed by a conversation with Professor Ludwig in 1884. Speaking of the state of English physiology, he lamented the lapse of a favourite English pupil from science to practice; but, he added, "while sorry for him, I am glad for the profession in England." He held that the clinical physicians of that country had received a very positive impress from the work of their early years in physiology and the natural sciences. I was surprised at the list of names which he cited; among them I remember Bowman, Paget, Savory and Lister. Ludwig attributed this feature in part to the independent character of the schools in England, to the absence of the University element so important in medical life in Germany, but, above all, to the practical character of the English mind, the better men preferring an active life in practice to a secluded laboratory career.

Thucydides it was who said of the Greeks that they possessed "the power of thinking before they acted, and of acting, too." The same is true in a high degree of the English race. To know just what has to be done, then to do it, comprises the whole philosophy of practical life. Sydenham—*Angliæ lumen*, as he has been well called—is the model practical physician of modern times. Linacre led Harvey back to Galen, Sydenham to Hippocrates. The one took Greek science, the other not so much Greek medicine as Greek methods, particularly intellectual fearlessness, and a certain knack of looking at things. Sydenham broke with authority and went to nature. It is an extraordinary fact that he could have been so emancipated from dogmas and theories of all sorts. He laid down the fundamental proposition, and acted upon it, that "all diseases should be described as objects of natural history." To do him justice we must remember, as Dr. John Brown says, "in the midst of what a mass of errors and prejudices, of theories actively mischievous, he was placed, at a time when the mania of hypothesis was at its height, and when the practical part of his art was overrun and stultified by vile and silly nostrums." Sydenham led us back to Hippocrates, I would that we could be led oftener to Sydenham! How necessary to bear in mind what he says about the method of the study of medicine. "In writing therefore, such a natural history of diseases, every merely philosophical hypothesis should be set aside, and the manifest and natural phenomena, however minute, should be noted with the utmost exactness. The usefulness of this procedure cannot be easily overrated, as compared with the subtle inquiries and trifling notions of modern writers, for can there be a shorter, or indeed any other way of coming at the morbific causes, or discovering the curative indications than by a certain perception of the peculiar symptoms? By these steps and helps it was that the father of physic, the great Hippocrates, came to

excel, his theory being no more than an exact description
or view of Nature. He found that Nature alone often
terminates diseases, and works a cure with a few simple
medicines, and often enough with no medicines at all."
Well indeed has a recent writer remarked, "Sydenham is
unlike every previous teacher of the principles and practice
of medicine in the modern world." He, not Linacre or
Harvey, is the model British physician in whom were concentrated all those practical instincts upon which we lay
such stress in the Anglo-Saxon character.

The Greek faculty which we possess of thinking and
acting has enabled us, in spite of many disadvantages, to
take the lion's share in the great practical advances in
medicine.   Three among the greatest scientific movements
of the century have come from Germany and France.
Bichat, Laënnec and Louis laid the foundation of modern
clinical medicine; Virchow and his pupils of scientific
pathology; while Pasteur and Koch have revolutionized
the study of the causes of disease; and yet, the modern
history of the art of medicine could almost be written in its
fulness from the records of the Anglo-Saxon race. We
can claim every practical advance of the very first rank—
vaccination, anæsthesia, preventive medicine and antiseptic
surgery, the "captain jewels in the carcanet" of the profession, beside which can be placed no others of equal lustre.

One other lesson of Sydenham's life needs careful conning.
The English Hippocrates, as I said, broke with authority.
His motto was

> Thou Nature art my Goddess; to thy law
> My services are bound.

Undue reverence for authority as such, a serene satisfaction with the *status quo*, and a fatuous objection to change
have often retarded the progress of medicine. In every

generation, in every country, there have been, and ever will be, *laudatores temporis acti*, in the bad sense of that phrase, not a few of them men in high places, who have lent the weight of a complacent conservatism to bolster up an ineffectual attempt to stay the progress of new ideas. Every innovator from Harvey to Lister has been made to feel its force.   The recently issued life of Thomas Wakley is a running commentary of this spirit, against the pricks of which he kicked so hard and so effectually.   But there are signs of a great change.   The old universities and the colleges, once the chief offenders, have been emancipated, and remain no longer, as Gibbon found them, steeped in port and prejudice.   The value of authority *per se* has lessened enormously, and we of Greater Britain have perhaps suffered as the pendulum has swung to the other extreme.   Practice loves authority, as announced in "the general and perpetual voice of men."   Science must ever hold with Epicharmus that a judicious distrust and wise scepticism are the sinews of the understanding.   And yet the very foundations of belief in almost everything relating to our art rest upon authority.   The practitioner cannot always be the judge; the responsibility must often rest with the teachers and investigators, who can only learn in the lessons of history the terrible significance of the word.   The fetters of a thousand years in the treatment of fever were shattered by Sydenham, shattered only to be riveted anew. How hard was the battle in this century against the entrenched and stubborn foe! Listen to the eloquent pleadings of Stokes, pleading as did Sydenham, against authority, and against the bleedings, the purgings and sweatings of fifty years ago.   "Though his hair be grey and his authority high, he is but a child in knowledge and his reputation an error.   On a level with a child, so far as correct appreciation of the great truths of medicine is concerned, he is very different in other respects, his powers of doing mischief are greater; he is far more dangerous. Oh! that men would stoop to learn, or at least cease to destroy." The potency of human authority among the powers that be was never better drawn than by the judicious Hooker in his section on this subject. "And this not only with 'the simpler sort,' but the learneder and wiser we are, the more such arguments in some cases prevail with us. The reason why the simpler sort are moved with authority is the conscience of their own ignorance; whereby it cometh to pass that having learned men in admiration, they rather fear to dislike them than know wherefore they should allow and follow their judgments. Contrariwise with them that are skilful authority is much more strong and forcible; because they only are able to discern how just cause there is why to some men's authority so much should be attributed. For which cause the name of Hippocrates (no doubt) were more effectual to persuade even such men as Galen himself than to move a silly empiric."[1]

Sydenham was called "a man of many doubts" and therein lay the secret of his great strength.

II

Passing now to the main question of the development of this British medicine in Greater Britain, I must at once acknowledge the impossibility of doing justice to it. I can only indicate a few points of importance, and I must confine my remarks chiefly to the American part of Greater Britain. We may recognize three distinct periods corresponding to three distinct waves of influence, the first from the early immigration to about 1820, the second from

[1] *Ecclesiastical Polity.* Book ii., vii. 2.

about 1820 to 1860. and the third from about 1860 to the present time.

The colonial settlements were contemporaneous with the revival of medicine in England. Fellow-students of Harvey at Cambridge might have sailed in the *Mayflower* and the *Arbella*. The more carefully planned expeditions usually enlisted the services of a well-trained physician, and the early records, particularly of the New England colonies, contain many interesting references to these college-bred men. Giles Firman, who settled in Boston in 1632, a Cambridge-man, seems to have been the first to give instruction in medicine in the new world. The parsons of that day had often a smattering of physic, and illustrated what Cotton Mather called an "angelical conjunction." He says: "Ever since the days of Luke, the Evangelist, skill in *Physick* has been frequently professed and practised by Persons whose more declared Business was the study of Divinity." Firman himself, finding physic "but a meane helpe," took orders. These English physicians in the New England colonies were scholarly, able men. Roger Chillingworth, in Hawthorne's *Scarlet Letter*, has depicted them in a sketch of his own life: "Made up of earnest, studious, thoughtful, quiet years, bestowed faithfully for the increase of knowledge, faithfully, too, for the advancement of human welfare—men, thoughtful for others, caring little for themselves, kind, just, true, and of constant if not warm affections,—" a singularly truthful picture of the old colonial physician.

Until the establishment of medical schools (University of Pennsylvania, 1763; King's College, afterwards Columbia, 1767; Harvard, 1782) the supply of physicians for the colonies came from Great Britain, supplemented by men trained under the old apprentice system, and of colonists who went to Edinburgh, Leyden and London for their medical education.   This latter group had a most powerful effect in moulding professional life in the prerevolutionary period.   They were men who had enjoyed not alone the instruction but often the intimate friendship of the great English and European physicians.   Morgan, Rush, Shippen, Bard, Wistar, Hosack and others had received an education comprising all that was best in the period, and had acquired the added culture which can only come from travel and wide acquaintance with the world.   Morgan, the founder of the medical school of the University of Pennsylvania, was away seven years, and before returning had taken his seat as a corresponding member of the French Academy of Surgery, besides having been elected a Fellow of the Royal Society. The War of Independence interrupted temporarily the stream of students, but not the friendship which existed between Cullen and Fothergill and their old pupils in America.   The correspondence of these two warm friends of the colonies testifies to the strong professional intimacy which existed at the time between the leaders of the profession in the old and new worlds.

But neither Boerhaave, Cullen nor Fothergill stamped colonial medicine as did the great Scotsman, John Hunter. Long, weary centuries separated Harvey from Galen; not a century elapsed from the death of the great physiologist to the advent of the man in whose phenomenal personality may be seen all the distinctive traits of modern medicine, and the range of whose mighty intellect has had few, if any, equals since Aristotle.   Hunter's influence on the profession of this continent, so deep and enduring, was exerted in three ways.   In the first place, his career as an army surgeon, and his writings on subjects of special interest to military men, carried his work and ways into innumerable campaigns in the long French wars and in the War of Independence. Hunter's works were reprinted in America as early as 1791 and 1793. In the second place, Hunter had a number of most distinguished students from the colonies, among whom were two who became teachers of wide reputation. William Shippen, the first Professor of Anatomy in the University of Pennsylvania, lived with Hunter on terms of the greatest intimacy. He brought back his methods of teaching and some measure of his spirit. With the exception of Hewson and Home, Hunter had no more distinguished pupil than Philip Syng Physick, who was his house surgeon at St. George's Hospital, and his devoted friend. For more than a generation Physick had no surgical compeer in America, and enjoyed a reputation equalled by no one save Rush. He taught Hunterian methods in the largest medical school in the country, and the work of his nephew (Dorsey) on Surgery is very largely Hunter modified by Physick. But in a third and much more potent way the great master influenced the profession of this continent. Hunter was a naturalist to whom pathological processes were only a small part of a stupendous whole, governed by law, which, however, could never be understood until the facts had been accumulated, tabulated and systematized. By his example, by his prodigious industry, and by his suggestive experiments he led men again into the old paths of Aristotle, Galen and Harvey. He made all thinking physicians naturalists, and he lent a dignity to the study of organic life, and re-established a close union between medicine and the natural sciences. Both in Britian and Greater Britain he laid the foundation of the great collections and museums, particularly those connected with the medical schools. The Wistar-Horner and the Warren museums originated with men who had been greatly influenced by Hunter. He was, moreover, the intellectual father of that interesting group of men on this side of the Atlantic who, while practising as physicians, devoted much time and labour to the study of Natural History.   In the latter part of the last century and during the first thirty years of this, the successful practitioner was very often a naturalist.   I wish that time permitted me to do justice to the long list of men who have been devoted naturalists and who have made contributions of great value.   Benjamin Smith Barton, David Hosack, Jacob Bigelow, Richard Harlan, John D. Godman, Samuel George Morton, John Collins Warren, Samuel L. Mitchill, J. Aiken Meigs and many others have left the records of their industry in their valuable works and in the Transactions of the various societies and academies.   In Canada, many of our best naturalists have been physicians, and collections in this city testify to the industry of Holmes and McCullough.

I was regretting the *humanities* a few minutes ago, and now I have to mourn the almost complete severance of medicine from the old natural history.   To a man the most delightful recollections of whose student life are the Saturdays spent with a preceptor who had a Hunterian appetite for specimens—anything from a trilobite to an acarus—to such a one across the present brilliant outlook comes the shadow of the thought that the conditions of progress will make impossible again such careers as those of William Kitchen Parker and William Carmichael McIntosh.

Until about 1820 the English profession of this continent knew little else than British medicine.   After this date in the United States the ties of professional union with the old country became relaxed, owing in great part to the increase in the number of home schools, and in part to the development of American literature.   To 1820 one hundred and fourteen native medical books of all kinds had been issued from the press, and one hundred and thirty-one reprints and translations, the former English, the latter, few in number, and almost exclusively French (Billings).

Turning for a few minutes to the condition of the profession in Canada during this period, I regret that I cannot speak of the many interesting questions relating to the French colonies. With the earliest settlers physicians had come, and among the Jesuits, in their devoted missions, there are records of *donnés* (laymen attached to the service), who were members of the profession. One of these, René Goupil, suffered martyrdom at the hands of the Iroquois.[1]

Between the fall of Quebec in 1759 and 1820, the English population had increased by the settlement of Upper Canada, chiefly by United Empire Loyalists from the United States, and after the war of 1812 by settlers from the old country. The physicians in the sparsely settled districts were either young men who sought their fortunes in the new colony or were army surgeons, who had remained after the revolutionary war or the war of 1812. The military element gave for some years a very distinctive stamp to the profession. These surgeons were men of energy and ability, who had seen much service, and were accustomed to order, discipline and regulations. Sabine, in his *American Loyalists*, refers to the Tory proclivities of the doctors, but says that they were not so much disturbed as the lawyers and clergymen. Still a good many of them left their homes for conscience' sake, and Canniff, in his *Medical Profession in Upper Canada*, gives a list of those known to have been among the United Empire Loyalists.

The character of the men who controlled the profession of the new colony is well shown by the proceedings of

[1] Parkman. *Jesuits in North America.*

the Medical Board which was organized in 1819. Drs.
Macaulay and Widmer, both army surgeons, were the chief
members. The latter, who has well been termed the father
of the profession in Upper Canada, a man of the very highest
character, did more than anyone else to promote the progress of the profession; and throughout his long career his
efforts were always directed in the proper channels. In
looking through Canniff's most valuable work one is much
impressed by the sterling worth and mettle of these old
army surgeons who in the early days formed the larger part
of the profession. The minutes of the Medical Board
indicate with what military discipline the candidates were
examined, and the percentage of rejections has probably
never been higher in the history of the province than it was
in the first twenty years of the existence of the Board.

One picture on the canvas of those early days lingers in
the memory, illustrating all the most attractive features
of a race which has done much to make this country what
it is to-day. Widmer was the type of the dignified old
army surgeon, scrupulously punctilious and in every detail
regardful of the proprieties of life. "Tiger" Dunlop may
be taken as the very incarnation of that restless roving spirit
which has driven the Scotch broadcast upon the world.
After fighting with the Connaught Rangers in the war of
1812, campaigning in India, clearing the Saugur of tigers—
hence his soubriquet "Tiger," lecturing on Medical Jurisprudence in Edinburgh, writing for *Blackwood*, editing the
British Press and the *Telescope*, introducing Beck's *Medical
Jurisprudence* to English readers, and figuring as director
and promoter of various companies, this extraordinary
character appears in the young colony as "Warden of the
Black Forest" in the employ of the Canada Company.
His life in the backwoods at Gairbraid, his *Noctes Ambrosianæ*

Canadenses, his famous "Twelve apostles," as he called his
mahogany liquor stand (each bottle a full quart), his active
political life, his remarkable household, his many eccentricities—are they not all portrayed to the life in the recently
issued *In the days of the Canada Company?*

III

Turning now to the second period, we may remark in
passing that the nineteenth century did not open very
auspiciously for British medicine.   Hunter had left no
successor, and powerful as had been his influence it was
too weak to stem the tide of abstract speculation, with which
Cullen, Brown, and others flooded the profession.   No more
sterile period exists than the early decades of this century.
Willan (a great naturalist in skin diseases) with a few others
saved it from utter oblivion.   The methods of Hippocrates,
of Sydenham, and of Hunter had not yet been made
available in everyday work.

The awakening came in France, and such an awakening!
It can be compared with nothing but the renaissance in
the sixteenth and seventeenth centuries, which gave us
Vesalius and Harvey.   "Citizen" Bichat and Broussais
led the way, but Laënnec really created clinical medicine
as we know it to-day.   The discovery of auscultation was
only an incident, of vast moment it is true, in a systematic
study of the correlation of symptoms with anatomical
changes.   Louis, Andral, and Chomel, extended the reputation of the French school which was maintained to the full
until the sixth decade, when the brilliant Trousseau ended
for a time a long line of Paris teachers, whose audience had
been world-wide.   The revival of medicine in Great Britain
was directly due to the French.   Bright and Addison,
Graves and Stokes, Forbes and Marshall Hall, Latham and

Bennett were profoundly affected by the new movement. In the United States Anglican influence did not wane until after 1820. Translations of the works of Bichat appeared as early as 1802, and there were reprints in subsequent years, but it was not until 1823 that the first translation (a reprint of Forbes' edition) of Laënnec was issued. Broussais' works became very popular in translations after 1830, and in the journals from this time on the change of allegiance became very evident. But men rather than books diverted the trend of professional thought. After 1825, American students no longer went to Edinburgh and London, but to Paris, and we can say that between 1830 and 1860, every teacher and writer of note passed under the Gallic yoke. The translations of Louis' works and the extraordinary success of his American pupils, a band of the ablest young men the country had ever seen, added force to the movement. And yet this was a period in which American medical literature was made up largely of pirated English books, and the systems, encyclopedias, and libraries, chiefly reprints, testify to the zeal of the publishers. Stokes, Graves, Watson, Todd, Bennett, and Williams, furnished Anglican pap to the sucklings, as well as strong meat to the full grown. In spite of the powerful French influence the text books of the schools were almost exclusively English.

In Canada the period from 1820 to 1860 saw the establishment of the English universities and medical schools. In Montreal the agencies at work were wholly Scotch. The McGill Medical School was organized by Scotchmen, and from its inception has followed closely Edinburgh methods. The Paris influence, less personal, was exerted chiefly through English and Scotch channels. The Upper Canada schools were organized by men with English affiliations, and the traditions of Guy's, St. Bartholomew's, St. Thomas's,

St. George's, and of the London Hospital, rather than those of Edinburgh, have prevailed in Toronto and Kingston.

The local French influence on British medicine in Canada has been very slight.   In the early decades of the century, when the cities were smaller, and the intercourse between the French and English somewhat closer, the reciprocal action was more marked.   At that period English methods became somewhat the vogue among the French; several very prominent French Canadians were Edinburgh graduates.   Attempts were made in the medical journals to have communications in both languages, but the fusion of the two sections of the profession was no more feasible than the fusion of the two nationalities, and the development has progressed along separate lines.

The third period dates from about 1860 when the influence of German medicine began to be felt.   The rise of the Vienna school was for a long time the only visible result in Germany of the French renaissance.   Skoda, the German Laënnec and Rokitansky, the German Morgagni, influenced English and American thought between 1840 and 1860, but it was not until after the last date that Teutonic medicine began to be felt as a vitalizing power, chiefly through the energy of Virchow.   After the translation of the *Cellular Pathology* by Chance (1860) the way lay clear and open to every young student who desired inspiration.   There had been great men in Berlin before Virchow, but he made the town on the Spree a Mecca for the faithful of all lands. From this period we can date the rise of German influence on the profession of this continent.   It came partly through the study of pathological histology, under the stimulus given by Virchow, and partly through the development of the specialties, particularly diseases of the eye, of the skin and of the larynx.   The singularly attractive courses of

Hebra, the organization on a large scale in Vienna of a system of graduate teaching designed especially for foreigners and the remarkable expansion of the German laboratories combined to divert the stream of students from France. The change of allegiance was a deserved tribute to the splendid organization of the German universities, to the untiring zeal and energy of their professors and to their single-minded devotion to science for its own sake.

In certain aspects the Australasian Settlements present the most interesting problems of Greater Britain. More homogeneous, thoroughly British, isolated, distant, they must work out their destiny with a less stringent environment, than, for example, surrounds the English in Canada. The traditions are more uniform and of whatever character have filtered through British channels. The professional population of native-trained men is as yet small, and the proportion of graduates and licentiates from the English, Scotch and Irish colleges and boards guarantees a dominance of Old Country ideas. What the maturity will show cannot be predicted, but the vigorous infancy is full of crescent promise. On looking over the files of Australian and New Zealand journals, one is impressed with the monotonous similarity of the diseases in the antipodes to those of Great Britain and of this continent. Except in the matter of parasitic affections and snake-bites, the nosology presents few distinctive qualities. The proceedings of the four Intercolonial Congresses indicate a high level of professional thought. In two points Australia has not progressed as other parts of Greater Britain. The satisfactory regulation of practice, so early settled in Canada, has been beset with many difficulties. Both in the United States and in Australia the absence of the military element, which was so strong in Canada, may in part at least account for the great difference which has prevailed in this matter of the state licence. The other relates to the question of ethics, to which one really does not care to refer, were it not absolutely forced upon the attention in reading the journals. Elsewhere professional squabbles, always so unseemly and distressing, are happily becoming very rare, and in Great Britain, and on this side of the water, we try at any rate "to wash our dirty linen at home." In the large Australian cities, differences and dissensions seem lamentably common. Surely they must be fomented by the atrocious system of elections to the hospitals, which plunges the entire profession every third or fourth year into the throes of a contest, in which the candidates have to solicit the suffrages of from 2,000 to 4,000 voters! Well, indeed, might Dr. Batchelor, say, in his address at the fourth Intercolonial Congress: "It is a scandal that in any British community, much less in a community which takes pride in a progressive spirit, such a pernicious system should survive for an hour."

Of India, of "Vishnu-land," what can one say in a few minutes? Three thoughts at once claim recognition. Here in the dim dawn of history, with the great Aryan people, was the intellectual cradle of the world. To the Hindoos we owe a debt which we can at any rate acknowledge; and even in medicine, many of our traditions and practices may be traced to them, as may be gathered from that most interesting *History of Aryan Medical Science*, by the Thakore Saheb of Gondal.

Quickly there arises the memory of the men who have done so much for British medicine in that great empire. Far from their homes, far from congenial surroundings, and far from the stimulus of scientific influences, Annesley, Ballingall, Twining, Morehead, Waring, Parkes, Cunningham, Lewis, Vandyke Carter, and many others, have upheld

the traditions of Harvey and of Sydenham.   On the great
epidemic diseases how impoverished would our literature
be in the absence of their contributions!   But then there
comes the thought of "the petty done, the undone vast,"
when one considers the remarkable opportunities for study
which India has presented.   Where else in the world is
there such a field for observation in cholera, leprosy,
dysentery, the plague, typhoid fever, malaria, and in a
host of other less important maladies.   And what has the
British Government done towards the scientific investigation of the diseases of India?   Until recently little or nothing, and the proposal to found an institute for the scientific
study of disease has actually come from the native chiefs!
The work of Dr. Hankin and of Professor Haffkine, and the
not unmixed evil of the brisk epidemic of plague in Bombay,
may arouse the officials to a consciousness of their shortcomings.   While sanitary progress has been great as shown
in a reduction of the mortality from sixty-nine per mille
before 1857 to fifteen per mille at present, many problems
are still urgent, as may be gathered from reading Dr.
Harvey's Presidental address and the proceedings of the
Indian Medical congress.   That typhoid fever can be called
the "scourge of India," and that the incidence of the disease
should remain so high among the troops point to serious
sanitary defects as yet unremedied.   As to the prevalence
of veneral disease among the soldiers—an admission of
nearly 500 per mille tells its own tale.

On reading the journals and discussions one gets the
impression that matters are not as they should be in India.
There seems to be an absence of proper standards of authority.   Had there been in each presidency during the past
twenty years thoroughly equipped government laboratories
in charge of able men, well trained in modern methods, the con-

tributions to our knowledge of epidemic diseases might have been epoch-making, and at any rate we should have been spared the crudeness which is evident in the work (particularly in that upon malaria) of some zealous but badly trained men.

In estimating the progress of medicine in the countries comprising Greater Britain, the future rather than the present should be in our minds. The strides which have been taken during the past twenty years are a strong warrant that we have entered upon a period of exceptional development. When I see what has been accomplished in this city in the short space of time since I left, I can scarcely credit my eyes: the reality exceeds the utmost desire of my dreams. The awakening of the profession in the United States to a consciousness of its responsibilities and opportunities has caused unparalleled changes, which have given an impetus to medical education and to higher lines of medical work which has already borne a rich harvest. Within two hundred years who can say where the intellectual centre of the Anglo-Saxon race will be? The Mother Country herself has only become an intellectual nation of the first rank within a period altogether too short to justify a prediction that she has reached the zenith. She will probably reverse the history of Hellas, in which the mental superiority was at first with the colonies. At the end of the twentieth century, ardent old-world students may come to this side "as o'er a brook," seeking inspiration from great masters, perhaps in this very city; or the current may turn towards the schools of the great nations of the south. Under new and previously unknown conditions, the Africander, the Australian, or the New Zealander may reach a development before which even "the glory that was Greece" may pale. Visionary as this may appear, it is not one whit more improbable to-day than would have been a prophecy made in 1797 that such a gathering as the present would be possible within a century on the banks of the St. Lawrence.

Meanwhile, to the throbbing vitality of modern medicine the two great meetings held this month, in lands so widely distant, bear eloquent testimony. Free, cosmopolitan, no longer hampered by the dogmas of schools, we may feel a just pride in a profession almost totally emancipated from the bondage of error and prejudice. Distinctions of race, nationality, colour, and creed are unknown within the portals of the temple of Æsculapius. Dare we dream that this harmony and cohesion so rapidly developing in medicine, obliterating the strongest lines of division, knowing no tie of loyalty, but loyalty to truth—dare we hope, I say, that in the wider range of human affairs a similar solidarity may ultimately be reached? Who can say that the forges of Time will weld no links between man and man stronger than those of religion or of country? Some Son of Beor, touched with prophetic vision, piercing the clouds which now veil the eternal sunshine of the mountain top—some spectator of all time and all existence (to use Plato's expression)—might see in this gathering of men of one blood and one tongue a gleam of hope for the future, of hope at least that the great race so dominant on the earth to-day may progress in the bonds of peace—a faint glimmer perhaps of the larger hope of humanity, of that day when "the common sense of most shall hold a fretful 'world' in awe." There remains for us, Greater Britons of whatsoever land, the bounden duty to cherish the best traditions of our fathers, and particularly of the men who gave to British medicine its most distinctive features, of the men, too, who found for us the light and liberty of Greek thought—Linacre, Harvey and Sydenham, those ancient founts of inspiration and models for all time in Literature, Science and Practice.

XI
AFTER TWENTY-FIVE YEARS

For some we loved, the loveliest and the best
That from his Vintage rolling Time has prest,
    Have drunk their Cup a Round or two before,
And one by one crept silently to rest.

OMAR KHAYYAM.

XI

AFTER TWENTY-FIVE YEARS[1]

I

FROM two points of view alone have we a wide and satisfactory view of life—one, as, amid the glorious tints of the early morn, ere the dew of youth has been brushed off, we stand at the foot of the hill, eager for the journey; the other, wider, perhaps less satisfactory, as we gaze from the summit, at the lengthening shadows cast by the setting sun. From no point in the ascent have we the same broad outlook, for the steep and broken pathway affords few halting places with an unobscured view. You remember in the ascent of the Mountain of Purgatory, Dante, after a difficult climb, reached a high terrace encircling the hill, and sitting down turned to the East, remarking to his conductor—"all men are delighted to look back." So on this occasion, from the terrace of a quarter of a century, I am delighted to look back, and to be able to tell you of the prospect.

Twenty-five years ago this Faculty, with some hardihood, selected a young and untried man to deliver the lectures on the Institutes of Medicine. With characteristic generosity the men who had claims on the position in virtue of service in the school, recognizing that the times were changing, stepped aside in favour of one who had had the advantage of post-graduate training in the subjects to be taught. The experiment of the Faculty, supplemented on my part by

[1]McGill College, Montreal, 1899.

191

enthusiasm, constitutional energy, and a fondness for the day's work, led to a certain measure of success. I have tried to live over again in memory those happy early days, but by no possible effort can I recall much that I would fain remember. The dust of passing years has blurred the details, even in part the general outlines of the picture. The blessed faculty of forgetting is variously displayed in us. In some, as in our distinguished countryman, John Beattie Crozier, it is absent altogether, and he fills chapter after chapter with delightful reminiscences and descriptions of his experiences and mental states.[1] At corresponding periods—we are about the same age—my memory hovers like a shade about the magic circle which Ulysses drew in Hades, but finds no Tiresias to lift the veil with which oblivion has covered the past. Shadowy as are these recollections, which,

> be they what they may
> Are yet the fountain light of all our day,
> Are yet a master light of all our seeing,

they are doubly precious from their association with men who welcomed me into the Faculty, now, alas, a sadly reduced remnant. To them—to their influence, to their example, to the kindly encouragement I received at their hands—I can never be sufficiently grateful. Faithfulness in the day of small things may be said to have been the distinguishing feature of the work of the Faculty in those days. The lives of the senior members taught us youngsters the lesson of professional responsibility, and the whole tone of the place was stimulating and refreshing. It was an education in itself, particularly in the amenities of faculty and professional life, to come under the supervision of two such Deans as Dr. George Campbell and Dr. Palmer

[1] *My Inner Life*, Longmans, 1898.

Howard.   How delightful it would be to see the chairs which
they adorned in the school endowed in their memories and
called by their names!

One recollection is not at all shadowy—the contrast in
my feelings to-day only serves to sharpen the outlines.   My
first appearance before the class filled me with a tremulous
uneasiness and an overwhelming sense of embarrassment.
I had never lectured, and the only paper I had read before
a society was with all the possible vaso-motor accompaniment.   With a nice consideration my colleagues did not
add to my distress by their presence, and once inside the
lecture room the friendly greeting of the boys calmed my
fluttering heart, and, as so often happens, the ordeal was
most severe in anticipation.   One permanent impression
of the session abides—the awful task of the preparation of
about one hundred lectures.   After the ten or twelve with
which I started were exhausted I was on the treadmill for
the remainder of the session.   False pride forbade the
reading of the excellent lectures of my predecessor, Dr.
Drake, which, with his wonted goodness of heart, he had
offered.   I reached January in an exhausted condition, but
relief was at hand.   One day the post brought a brand-new
work on physiology by a well-known German professor,
and it was remarkable with what rapidity my labours of
the last half of the session were lightened.   An extraordinary improvement in the lectures was noticed; the students
benefited, and I gained rapidly in the facility with which I
could translate from the German.

Long before the session was over I had learned to appreciate the value of the position entrusted to me, and sought
the means to improve the methods of teaching.   I had had
the advantage of one of the first systematic courses on
practical physiology given at University College, London,

a good part of which consisted of lessons and demonstrations in histology. In the first session, with but a single microscope, I was only able to give the stock display of the circulation of the blood, ciliary action, etc., but a fortunate appointment as physician to the smallpox department of the General Hospital carried with it a salary which enabled me to order a dozen Hartnack microscopes and a few bits of simple apparatus. This is not the only benefit I received from the old smallpox wards, which I remember with gratitude, as from them I wrote my first clinical papers. During the next session I had a series of Saturday demonstrations, and gave a private course in practical histology. One grateful impression remains—the appreciation by the students of these optional and extra hours. For several years I had to work with very scanty accomodation, trespassing in the chemical laboratory in winter, and in summer using the old cloak room downstairs for the histology. In 1880 I felt very proud when the faculty converted one of the lecture rooms into a physiological laboratory and raised a fund to furnish and equip it. Meanwhile I had found time to take my bearings. From the chair of the Institutes of Medicine both physiology and pathology were taught. It had been a time-honoured custom to devote twenty lectures of the course to the latter, and as my colleagues at the Montreal General Hospital had placed the post-mortem room at my disposal I soon found that my chief interest was in the pathological part of the work. In truth, I lacked the proper technique for practical physiology. For me the apparatus never would go right, and I had not a *Diener* who could prepare even the simplest experiments. Alas! there was money expended (my own usually, I am happy to say, but sometimes my friends', as I was a shocking beggar!) in apparatus that I never could set up, but over which the freshmen firmly believed that I spent sleepless nights in elaborate researches. Still one could always get the blood to circulate, cilia to wave and the fibrin to digest.   I do not think that any member of the ten successive classes to which I lectured understood the structure of a lymphatic gland, or of the spleen, or of the placental circulation.   To those structures I have to-day an ingrained hatred, and I am always delighted when a new research demonstrates the folly of all preceding views of their formation.   Upon no subjects had I harder work to conceal my ignorance.   I have learned since to be a better student, and to be ready to say to my fellow students "I do not know."   Four years after my college appointment the Governors of the Montreal General Hospital elected me on the visiting staff.   What better fortune could a young man desire!   I left the same day for London with my dear friend, George Ross, and the happy days we had together working at clinical medicine did much to wean me from my first love.   From that date I paid more and more attention to pathology and practical medicine, and added to my courses one in morbid anatomy, another in pathological histology, and a summer class in clinical medicine.   I had become a pluralist of the most abandoned sort, and at the end of ten years it was difficult to say what I did profess: I felt like the man in Alcibiades II. to whom are applied the words of the poet:—

> Full many a thing he knew;
> But knew them all badly.

Weakened in this way, I could not resist when temptation came to pastures new in the fresh and narrower field of clinical medicine.

After ten years of hard work I left this city a rich man not in this world's goods, for such I have the misfortune—or the good fortune—lightly to esteem, but rich in the goods which neither rust nor moth have been able to corrupt,—in treasures of friendship and good fellowship, and in those treasures of widened experience and a fuller knowledge of men and manners which contact with the bright minds in the profession ensures. My heart, or a good bit of it at least, has stayed with those who bestowed on me these treasures. Many a day I have felt it turn towards this city to the dear friends I left there, my college companions, my teachers, my old chums, the men with whom I lived in closest intimacy, and in parting from whom I felt the chordæ tendineæ grow tense.

II

Twenty-five years ago the staff of this school consisted of the historic septenary, with one demonstrator. To-day I find on the roll of the Faculty 52 teachers. Nothing emphasizes so sharply the character of the revolution which has gradually and silently replaced in great part for the theoretical, practical teaching, for the distant, cold lecture of the amphitheatre the elbow to elbow personal contact of the laboratory. The school, as an organization, the teacher and the student have been profoundly influenced by this change.

When I joined the faculty its finances were in a condition of delightful simplicity, so simple indeed that a few years later they were intrusted to my care. The current expenses were met by the matriculation and graduation fees and the government grant, and each professor collected the fees and paid the expenses in his department. To-day the support of the laboratories absorbs a much larger sum than the entire income of the school in 1874. The greatly increased accommodation required for the practical teaching has made endowment a vital necessity. How nobly, by spontaneous gifts and in generous response to appeals, the citizens have aided the efforts of this faculty I need not remind you. Without it McGill could not have kept pace with the growing demands of modern methods. Upon one feature in the organization of a first-class school permit me to dwell for a moment or two. The specialization of to-day means a group of highly trained experts in the scientific branches, men whose entire energies are devoted to a single subject. To attain proficiency of this sort much time and money are required. More than this, these men are usually drawn from our very best students, with minds above the average. For a majority of them the life devoted to science is a sacrifice; not, of course, that it is so felt by them, since the very essence of success demands that in their work should lie their happiness. I wish that the situation could be duly appreciated by the profession at large, and by the trustees, governors and the members of the faculties throughout the country. Owing these men an enormous debt, since we reap where they have sown, and garner the fruits of their husbandry, what do we give them in return? Too often beggarly salaries and an exacting routine of teaching which saps all initiative. Both in the United States and Canada the professoriate as a class, the men who live by college teaching, is wretchedly underpaid. Only a few of the medical schools have reached a financial position which has warranted the establishment of thoroughly equipped laboratories, and fewer still pay salaries in any way commensurate with the services rendered. I am fully aware that with cobwebs in the purse not what a faculty would desire has only too often to be done, but I have not referred to the matter without full knowledge, as there are schools with large incomes in which there has been of late a tendency to cut down salaries and to fill vacancies too much on Wall Street principles. And not for relief of the pocket alone would I plead. The men in charge of our Canadian laboratories are overworked in teaching. A well organized staff of assistants is very difficult to get, and still more difficult to get paid. The salary of the professor should be in many cases that of the first assistant. When the entire energy of a laboratory is expended on instruction, research, a function of equal importance, necessarily suffers. Special endowments are needed to meet the incessant and urgent calls of the scientific staff. It is gratifying to know that certain of the bequests to this school have of late been of this kind, but I can safely say that no department is as yet fully endowed. Owing to faulty conditions of preliminary education the medical school has to meet certain illegitimate expenses. No one should be permitted to register as a medical student who has not a good preliminary training in chemistry. It is an anomaly that our schools should continue to teach general chemistry, to the great detriment of the subject of medical chemistry, which alone belongs in the curriculum. Botany occupies a similar position.

But *the* laboratories of this medical school are not those directly under its management. McGill College turned out good doctors when it had no scientific laboratories, when the Montreal General Hospital and the University Maternity were its only practical departments. Ample clinical material and good methods of instruction gave the school its reputation more than fifty years ago. Great as has been the growth of the scientific half of the school, the all-important practical half has more than kept pace. The princely endowment of the Royal Victoria Hospital by our large-hearted Canadian Peers has doubled the clinical facilities of this school, and by the stimulus of a healthy rivalry has

put the Montreal General Hospital into a condition of
splendid efficiency.   Among the many changes which have
occurred within the past twenty-five years, I would place
these first in order of importance, since they assure the
continued success of McGill as a school of practical
medicine.

Equally with the school as an organization, the teacher
has felt deeply the changed conditions in medical education,
and many of us are much embarrassed to know what and
how to teach.   In a period of transition it is not easy to get
orientirt.   In some subjects fortunately there is but the
single difficulty—what to teach.   The phenomenal strides
in every branch of scientific medicine have tended to over-
load it with detail.   To winnow the wheat from the chaff
and to prepare it in an easily digested shape for the tender
stomachs of first and second year students taxes the
resources of the most capable teacher.   The devotion to a
subject, and the enthusiasm and energy which enables a
man to keep abreast with its progress, are the very qualities
which often lead him into pedagogic excesses.   To reach a
right judgment in these matters is not easy, and after all
it may be said of teaching as Izaak Walton says of angling,
"Men are to be born so, I mean with inclinations to it."
For many it is very hard to teach down to the level of
beginners.   The Rev. John Ward, Vicar of Stratford-on-
Avon, shortly after Shakespeare's day made an uncompli-
mentary classification of doctors which has since become
well-known:—"first, those that can talk but doe nothing;
secondly, some that can doe but not talk; third, some that
can both doe and talk; fourthly, some that can neither doe
nor talk —and these get most monie."[1]   Professors similarly
may be divided into four classes.   There is, first, the man

[1] *Diary of the Rev. John Ward*, ed. Dr. Charles Severn, Lond., 1839.

who can think but who has neither tongue nor technique. Though useless for the ordinary student, he may be the leaven of a faculty and the chief glory of his university. A second variety is the phonographic professor, who can talk but who can neither think nor work. Under the old régime he repeated year by year the same lecture. A third is the man who has technique but who can neither talk nor think; and a fourth is the rare professor who can do all three—think, talk and work. With these types fairly represented in a faculty, the diversities of gifts only serving to illustrate the wide spirit of the teacher, the Dean at least should feel happy.

But the problem of all others which is perplexing the teacher to-day is not so much what to teach, but how to teach it, more especially how far and in what subjects the practical shall take the place of didactic teaching. All will agree that a large proportion of the work of a medical student should be in the laboratory and in the hospital. The dispute is over the old-fashioned lecture, which has been railed against in good set terms, and which many would like to see abolished altogether. It is impossible, I think to make a fixed rule, and teachers should be allowed a wide discretion. With the large classes of many schools the abolition of the didactic lecture would require a total reconstruction of the curriculum and indeed of the faculty. Slowly but surely practical methods are everywhere taking the place of theoretical teaching, but there will, I think, always be room in a school for the didactic lecture. It is destined within the next ten years to be much curtailed, and we shall probably, as is usual, go to extremes, but there will always be men who can present a subject in ⸱. more lucid and attractive manner than it can be given in a book. Sir William Gairdner once remarked that the reason why

the face and voice of the teacher had so much more power
than a book is that one has a more living faith in him.
Years ago Murchison (than whom Great Britain certainly
never had a more successful teacher of medicine) limited
the lecture in medicine to the consideration of rare cases,
and the prominent features of a group of cases, and to questions of prognosis which cannot be discussed at the bedside.
For the past four years in the subject of medicine I have
been making an experiment in teaching only by a weekly
examination on a set topic, by practical work in the wards,
in the out-patient room and the clinical laboratory, and by
a weekly consideration in the amphitheatre of the acute
diseases of the season. With a small class I have been
satisfied with the results, but the plan would be difficult to
carry out with a large body of students.

The student lives a happy life in comparison with that
which fell to our lot thirty years ago.   Envy, not sympathy,
is my feeling towards him. Not only is the *menu* more
attractive, but it is more diversified and the viands arc
better prepared and presented. The present tendency to
stuffing and cramming will be checked in part when you
cease to mix the milk of general chemistry and botany with
the proper dietary of the medical school. Undoubtedly
the student tries to learn too much, and we teachers try to
teach him too much—neither, perhaps with great success.
The existing evils result from neglect on the part of the
teacher, student and examiner of the great fundamental
principle laid down by Plato—that education is a life-long
process, in which the student can only make a beginning
during his college course. The system under which we
work asks too much of the student in a limited time. To
cover the vast field of medicine in four years is an impossible
task. We can only instil principles, put the student in the

right path, give him methods, teach him how to study, and early to discern between essentials and non-essentials. Perfect happiness for student and teacher will come with the abolition of examinations, which are stumbling blocks and rocks of offence in the pathway of the true student. And it is not so Utopian as may appear at first blush. Ask any demonstrator of anatomy ten days before the examinations, and he should be able to give you a list of the men fit to pass. Extend the personal intimate knowledge such as is possessed by a competent demonstrator of anatomy into all the other departments, and the degree could be safely conferred upon certificates of competency, which would really mean a more thorough knowledge of a man's fitness than can possibly be got by our present system of examination. I see no way of avoiding the necessary tests for the license to practise before the provincial or state boards, but these should be of practical fitness only, and not, as is now so often the case, of a man's knowledge of the entire circle of the medical sciences.

III

But what is most important in an introductory lecture remains to be spoken, for dead indeed would I be to the true spirit of this day, were I to deal only with the questions of the curriculum and say nothing to the young men who now begin the serious work of life. Personally, I have never had any sympathy with the oft-repeated sentiment expressed originally by Abernethy, I believe, who, seeing a large class of medical students, exclaimed, "Good God, gentlemen! whatever will become of you?" The profession into which you enter to-day guarantees to each and every one of you a happy, contented, and useful life. I do not know of any other of which this can be said with greater

assurance. Many of you have been influenced in your
choice by the example and friendship of the doctor in your
family, or some country practitioner in whom you have
recognized the highest type of manhood and whose unique
position in the community has filled you with a laudable
ambition. You will do well to make such an one your exemplar, and I would urge you to start with no higher ambition than to join the noble band of general practitioners.
They form the very sinews of the profession—generous-
hearted men, with well-balanced, cool heads, not scientific
always, but learned in the wisdom not of the laboratories
but of the sick room. This school can take a greater pride
in her graduates scattered throughout the length and
breadth of the continent than in her present splendid
equipment; they explain in great part the secret of her
strength.

I was much interested the other day in reading a letter
of John Locke to the Earl of Peterborough who had consulted him about the education of his son. Locke insisted
that the main point in education is to get "a relish of knowledge." "This is putting life into a pupil." Get early
this relish, this clear, keen joyance in work, with which
langour disappears and all shadows of annoyance flee away.
But do not get too deeply absorbed to the exclusion of all
outside interests. Success in life depends as much upon the
man as on the physician. Mix with your fellow students,
mingle with their sports and their pleasures. You may
think the latter rash advice, but now-a-days even the pleasures of a medical student have become respectable, and I
have no doubt that the "footing supper," which in old
Coté street days was a Bacchanalian orgie, has become a
love feast in which even the Principal and the Dean might
participate. You are to be members of a polite as well as

of a liberal profession and the more you see of life outside the narrow circle of your work the better equipped will you be for the struggle. I often wish that the citizens in our large educational centres would take a little more interest in the social life of the students, many of whom catch but few glimpses of home life during their course.

As to your method of work, I have a single bit of advice, which I give with the earnest conviction of its paramount influence in any success which may have attended my efforts in life—*Take no thought for the morrow.* Live neither in the past nor in the future, but let each day's work absorb your entire energies, and satisfy your widest ambition. That was a singular but very wise answer which Cromwell gave to Bellevire—"No one rises so high as he who knows not whither he is going," and there is much truth in it. The student who is worrying about his future, anxious over the examinations, doubting his fitness for the profession, is certain not to do so well as the man who cares for nothing but the matter in hand, and who knows not whither he is going!

While medicine is to be your vocation, or calling, see to it that you have also an avocation—some intellectual pastime which may serve to keep you in touch with the world of art, of science, or of letters. Begin at once the cultivation of some interest other than the purely professional. The difficulty is in a selection and the choice will be different according to your tastes and training. No matter what it is—but have an outside hobby. For the hard working medical student it is perhaps easiest to keep up an interest in literature. Let each subject in your year's work have a corresponding outside author. When tired of anatomy refresh your mind with Oliver Wendell Holmes; after a worrying subject in physiology, turn to the great idealists,

to Shelley or Keats for consolation; when chemistry dis-
tresses your soul, seek peace in the great pacifier, Shakespeare; and when the complications of pharmacology are
unbearable, ten minutes with Montaigne will lighten the
burden.   To the writings of one old physician I can urge
your closest attention.   There have been, and, happily,
there are still in our ranks notable illustrations of the intimate relations between medicine and literature, but in the
group of literary physicians Sir Thomas Browne stands
preeminent.   The Religio Medici, one of the great English
classics, should be in the hands—in the hearts too—
of every medical student.   As I am on the confessional to-day,
I may tell you that no book has had so enduring an influence
on my life.   I was introduced to it by my first teacher, the
Rev. W. A. Johnson, Warden and Founder of the Trinity
College School, and I can recall the delight with which I
first read its quaint and charming pages.   It was one of the
strong influences which turned my thoughts towards medicine as a profession, and my most treasured copy—the
second book I ever bought—has been a constant companion
for thirty-one years,—comes viæ vitæque.   Trite but true,
is the comment of Seneca—"If you are fond of books you
will escape the ennui of life, you will neither sigh for evening, disgusted with the occupations of the day—nor will
you live dissatisfied with yourself or unprofitable to others."

And, finally, every medical student should remember
that his end is not to be made a chemist or physiologist or
anatomist, but to learn how to recognize and treat disease,
how to become a practical physician.   Twenty years ago
during the summer session, I held my first class in clinical
medicine at the Montreal General Hospital, and on the title
page of a note book I had printed for the students I placed
the following sentence, which you will find the alpha and

omega of practical medicine, not that it by any means covers the whole field of his education:—

"The knowledge which a man can use is the only real knowledge, the only knowledge which has life and growth in it and converts itself into practical power. The rest hangs like dust about the brain or dries like rain drops off the stones." (Froude.)

XII
BOOKS AND MEN

How easily, how secretly, how safely in books do we make bare without shame the poverty of human ignorance! These are the masters that instruct us without rod and ferrule, without words of anger, without payment of money or clothing. Should ye approach them, they are not asleep; if ye seek to question them, they do not hide themselves; should ye err, they do not chide; and should ye show ignorance, they know not how to laugh. O Books! ye alone are free and liberal. Ye give to all that seek, and set free all that serve you zealously.

RICHARD DE BURY, *Philobiblon*, Grolier Club Edition, vol. ii. p. 22

Books delight us when prosperity sweetly smiles; they stay to comfort us when cloudy fortune frowns. They lend strength to human compacts, and without them grave judgments may not be propounded.

Ibid. p. 113.

For Books are not absolutely dead things, but do contain a potency of life in them to be as active as that soul was whose progeny they are; nay, they do preserve as in a vial the purest efficacy and extraction of that living intellect that bred them.

JOHN MILTON, *Areopagitica.*

XII

BOOKS AND MEN[1]

THOSE of us from other cities who bring congratu
lations this evening can hardly escape the tinglings
of envy when we see this noble treasure house; but in my
own case the bitter waters of jealousy which rise in my
soul are at once diverted by two strong sensations. In the
first place I have a feeling of lively gratitude towards this
library. In 1876 as a youngster interested in certain
clinical subjects to which I could find no reference in our
library at McGill, I came to Boston, and I here found what
I wanted, and I found moreover a cordial welcome and
many friends. It was a small matter I had in hand but I
wished to make it as complete as possible, and I have always felt that this library helped me to a good start. It
has been such a pleasure in recurring visits to the library to
find Dr Brigham in charge, with the same kindly interest
in visitors that he showed a quarter of a century ago.
But the feeling which absorbs all others is one of deep
satisfaction that our friend, Dr. Chadwick, has at last seen
fulfilled the desire of his eyes. To few is given the tenacity
of will which enables a man to pursue a cherished purpose
through a quarter of a century—"*Ohne Hast, aber ohne
Rast*" ('tis his favourite quotation); to fewer still is the
fruition granted. Too often the reaper is not the sower.
Too often the fate of those who labour at some object for
the public good is to see their work pass into other hands,
and to have others get the credit for enterprises which they

[1] Boston Medical Library, 1901.

have initiated and made possible. It has not been so with our friend, and it intensifies a thousandfold the pleasure of this occasion to feel the fitness, in every way, of the felicitations which have been offered to him.

It is hard for me to speak of the value of libraries in terms which would not seem exaggerated. Books have been my delight these thirty years, and from them I have received incalculable benefits. To study the phenomena of disease without books is to sail an uncharted sea, while to study books without patients is not to go to sea at all. Only a maker of books can appreciate the labours of others at their true value. Those of us who have brought forth fat volumes should offer hecatombs at these shrines of Minerva Medica. What exsuccous, attenuated offspring they would have been but for the pabulum furnished through the placental circulation of a library. How often can it be said of us with truth, "*Das beste was er ist verdankt er Andern!*"

For the teacher and the worker a great library such as this is indispensable. They must know the world's best work and know it at once. They mint and make current coin the ore so widely scattered in journals, transactions and monographs. The splendid collections which now exist in five or six of our cities and the unique opportunities of the Surgeon-General's Library have done much to give to American medicine a thoroughly eclectic character.

But when one considers the unending making of books, who does not sigh for the happy days of that thrice happy Sir William Browne[1] whose pocket library sufficed for

---

[1] In one of the Annual Orations at the Royal College of Physicians he said: "Behold an instance of human ambition! not to be satisfied but by the conquest, as it were, of three worlds, lucre in the country, honour in the college, pleasure in the medicinal springs."

his life's needs, drawing from a Greek testament his divinity, from the aphorisms of Hippccrates his medicine, and from an Elzevir Horace his good sense and vivacity. There should be in connection with every library a corps of instructors in the art of reading, who would, as a labour of love, teach the young idea how to read. An old writer says that there are four sorts of readers: "Sponges which attract all without distinguishing; Howre-glasses which receive and powre out as fast; Bagges which only retain the dregges of the spices and let the wine escape, and Sives which retaine the best onely." A man wastes a great many years before he reaches the "sive" stage.

For the general practitioner a well-used library is one of the few correctives of the premature senility which is so apt to overtake him. Self-centred, self-taught, he leads a solitary life, and unless his every-day experience is controlled by careful reading or by the attrition of a medical society it soon ceases to be of the slightest value and becomes a mere accretion of isolated facts, without correlation. It is astonishing with how little reading a doctor can practise medicine, but it is not astonishing how badly he may do it. Not three months ago a physician living within an hour's ride of the Surgeon-General's Library brought to me his little girl, aged twelve. The diagnosis of infantile myxœdema required only a half glance. In placid contentment he had been practising twenty years in "Sleepy Hollow" and not even when his own flesh and blood was touched did he rouse from an apathy deep as Rip Van Winkle's sleep. In reply to questions: No, he had never seen anything in the journals about the thyroid gland; he had seen no pictures of cretinism or myxœdema; in fact his mind was a blank on the whole subject. He had not been a reader, he said, but he was a practical man with very

little time. I could not help thinking of John Bunyan's
remarks on the elements of success in the practice of
medicine. "Physicians," he says, "get neither name nor
fame by the pricking of wheals or the picking out thistles,
or by laying of plaisters to the scratch of a pin; every old
woman can do this. But if they would have a name and
a fame, if they will have it quickly, they must do some
great and desperate cures. Let them fetch one to life
that was dead, let them recover one to his wits that was
mad, let them make one that was born blind to see, or let
them give ripe wits to a fool—these are notable cures, and
he that can do thus, if he doth thus first, he shall have the
name and fame he deserves; he may lie abed till noon."
Had my doctor friend been a reader he might have done
a great and notable cure and even have given ripe wits to
a fool!   It is in utilizing the fresh knowledge of the journals
that the young physician may attain quickly to the name
and fame he desires.

There is a third class of men in the profession to whom
books are dearer than to teachers or practitioners—a small,
a silent band, but in reality the leaven of the whole lump.
The profane call them bibliomaniacs, and in truth they
are at times irresponsible and do not always know the
difference between *meum* and *tuum*. In the presence of
Dr. Billings or of Dr. Chadwick I dare not further characterize them. Loving books partly for their contents,
partly for the sake of the authors, they not alone keep
alive the sentiment of historical continuity in the profession, but they are the men who make possible such gatherings as the one we are enjoying this evening. We need
more men of their class, particularly in this country, where
every one carries in his pocket the tape-measure of utility.
Along two lines their work is valuable. By the historical

method alone can many problems in medicine be approached profitably. For example, the student who dates his knowledge of tuberculosis from Koch may have a very correct, but he has a very incomplete, appreciation of the subject. Within a quarter of a century our libraries will have certain alcoves devoted to the historical consideration of the great diseases, which will give to the student that mental perspective which is so valuable an equipment in life. The past is a good nurse, as Lowell remarks, particularly for the weanlings of the fold.

> 'Tis man's worst deed
> To let the things that have been, run to waste
> And in the unmeaning Present sink the Past.

But in a more excellent way these *laudatores temporis acti* render a royal service. For each one of us to-day, as in Plato's time, there is a higher as well as a lower education. The very marrow and fatness of books may not suffice to save a man from becoming a poor, mean-spirited devil, without a spark of fine professional feeling, and without a thought above the sordid issues of the day. The men I speak of keep alive in us an interest in the great men of the past and not alone in their works, which they cherish, but in their lives, which they emulate. They would remind us continually that in the records of no other profession is there to be found so large a number of men who have combined intellectual pre-eminence with nobility of character. This higher education so much needed to-day is not given in the school, is not to be bought in the market place, but it has to be wrought out in each one of us for himself; it is the silent influence of character on character and in no way more potent than in the contemplation of the lives of the great and good of the past, in no way more than in "the touch divine of noble natures gone."

I should like to see in each library a select company of
the Immortals set apart for special adoration. Each country might have its representatives in a sort of alcove of
Fame, in which the great medical classics were gathered.
Not necessarily books, more often the epoch-making contributions to be found in ephemeral journals. It is too
early, perhaps, to make a selection of American medical
classics, but it might be worth while to gather suffrages
in regard to the contributions which ought to be placed
upon our Roll of Honour. A few years ago I made out a list
of those I thought the most worthy which I carried down to
1850, and it has a certain interest for us this evening. The
native modesty of the Boston physician is well known,
but in certain circles there has been associated with it a
curious psychical phenomenon, a conviction of the utter
worthlessness of the *status praesens* in New England, as
compared with conditions existing elsewhere. There is a
variety to-day of the Back Bay Brahmin who delights
in cherishing the belief that medically things are everywhere better than in Boston, and who is always ready to
predict "an Asiatic removal of candlesticks," to borrow
a phrase from Cotton Mather. Strange indeed would it
have been had not such a plastic profession as ours felt
the influences which moulded New England into the intellectual centre of the New World. In reality, nowhere
in the country has the profession been adorned more plen-
tifully with men of culture and of character—not volu-
minous writers or exploiters of the products of other men's
brains—and they manage to get a full share on the Roll
of Fame which I have suggested. To 1850, I have counted
some twenty contributions of the first rank, contributions
which for one reason or another deserve to be called American medical classics. New England takes ten. But in

medicine the men she has given to the other parts of the
country have been better than books.   Men like Nathan
R. Smith, Austin Flint, Willard Parker, Alonzo Clark,
Elisha Bartlett, John C. Dalton, and others carried away
from their New England homes a love of truth, a love of
learning and above all a proper estimate of the personal
character of the physician.

Dr. Johnson shrewdly remarked that ambition was
usually proportionate to capacity, which is as true of a
profession as it is of a man.   What we have seen to-night
reflects credit not less on your ambition than on your
capacity.   A library after all is a great catalyser, accelerat-
ing the nutrition and rate of progress in a profession, and
I am sure you will find yourselves the better for the sacrifice you have made in securing this home for your books,
this workshop for your members.

XIII
MEDICINE IN THE NINETEENTH CENTURY

Even where the milder zone afforded man
A seeming shelter, yet contagion there,
Blighting his being with unnumbered ills,
Spread like a quenchless fire; nor truth availed
Till late to arrest its progress, or create
That peace which first in bloodless victory waved
Her snowy standard o'er this favoured clime.
. . . . Happiness
And Science dawn though late upon the earth;
Peace cheers the mind, health renovates the frame;
Disease and pleasure cease to mingle here,
Reason and passion cease to combat there;
Whilst mind unfettered o'er the earth extends
Its all-subduing energies, and wields
The sceptre of a vast dominion there.

SHELLEY, *The Daemon of the World.*

XIII

MEDICINE IN THE NINETEENTH CENTURY[1]

FOR countless generations the prophets and kings of humanity have desired to see the things which men have seen, and to hear the things which men have heard in the course of the wonderful nineteenth century. To the call of the watchers on the towers of progress there had been the one sad answer—the people sit in darkness and in the shadow of death. Politically, socially, and morally the race had improved, but for the unit, for the individual, there was little hope. Cold philosophy shed a glimmer of light on his path, religion in its various guises illumined his sad heart, but neither availed to lift the curse of suffering from the sin-begotten son of Adam. In the fulness of time, long expected, long delayed, at last Science emptied upon him from the horn of Amalthea blessings which cannot be enumerated, blessings which have made the century forever memorable; and which have followed each other with a rapidity so bewildering that we know not what next to expect. To us in the medical profession, who deal with this unit, and measure progress by the law of the greatest happiness to the greatest number, to us whose work is with the sick and suffering, the great boon of this wonderful century, with which no other can be compared, is the fact that the leaves of the tree of Science have been for the healing of the nations.

[1] Johns Hopkins Historical Club, January, 1901; and published in the New York *Sun*.

Measure as we may the progress of the world—materially, in the advantages of steam, electricity, and other mechanical appliances; sociologically, in the great improvement in the conditions of life; intellectually, in the diffusion of education; morally, in a possibly higher standard of ethics—there is no one measure which can compare with the decrease of physical suffering in man, woman, and child when stricken by disease or accident. This is the one fact of supreme personal import to every one of us. This is the Promethean gift of the century to man.

THE GROWTH OF SCIENTIFIC MEDICINE

The century opened auspiciously, and those who were awake saw signs of the dawn. The spirit of Science was brooding on the waters. In England the influence of John Hunter stimulated the younger men to the study of the problems of anatomy and pathology. On the Continent the great Boerhaave—the Batavian Hippocrates—had taught correct ways in the study of the clinical aspects of disease, and the work of Haller had given a great impetus to physiology. The researches of Morgagni had, as Virchow has remarked, introduced anatomical thinking into medicine. But theories still controlled practice. Under the teaching of Cullen, the old idea that humours were the seat of disease had given place to a neuropathology which recognized the paramount influence of the nervous system in disease. His colleague at Edinburgh, Brown, brought forward the attractive theory that all diseases could be divided into two groups, the one caused by excess of excitement—the sthenic—the other by deficiency—the asthenic—each having its appropriate treatment, the one by depletion, the other by stimulation. In a certain measure Hahnemann's theory of homœopathy was a reaction against the prevalent theories of the day, and has survived through the century, though in a much modified form. Some of his views were as follows:

"The only vocation of the physician is to heal; theoretical knowledge is of no use. In a case of sickness he should only know what is curable and the remedies. Of the diseases he cannot know anything except the symptoms. There are internal changes, but it is impossible to learn what they are; symptoms alone are accessible; with their removal by remedies the disease is removed. Their effects can be studied in the healthy only. They act on the sick by causing a disease similar to that which is to be combated, and which dissolves itself into this similar affection. The full doses required to cause symptoms in the well are too large to be employed as remedies for the sick. The healing power of a drug grows in an inverse proportion to its substance. He says, literally: 'Only potencies are homœopathic medicines.' 'I recognize nobody as my follower but him who gives medicine in so small doses as to preclude the perception of anything medicinal in them by means either of the senses or of chemistry.' 'The pellets may be held near the young infant when asleep.' 'Gliding the hand over the patient will cure him, provided the manipulation is done with firm intention to render as much good with it as possible, for its power is in the benevolent will of the manipulator.' Such is the homœopathy of Hahnemann, which is no longer recognized in what they call homœopathy to-day."— (A. Jacobi.)

The awakening came in France. In 1801 Bichat, a young man, published a work on general anatomy, in which he placed the seat of disease, not in the organs, but in the tissues or fabrics of which they were composed.

which gave an extraordinary impetus to the investigation of pathological changes. Meanwhile, the study of the appearances of organs and bodies when diseased (morbid anatomy), which had been prosecuted with vigor by Morgagni in the eighteenth century, had been carried on actively in Great Britain and on the Continent, and the work of Broussais stimulated a more accurate investigation of local disorders. The discovery by Laënnec of the art of auscultation, by which, through changes in the normal sounds within the chest, various diseases of the heart and lungs could be recognized, gave an immense impetus to clinical research. The art of percussion, discovered by Auenbrugger in the eighteenth century, and reintroduced by Corvisart, contributed not a little to the same. Laënnec's contributions to the study of diseases of the lungs, of the heart, and of the abdominal organs really laid the foundation of modern clinical medicine. A little later Bright published his researches on diseases of the kidneys, from which we date our knowledge of this important subject. One of the most complicated problems of the first half of the century related to the differentiation of the fevers. The eruptive fevers, measles, scarlet fever, and small-pox were easily recognized, and the great group of malarial fevers was well known; but there remained the large class of continued fevers, which had been a source of worry and dispute for many generations. Louis clearly differentiated typhoid fever, and by the work of his American pupils, W. W. Gerhard and Alfred Stillé, of Philadelphia, and George B. Shattuck, of Boston, typhus and typhoid fevers were defined as separate and independent affections. Relapsing fever, yellow fever, dengue, etc., were also distinguished. The work of Graves and Stokes, of Dublin; of Jenner and Budd, in England; of Drake, Dicksen, and Flint, in America, supplemented the labours of the French physicians, and by the year 1860 the profession had reached a sure and safe position on the question of the clinical aspects of fevers.

The most distinguishing feature of the scientific medicine of the century has been the phenomenal results which have followed *experimental investigations*. While this method of research is not new, since it was introduced by Galen, perfected by Harvey, and carried on by Hunter, it was not until well into the middle of the century that, by the growth of research laboratories, the method exercised a deep influence on progress. The lines of experimental research have sought to determine the functions of the organs in health, the conditions under which perversion of these functions occurs in diseases, and the possibility of exercising protective and curative influences on the processes of disease.

The researches of the physiological laboratories have enlarged in every direction our knowledge of the great functions of life—digestion, assimilation, circulation, respiration, and excretion. Perhaps in no department have the results been more surprising than in the growth of our knowledge of the functions of the brain and nerves. Not only has experimental science given us clear and accurate data upon the localization of certain functions of the brain and of the paths of sensatory and of motor impulses, but it has opened an entirely new field in the diagnosis and treatment of the diseases of these organs, in certain directions of a most practical nature, enabling us to resort to measures of relief undreamed of even thirty years ago.

The study of physiology and pathology within the past half-century has done more to emancipate medicine from routine and the thraldom of authority than all the work of all the physicians from the days of Hippocrates to Jenner, and we are as yet but on the threshold.

THE GROWTH OF SPECIALISM

The restriction of the energies of trained students to narrow fields in science, while not without its faults, has been the most important single factor in the remarkable expansion of our knowledge. Against the disadvantages in a loss of breadth and harmony there is the compensatory benefit of a greater accuracy in the application of knowledge in specialism, as is well illustrated in the cultivation of special branches of practice. Diseases of the skin, of the eye, of the ear, of the throat, of the teeth, diseases of women, and of children are now studied and practised by men who devote all their time to one limited field of work. While not without minor evils, this custom has yielded some of the great triumphs of the profession. Dentistry, ophthalmology, and gynæcology are branches which have been brought to a state of comparative perfection, and very largely by the labours of American physicians. In the last-named branch the blessings which have been brought to suffering women are incalculable, not only as regards the minor ailments of life, but in the graver and more critical accidents to which the sex is liable.

One of the most remarkable and beneficial reforms of the nineteenth century has been in the attitude of the profession and the public to the subject of insanity, and the gradual formation of a body of men in the profession who labour to find out the cause and means of relief of this most distressing of all human maladies. The reform movement inaugurated by Tuke in England, by Rush in the United States, by Pinel and Esquirol in France, and by Jacobi and Hasse in Germany, has spread to all civilized countries, and has led not only to an amelioration and improvement in the care of the insane, but to a scientific study of the subject which has already been productive of much good. In this country, while the treatment of the insane is careful and humanitarian, the unfortunate affiliation of insanity with politics is still in many States a serious hindrance to progress.

It may be interesting to take a glance at the state of medicine in this country at the opening of the century. There were only three schools of medicine, the most important of which were the University of Pennsylvania and the Harvard. There were only two general hospitals. The medical education was chiefly in the hands of the practitioners, who took students as apprentices for a certain number of years. The well-to-do students and those wishing a better class of education went to Edinburgh or London. There were only two or three medical journals, and very few books had been published in the country, and the profession was dependent entirely upon translations from the French and upon English works. The only medical libraries were in connexion with the Pennsylvania Hospital and the New York Hospital. The leading practitioners in the early years were Rush and Physick, in Philadelphia; Hosack and Mitchill, in New York; and James Jackson and John Collins Warren, in Boston. There were throughout the country, in smaller places, men of great capabilities and energy, such as Nathan Smith, the founder of the Medical Schools of Dartmouth and of Yale, and Daniel Drake in Cincinnati. After 1830 a remarkable change took place in the profession, owing to the leaven of French science brought back from Paris by American students. Between 1840 and 1870 there was a great increase in the number of medical schools, but the general standard of education was low—lower, indeed, than had ever before been reached in the medical profession. The private schools multiplied rapidly, diplomas were given on short two-year sessions, and nothing contributed more to the degeneration of the profession than this competition and rivalry between ill-equipped medical schools. The reformation, which started at Harvard shortly after 1870, spread over the entire country, and the rapid evolution of the medical school has been one of the most striking phenomena in the history of medicine in the century. University authorities began to appreciate the fact that medicine was a great department of knowledge, to be cultivated as a science and promoted as an art. Wealthy men felt that in no better way could they contribute to the progress of the race than by the establishment of laboratories for the study of disease and hospitals for the care of the sick poor. The benefactions of Johns Hopkins, of Sims, of Vanderbilt, of Pierpont Morgan, of Strathcona, of Mount-Stephen, of Payne, and of Levi C. Lane and others have placed scientific medicine on a firm basis.

THE GROWTH OF PREVENTIVE MEDICINE

Sanitary science, hygiene, or preventive medicine may claim to be one of the brightest spots in the history of the nineteenth century. Public hygiene was cultivated among the Egyptians, and in the Mosaic law it reached a remarkable organization. The personal hygiene of the Greeks was embraced in the saying, "The fair mind in the fair body," and the value of exercise and training was fully recognized. The Romans, too, in public and private hygiene, were our superiors in the matter of water supply and baths. But modern sanitary science has a much wider scope and is concerned with the causes of disease quite as much as with the conditions under which these diseases prevail. The foundations of the science were laid in the last century with Jenner's discovery of vaccination. Howard, too, had grasped the association of fever with overcrowding in the jails, while the possibility of the prevention of scurvy had been shown by Captain Cook and by Sir Gilbert Blane.

Preventive medicine was a blundering, incomplete science until bacteriology opened unheard-of possibilities for the prevention of disease. Before discussing some of the victories of preventive medicine it will be well to take a brief survey of the growth of the following subject:

SCIENCE OF BACTERIOLOGY

From the brilliant overthrow by Pasteur, in 1861, and by Koch and Cohn, in 1876, of the theory of spontaneous generation, we may date its modern growth. Wrapped up in this theory of spontaneous generation, upon which speculation raged centuries before the invention of the microscope, lies the history of bacteriology.

The ancient Greek and Roman philosophers wrestled with the question, and very interesting views of the relation of germ life to disease are preserved to us in their manuscripts. With the invention of the microscope we can mark the first positive step towards the goal of to-day. A Jesuit priest, Kircher, in 1671 was the first to investigate putrefying meat, milk, and cheese with the crude microscope of his day, and left us indefinite remarks concerning "very minute living worms" found therein. Four years after Kircher a Dutch linen merchant, Antonius von Leeuwenhoek, by improving the lenses of the microscope, saw in rain-water, putrefying fluids, intestinal contents, and saliva, minute, moving, living particles, which he called "animalculæ." In medical circles of his day these observations aroused the keenest interest, and the theory that these "animalculæ" might be the cause of all disease was eagerly discussed. Plenciz, of Vienna, after much observation of various fluids, putrefying and otherwise, wrote in 1762 that it was his firm belief that the phenomena of diseases and the decomposition of animal fluids were wholly caused by these minute living things.

Notwithstanding such assertions, from his day on until Pasteur, Koch, and Cohn finally proved its misconceptions in 1876, the theory of spontaneous generation held the upper hand in all discussions upon the question.

The stimulus to research as to the causes of disease along the line of bacterial origin did not entirely cease to be felt, and the names of Pollender and Davaine are linked together in the first undoubted discovery of micro-organisms in disease, when the cause of anthrax, a disease of cattle, was solved in 1863. Following closely upon Davaine's researches, the primary causes of wound infection were worked out, and to the efforts of the British surgeon Lister are due the great advances of modern surgery.

In rapid succession the presence of bacteria was clearly demonstrated in relapsing fever, leprosy, and typhoid fever; but far eclipsing all former discoveries, on account of the magnitude of the difficulties encountered and overcome, were the brilliant demonstrations of the cause of consumption and allied diseases, and that of Asiatic cholera, by Dr. Robert Koch in 1882 and in 1884 respectively.

From that time onward innumerable workers have satisfied the critical scientific world as to the causes of pneumonia, diphtheria, tetanus, influenza, and bubonic plague, besides many diseases of cattle, horses, sheep, and other animals and insects.

Having glanced hastily at the history of bacteriology, we may next consider some facts concerning the germs themselves. What are they? To the lay mind the words germ, microbe, bacterium, and bacillus often convey confused ideas of invisible, wriggling, worm-like creatures, enemies of mankind, ever on the watch to gain a stealthy entrance into our bodies, where they wreak harm and death. Scientifically considered, however, they are the smallest of living things yet known. They are not animals, but are members of the vegetable kingdom, and are possessed of definite yet varying shapes. They consist of a jelly-like substance called protoplasm, which is covered in and held in place by a well-formed membrane of a relatively hard and dense character, exactly similar in composition to the woody fibre of trees.

According to their shape the bacteria are divided into three chief groups, called respectively cocci, bacilli, and spirilla. The cocci are spherical bodies and may exist singly or in pairs, in fours, in clusters, or in chains. In this group we find the smallest bacteria known, many of them not over 1–150,000 of an inch in diameter. The bacilli are rod-like bodies, varying much in size in different species and in members of the same species. They are larger than the cocci, measuring in length from 1-25,000 of an inch to 1-4,000, and in breadth from 1-125,000 to 1-16,000 of an inch. Many varieties are possessed of organs of locomotion called flagella.

The spirilla resemble the bacilli, except that they are twisted into corkscrew shapes, or have gently undulating outlines. Upon an average they are much longer than the bacilli, one species being very long, measuring about

1-600 of an inch.   As seen in the natural state bacteria
are found to be colourless, but it is by the application of
various aniline dyes that they are usually studied.   These
minute plants increase by a simple method of division
into two equal parts, or by a more complex process of
forming a seed—the so-called spore—which later on
develops into the adult form.   Under favourable conditions
they are able to multiply at an enormous rate; for instance,
it has been calculated that a bacillus, dividing once every
hour would at the end of twenty-four hours have increased
to seventeen millions; and if the division continued at the
same rate we should find at the end of the third day an
incalculable number of billions, whose weight would be
nearly seven thousand five hundred tons!

But, fortunately for our welfare, nature by various
means renders the possibility of such a happening entirely
beyond the slightest chance of realization, her greatest
barrier being the lack of an adequate food supply.

The distribution in nature of bacteria is well-nigh universal, occurring as they do in the air we breathe, the
water and milk we drink, upon the exposed surfaces of
man and animals, and in their intestinal tracts, and in
the soil to a depth of about nine feet.   But it has been
noted that at very high altitudes and in glacier ice none
exist, while in the Arctic regions and at sea far from land
their numbers are very few.

The conditions governing their growth involve many
complex problems, but a few of the chief factors concerned
are moisture, air, food, temperature, and light.   All bacteria must have moisture, else they die sooner or later,
the period of survival depending upon the hardness of
the species, and none can multiply without it.   A supply
of air is by no means essential to all germs.   To some it is

absolutely necessary, and such germs are called aerobes. To others air is wholly detrimental, and they constitute the anaerobes, while to the majority of bacteria air supply is a matter of indifference, and in consequence they are grouped under the term facultative anaerobes.

The food supply of many consists of dead animal and vegetable materials, a few require living tissues, while a small number can exist wholly upon mineral salts, or even the nitrogen of the air. The lowest temperature at which some bacteria can multiply is the freezing-point of water, and the highest 170 degrees Fahrenheit. However, the average range of temperature suitable to the majority lies between 60 and 104 degrees Fahrenheit, 98 2-5 degrees Fahrenheit being the most suitable for the growth of disease-producing germs. Light, ordinarily diffused daylight, or its absence, is a matter of no moment to most germs, but direct sunlight is a destroyer of all bacteria.

The study of the life histories of these diminutive plants excites the wonder of those who make observations upon them. It is truly marvellous to know that these bacteria can accomplish in their short lives of possibly a few hours or days feats which would baffle the cleverest of chemists if given years of a lifetime to work upon. They give to the farmer the good quality of his crops, to the dairyman superior butter and cheese; they assist in large measure in freeing our rivers and lakes from harmful pollutions. Here it should be strongly emphasized that those bacteria which cause disease are only of a few species, all others contributing to our welfare in countless ways.

Quite as astonishing is the discovery that within the root-knobs of peas and beans live bacteria which by splitting up mineral salts containing nitrogen, and by absorbing nitrogen from the air, give it over to the plant so that it is enabled to grow luxuriantly, whereas, without their presence, the tiller of the soil might fertilize the ground in vain. It is quite possible that not alone peas and beans, but all grasses and plants and trees depend upon the presence of such germs for their very existence, which in turn supply man and animals with their means of existence. Hence we see that these nitrifying bacteria, as they are called, if swept out of existence, would be the cause of cessation of all life upon the globe. And arguing backward, one prominent authority states it as his belief that the first of all life on this earth were those lowly forms of plants which only required the nitrogen of air or salts to enable them to multiply.

Limiting observation now to the sphere of medicine, it will be readily perceived that the presence of bacterial life in a causative relation to disease is an object of paramount regard. The following paragraphs will briefly treat of the diseases associated with micro-organisms and the common modes of infection in each, the chain of events subsequent to an infection, and the possibilities of protection or cure by means of substances elaborated in the body of an individual or animal recently recovered from an infectious disease:

Anthrax.—A disease chiefly of cattle and sheep, occasionally of man, is caused by the *Bacillus anthracis*, discovered in 1849–50 by Pollender and Davaine. It enters the body through abrasions of the skin, by inhalation of the spores, or seeds, into the lungs, or by swallowing infected material.

Leprosy.—This disease is caused by a bacillus known as *Bacillus lepræ*, which was discovered by Hansen in 1879. It is doubtful if it has been grown outside the body. It is supposed to enter by abrasions of the skin, but it is very feebly contagious, notwithstanding popular ideas as to its supposedly highly contagious nature.

Tuberculosis.—All forms of this disease, among which is ordinary consumption, are caused by a bacillus closely resembling that of leprosy. It was discovered by Koch in 1880–82, and named *Bacillus tuberculosis.* The ways of infection are by inhaling the dried sputum of consumptives, drinking infected cow's milk, or eating infected meat.

Typhoid Fever.—A disease of human beings only. Eberth in 1880 discovered the germ causing it and called it *Bacillus typhosus.* It gains entrance to our bodies chiefly in the milk and water we drink, which comes from infected sources; a rarer method is by inhalation of infected air.

Diphtheria.—A disease of human beings chiefly. It is caused by a bacillus which was described in 1883–84 by Klebs and Loeffler, and is known as *Bacillus diphtheriae,* or Klebs-Loeffler bacillus. Its mode of entry is by inhaling infected air, or by drinking or eating infected milk or food.

Cholera.—This disease is peculiar to human beings. Its native home is on the banks of the river Ganges in India, where Koch in 1884 was able to isolate its causative spirillum. Man is infected by drinking contaminated water or by contact.

Lockjaw, or Tetanus.—Afflicts men, horses, and dogs. The *Bacillus tetani* is the most deadly of all known bacteria. It enters the body by wounds. It was discovered in 1884 by Nicolaier.

Influenza, or the Grip.—Caused by one of the smallest-known bacilli; discovered in 1892 by Canon and Pfeiffer. Infection spreads by the scattering about by air-currents of the dried nasal and bronchial secretion of those suffering from the disease, and its portal of entry is by the nose and bronchial tubes.

Pneumonia.—Caused by a coccus which grows in pairs and small chains. It enters the body by means of the respiratory tract. It is present in the saliva of twenty per cent. of healthy persons. Proved by Fraenkel in 1886 to be the cause of this disease.

Bubonic Plague.—In 1849 Kitasato and Yersin isolated a small bacillus in a large number of cases and proved it to be the cause. It enters the body by means of wounds of the skin, and through bites of fleas from infected rats, which are said to be one of the chief factors in spreading this dread malady.

Yellow Fever.—The cause of this disease is still under discussion.

Such are a few of the infectious diseases which we can readily attribute to the presence of definite micro-organisms in respective cases. But strange as it may seem, the most typical of all infectious diseases, small-pox, scarlet fever, measles, and hydrophobia, have as yet not yielded up their secrets. This is possibly due to the minute size of the micro-organisms concerned, which makes it beyond the power of the best microscope to demonstrate them. In this connexion it has recently been shown by Roux and Nocard that in the case of the disease known as pleuropneumonia of cattle the causative agent is so very small as just to be barely visible. Again, it is quite possible that these diseases may be caused by living things we know nothing about, which may be quite dissimilar from the bacteria.

INFECTION—ITS PROCESSES AND RESULTS

In the foregoing list of diseases associated with specific bacteria, attention has been drawn to the common modes of infection, or, as they are technically called, "portals of entry," and it now remains to touch upon the main factors, processes, and results following upon the entry into the body of such disease-producing microbes.

It is a well-known fact that the normal blood has of itself to a considerable extent the power of killing germs which may wander into it through various channels. Likewise the tissue cells of the body in general show similar action depending upon the different cell groups, state of health, general robustness, and period of life. The germ-killing power varies in different individuals, though each may be quite healthy. Considered as a whole, this power possessed by the body against germs is known as "general resistance." And when by any means this power of resistance is lost or diminished, we run grave risks of incurring disease.

Granted a case of infection, let us now trace up briefly what occurs. Between the period when the bacteria gain a lodgment and that in which the disease assumes a noticeable form, the patient simply feels out of sorts. It is during this stage that the blood and tissues are deeply engaged in the attempt to repel the attacks of the invading microbes.

With varying speed the germs multiply throughout the body generally, or may be at first localized, or even, as in lockjaw, remain localized throughout the entire disease. Multiplying in the tissues, they generate in increasing amounts their noxious poisons, which soon cause profound changes throughout the body; the patient becomes decidedly ill, and shows the signs of an unmistakable infection.

Does the body now give up the fight entirely? No; on the contrary, the white blood-cells, the wandering cells, and the cells of the tissues most affected still carry on an unequal fight. From the lymphatic glands and spleen, armies of white cells rush to the fray and attempt to eat up and destroy the foe, but possibly in vain; the disease runs its course, to end either in death or recovery.

How, then, in cases of recovery, are the microbes finally overcome?

This question involves many complex processes which at present are by no means thoroughly understood, but we will concern ourselves with the simple principles.

It has been previously mentioned that once the bacteria get a good foothold the body is subjected to the action of generated poisons, which are known as toxins. They give rise to such symptoms as loss of appetite, headache, fever, pains and aches, and even a state of stupor or unconsciousness. In addition to the active warfare of the white blood-cells, groups of cells throughout the body, after recovering from the first rude shock of the toxins, begin to tolerate their presence, then effect a change in the chemical constitution of the toxins, and finally elaborate substances which antagonize the toxins and destroy their action altogether, thus lending aid to the warrior cells, which at last overcome the invading microbes. Recovery is brought about, and a more or less permanent degree of immunity against the special form of disease ensues.

Now if we could use these antagonizing substances, or, as they are called, antitoxins, upon other men or animals sick with a similar disease, would their bodies be at once strengthened to resist and finally overcome the disease? Yes, in a certain majority of cases they would, and this is exactly what scientific observers have noted, worked out, and have successfully applied. A new art in the healing of disease, which is spoken of broadly as serum-therapy, or medication by curative or protective serums, has thus been discovered.

The first observers in this new field were Pasteur and Raynaud in France in 1877–78, and Salmon and Smith in this country in 1886. Raynaud, by injecting serum from a calf which had had an attack of cow-pox, prevented the appearance of the disease in a calf freshly inoculated with the virulent material of the disease. Pasteur, by using feebly infective germs of fowl cholera, conferred immunity upon healthy fowls against the disease, and was able to cure those which were ill. Salmon and Smith injected small and repeated amounts of the elaborated toxins or poisons of the bacillus of hog cholera into healthy swine, and were able to confer immunity upon them.

However, it was not until Behring in 1892 announced his discovery of an antitoxin serum for diphtheria, along with an undisputed proof of its value in treatment, that the attention of the scientific world was finally aroused and stimulated to the appreciation of the great possibilities of serum-therapy.

Strange as it may seem, much opposition arose to this new method of treatment, not alone from the lay portions of the community, but even from the ranks of the medical profession itself. This opposition was due in part to misconceptions of the principles involved in the new doctrine, and in part to the falsely philanthropic prejudices of the pseudo-scientific sections of both parties. But by the perserving work of the enthusiastic believers in serum-therapy, positive conviction has now replaced misconception and prejudice in the minds of the majority of its former opponents.

The accumulation of statistical evidence, even where all allowance is made for doubtful methods of compilation, shows that the aggregate mortality of diphtheria has been reduced fully fifty per cent. since the introduction of antitoxic treatment by Behring in 1892.

Since the method of preparation of the commercial diphtheria antitoxin illustrates the general principles involved in the search for the production of curative or protective serums for infectious diseases in general, a summary of the steps in its manufacture will now be given.

A race of diphtheria bacilli, which has been found to yield a poison of great virulence in alkaline beef broth, is grown for a week or ten days in this medium. The toxin is then separated and its virulence exactly determined. It is preserved in sterile rec≥ptacles for immediate or future use. The next step is the inoculation of a suitable animal with the toxin. Of all animals the horse has been found to meet nearly every requirement. Such an animal, in a state of perfect health, receives an injection of twenty cubic centimetres of toxin, along with ten or fifteen of standard antitoxin, beneath the skin of the neck or forequarters, upon three separate occasions at intervals of five days. After this it receives increasing doses of toxin, alone, at intervals of six to eight days, until, at the end of two months, it is able to stand with little discomfort doses of such strength that if given in the first stage these doses would have quickly caused death.

At this period the horse is bled to a small extent, and its serum tested to ascertain if prospects are good for the production by the animal of a high grade of antitoxin. If satisfactory progress has been made, the injections are continued for another month, when, as a rule, the maximal degree of antitoxic power in the serum will have been attained.

The horse is now bled to the proper extent, the blood being received in a sterile jar and placed in an ice-box. Here it coagulates, and the serum separates from it. When the separation of clot and serum is complete, the latter is drawn off, taken to the laboratory, and standardized. This being finished, an antiseptic fluid is added to preserve the serum from decomposition.   It is then bottled, labelled, and sent out for use.

In similar fashion tetanus antitoxin is prepared; and quite recently Calmette has produced an antitoxic serum for use in snake bite, by injecting horses with minute increasing doses of snake venom.   His experiments have given some remarkable results, not only in laboratory work, but also in cases of actual snake bite occurring in man.   Thus bacteriological scientists, after years of laborious work, in the face of much criticism and severe denunciation, may confidently announce that they have in their possession a magic key to one of nature's secret doors.   The lock has been turned. The door stands partly open, and we are permitted a glimpse of the future possibilities to be attained in the great fight against disease.

PREVENTIVE MEDICINE

The following are some of the diseases which have been remarkably controlled through preventive medicine:

Small-pox.—While not a scourge of the first rank, like the plague or cholera, at the outset of the nineteenth century variola was one of the most prevalent and dreaded of all diseases.   Few reached adult life without an attack. To-day, though outbreaks still occur, it is a disease thoroughly controlled by vaccination.   The protective power of the inoculated cow-pox is not a fixed and constant quantity.   The protection may be for life, or it may last only for a year or two.   The all-important fact is this: That efficiently vaccinated persons may be exposed with impunity, and among large bodies of men (e.g., the German army), in which revaccination is practised, small-pox is unknown. Of one hundred vaccinated persons exposed to small-pox, possibly one might take the disease in a mild form; of one hundred unvaccinated persons so exposed, one alone might escape—from twenty-five to thirty would die. To be efficient, vaccination must be carried out systematically, and if all the inhabitants of this country were revaccinated at intervals small-pox would disappear (as it has from the German army), and the necessity for vaccination would cease. The difficulty arises from the constant presence of an unvaccinated remnant, by which the disease is kept alive. The Montreal experience in 1885 is an object-lesson never to be forgotten.

For eight or ten years vaccination had been neglected, particularly among the French-Canadians. On February 28, 1885, a Pullman car conductor, who came from Chicago, where the disease had been slightly prevalent, was admitted into the Hôtel Dieu. Isolation was not carried out, and on the 1st of April a servant in the hospital died of small-pox. Following her death the authorities of the hospital sent to their homes all patients who presented no symptoms of the disease. Like fire in dry grass, the contagion spread, and within nine months there died of small-pox three thousand one hundred and sixty-four persons. It ruined the trade of the city for the winter, and cost millions of dollars. There are no reasonable objections to vaccination, which is a simple process, by which a mild and harmless disease is introduced. The use of the animal vaccine does away with the possibility of introduction of other disorders, such as syphilis.

Typhus Fever.—Until the middle of the nineteenth century this disease prevailed widely in most of the large cities, particularly in Europe, and also in jails, ships, hospitals and camps. It was more widely spread than typhoid fever and much more fatal. Murchison remarks of it that a complete history of its ravages would be the history of Europe during the past three centuries and a half. Not one of the acute infections seems to have been more dependent upon filth and unsanitary conditions. With the gradual introduction of drainage and a good water supply, and the relief of over-crowding, the disease has almost entirely disappeared, and is rarely mentioned now in the bills of mortality, except in a few of the larger and more unsanitary cities. The following figures illustrate what has been done in England within sixty years: In 1838 in England twelve hundred and twenty-eight persons died of fever (typhus and typhoid) per million of living. Twenty years later the figures were reduced to nine hundred and eighteen; in 1878 to three hundred and six of typhoid and to thirty-six of typhus fever. In 1892 only one hundred and thirty-seven died of typhoid fever and only three of typhus per million living!

Typhoid Fever.—While preventive medicine can claim a great victory in this disease also, it is less brilliant, since the conditions which favour its prevalence are not those spe-cially relating to overcrowding as much as to imperfect water supply and the contamination of certain essential foods, as milk. It has been repeatedly demonstrated that, with a pure water supply and perfect drainage, typhoid fever almost disappears from a city. In Vienna, after the introduction of good water, the rate of mortality from typhoid fever fell from twelve per ten thousand of the inhabitants to about one. In Munich the fall was still more remarkable; from above twenty-nine per ten thousand inhabitants in 1857 it fell to about one per ten thousand in 1887. That typhoid fever in this country is still a very prevalent disease depends mainly upon two facts: First, not only is the typhoid bacillus very resistant, but it may remain for a long time in the body of a person after recovery from typhoid fever, and such persons, in apparent good health, may be a source of contamination. With many of the conditions favouring the persistence and growth of the bacillus outside the body we are not yet familiar. The experience in the Spanish-American War illustrates how dangerous is the concentration together of large numbers of individuals. But, secondly, the essential factor in the widespread prevalence of typhoid fever in the United States, particularly in country districts, is the absence of anything like efficient rural sanitation. Many countries have yet to learn the alphabet of sanitation. The chief danger results from the impure water supplies of the smaller towns, while the local house epidemics are due to infected wells, and the milk outbreaks due to the infection of dairy farms.

The importance of scrupulously guarding the sources of supply was never better illustrated than in the well-known and oft-quoted epidemic in Plymouth, Pennsylvania. The town, with a population of eight thousand, was in part supplied with drinking-water from a reservoir fed by a mountain-stream. During January, February, and March, in a cottage by the side of and at a distance of from sixty to eighty feet from this stream, a man was ill with typhoid fever. The attendants were in the habit at night of throwing out the evacuations on the ground towards the stream. During these months the ground was frozen and covered with snow. In the latter part of March and early in April there was considerable rainfall and a thaw, in which a large part of the three months' accumulation of discharges was washed into the brook not sixty feet distant. At the very time of this thaw the patient had numerous and copious discharges. About the 10th of April cases of typhoid fever broke out in the town, appearing for a time at the rate of fifty a day. In all about twelve hundred were attacked

An immense majority of the cases were in the part of the town which received water from the infected reservoir.

The use of boiled water and of ice made from distilled water, the systematic inspection of dairies, the scrupulous supervision of the sources from which the water is obtained, an efficient system of sewage removal, and, above all, the most scrupulous care on the part of physicians and of nurses in the disinfection of the discharges of typhoid fever patients —these are the factors necessary to reduce to a minimum the incidence of typhoid fever.

Cholera.—One of the great scourges of the nineteenth century made inroads into Europe and America from India, its native home.   We have, however, found out the germ, found out the conditions under which it lives, and it is not likely that it will ever again gain a foothold in this country or Great Britain.   Since the last epidemic, 1873, the disease, though brought to this country on several occasions, ha\ always been held in check at the port of entry.   It is communicated almost entirely through infected water, and the virulence of an epidemic in any city is in direct propor- tion to the imperfection of the water supply.   This was shown in a remarkable way in the Hamburg epidemic of 1892.   In Altona, which had a filtration plant, there were only five hundred and sixteen cases, many of them refugees from Hamburg.   Hamburg, where the unfiltered water of the Elbe was used, had some eighteen thousand cases, with nearly eight thousand deaths.

Yellow Fever.—The cause of this disease is still under discussion.   It has an interest to us in this country from its continued prevalence in Cuba, and from the fact that at intervals it makes inroads into the Southern States, causing serious commercial loss.   The history of the disease in the other West India islands, particularly Jamaica, indicates the steps which must be taken for its prevention. Formerly yellow fever was as fatal a scourge in them as it is to-day in Cuba. By an efficient system of sanitation it has been abolished. The same can be done (and will be done) in Cuba within a few years. General Wood has already pointed out the way in the cleansing of Santiago.

The Plague.—One of the most remarkable facts in connexion with modern epidemics has been the revival of the bubonic plague, the most dreaded of all the great infections. During the nineteenth century the disease in Europe has been confined almost exclusively to Turkey and Southern Europe. Since 1894, when it appeared at Hong Kong, it has gradually spread, and there have been outbreaks of terrible severity in India. It has extended to certain of the Mediterranean ports, and during the past summer it reached Glasgow, where there has been a small outbreak. On this hemisphere there have been small outbreaks in certain of the South American ports, cases have been brought to New York, and there have been to November 1 twenty-one cases among the Chinese in San Francisco. Judging from the readiness with which it has been checked and limited in Australia, and in particular the facility with which the recent outbreak in Glasgow has been stamped out, there is very little risk that plague will ever assume the proportions which gave to it its terrible reputation as the "black death" of the Middle Ages. As I have already mentioned, the germ is known, and prophylactic inoculations have been made on a large scale in India, with a certain measure of success.

Tuberculosis.—In all communities the *white plague*, as Oliver Wendel Holmes calls it, takes the first rank as a killing disease. It has been estimated that of it one hundred and twenty thousand people die yearly in this country.

In all mortality bills tuberculosis of the lungs, or consumption, heads the list, and when to this is added tuberculosis of the other organs, the number swells to such an extent that this disease equals in fatality all the other acute infective diseases combined, if we leave out pneumonia. Less than twenty years ago we knew little or nothing of the cause of the disease. It was believed to be largely hereditary. Koch discovered the germ, and with this have come the possibilities of limiting its ravages.

The following points with reference to it may be stated: In a few very rare instances the disease is transmitted from parent to child. In a large proportion of all cases the disease is "caught." The germs are widely distributed through the sputum, which, when dry, becomes dust, and is blown about in all directions. Tubercle bacilli have been found in the dust of streets, houses, hospital wards, and much-frequented places. A single individual may discharge from the lungs countless myriads of germs in the twenty-four hours. Dr. Nuttall estimated from a patient in the Johns Hopkins Hospital, who had only moderately advanced consumption, that from one and a half to four and a third billions of germs were thrown off in the twenty-four hours. The consumptive, as has been well stated, is almost harmless, and only becomes harmful through bad habits. The germs are contained in the sputum, which, when dry, is widely scattered in the form of dust, and constitutes the great medium for the transmission of the disease. If expectorated into a handkerchief, the sputum dries quickly, particularly if it is put into the pocket or under the pillow. The beard or moustache of a consumptive is smeared with the germs. Even in the most careful the hands are apt to be soiled with the germs, and in those who are dirty and careless the furniture and materials which they handle readily become infected. Where the dirty habit prevails of spitting on the floor, a room, or the entire house, may contain numbers of germs. In the majority of all cases the infection in tuberculosis is by inhalation. This is shown by the frequency with which the disease is met in the lungs, and the great prevalence of tuberculosis in institutions in which the residents are restricted in the matter of fresh air and a free, open life. The disease prevails specially in cloisters, in jails and in asylums. Infection through milk is also possible; it is doubtful whether the disease is transmitted through meat. So widespread are the germs that post-mortem examination has shown that a very large number of persons show slight signs of the disease who have never during life presented any symptoms; in fact, some recent investigations would indicate that a very large proportion of all persons at the age of forty have somewhere in their bodies slight tuberculous lesions. This shows the importance of the individual predisposition, upon which the older writers laid so much stress, and the importance of maintaining the nutrition at its maximum.

One of the most remarkable features of modern protective medicine is the widespread interest that has been aroused in the crusade against tuberculosis. What has already been accomplished warrants the belief that the hopes of even the most enthusiastic may be realized. A positive decline in the prevalence of the disease has been shown in many of the larger cities during the past ten years. In Massachusetts, which has been a hot-bed of tuberculosis for many years, the death-rate has fallen from forty-two per ten thousand inhabitants in 1853 to twenty-one and eight-tenths per ten thousand inhabitants in 1895. In the city of Glasgow, in which the records have been very carefully kept, there has been an extraordinary fall in the death-rate from tuberculosis, and the recent statistics of New York City show, too, a similar remarkable diminution.

In fighting the disease our chief weapons are: First, education of the public, particularly of the poorer classes, who do not fully appreciate the chief danger in the disease. Secondly, the compulsory notification and registration of all cases of tuberculosis. The importance of this relates chiefly to the very poor and improvident, from whom after all, comes the greatest danger, and who should be under constant surveillance in order that these dangers may be reduced to a minimum. Thirdly, the foundation in suitable localities by the city and by the State of sanatoria for the treatment of early cases of the disease. Fourthly, provision for the chronic, incurable cases in special hospitals.

Diphtheria.—Since the discovery of the germ of this disease and our knowledge of the conditions of its transmission, and the discovery of the antitoxin, there has been a great reduction in its prevalence and an equally remarkable reduction in the mortality. The more careful isolation of the sick, the thorough disinfection of the clothing, the rigid scrutiny of the milder cases of throat disorder, a more stringent surveillance in the period of convalescence, and the routine examination of the throats of school-children—these are the essential measures by which the prevalence of the disease has been very markedly diminished. The great danger is in the mild cases, in which the disease has perhaps not been suspected, and in which the child may be walking about and even going to school. Such patients are often a source of widespread infection. The careful attention given by mothers to teeth and mouth of children is also an important factor. In children with recurring attacks of tonsillitis, in whom the tonsils are enlarged, the organs should be removed. Through these measures the incidence of the disease has been very greatly reduced.

Pneumonia.—While there has been a remarkable diminution in the prevalence of a large number of all the acute infections, one disease not only holds its own, but seems even to have increased in its virulence. In the mortality bills, pneumonia is an easy second to tuberculosis; indeed, in many cities the death-rate is now higher and it has become, to use the phrase of Bunyan, "the Captain of the men of death." It attacks particularly the intemperate, the feeble, and the old, though every year a large number of robust, healthy individuals succumb. So frequent is pneumonia at advanced periods of life that to die of it has been said to be the natural end of old men in this country. In many ways, too, it is a satisfactory disease, if one may use such an expression. It is not associated with much pain, except at the onset, the battle is brief and short, and a great many old persons succumb to it easily and peacefully.

We know the cause of the disease; we know only too well its symptoms, but the enormous fatality (from twenty to twenty-five per cent.) speaks only too plainly of the futility of our means of cure, and yet in no disease has there been so great a revolution in treatment. The patient is no longer drenched to death with drugs, or bled to a point where the resisting powers of nature are exhausted. We are not without hope, too, that in the future an antidote may be found to the toxins of the disease, and of late there have been introduced several measures of great value in supporting the weakness of the heart, a special danger in the old and debilitated.

Hydrophobia.—Rabies, a remarkable, and in certain countries a widespread, disease of animals, when transmitted to a man by the bite of rabid dogs, wolves, etc., is known as hydrophobia. The specific germ is unknown, but by a series of brilliant observations Pasteur showed (1) that the poison has certain fixed and peculiar properties in connexion with the nervous system; (2) that susceptible animals could be rendered refractory to the disease, or incapable of taking it, by a certain method of inoculation; and (3) that an animal unprotected and inoculated with a dose of the virus sufficient to cause the disease may, by the injection of proper anti-rabic treatment escape. Supported by these facts, Pasteur began a system of treatment of hydrophobia in man, and a special institute was founded in Paris for the purpose. When carried out promptly the treatment is successful in an immense majority of all cases, and the mortality in persons bitten by animals proved to be rabid, who have subsequently had the anti-rabic treatment, has been reduced to less than one-half per cent. The disease may be stamped out in dogs by careful quarantine of suspected animals and by a thoroughly carried out muzzling order.

Malaria.—Among the most remarkable of modern discoveries is the cause of malarial fever, one of the great maladies of the world, and a prime obstacle to the settlement of Europeans in tropical regions. Until 1880 the cause was quite obscure. It was known that the disease prevailed chiefly in marshy districts, in the autumn, and that the danger of infection was greatest in the evening and at night, and that it was not directly contagious. In 1880 a French army surgeon, Laveran, discovered in the red blood-corpuscles small bodies which have proved to be the specific germ of the disease. They are not bacteria, but little animal bodies resembling the amœba—tiny little portions of protoplasm. The parasite in its earliest form is a small, clear, ring-shaped body inside the red blood-corpuscle, upon which it feeds, gradually increasing in size and forming within itself blackish grains out of the colouring matter of the corpuscle. When the little parasite reaches a certain size it begins to divide or multiply, and an enormous number of these breaking up at the same time give off poison in the blood, which causes the paroxysms of fever. During what is known as the chill, in the intermittent fever, for example, one can always find these dividing parasites. Several different forms of the parasites have been found, corresponding to different varieties of malaria. Parasites of a very similar nature exist abundantly in birds. Ross, an army surgeon in India, found that the spread of this parasite from bird to bird was effected through the intervention of the mosquito. The parasites reach maturity in certain cells of the coats of the stomach of these insects, and develop into peculiar thread-like bodies, many of which ultimately reach the salivary glands, from which, as the insect bites, they pass with the secretion of the glands into the wound. From this as a basis, numerous observers have worked out the relation of the mosquito to malaria in the human subject.

Briefly stated, the disease is transmitted chiefly by certain varieties of the mosquito, particularly the *Anopheles*. The ordinary *Culex*, which is present chiefly in the Northern States, does not convey the disease. The *Anopheles* sucks the blood from a person infected with malaria, takes in a certain number of parasites, which undergo development in the body of the insect, the final outcome of which is numerous small, thread-like structures, which are found in numbers in the salivary glands. From this point, when the mosquito bites another individual, they pass into his blood, infect the system, and in this way the disease is transmitted. Two very striking experiments may be mentioned. The Italian observers have repeatedly shown that

Anopheles which have sucked blood from patients suffering from malaria, when sent to a non-malarial region, and there allowed to bite perfectly healthy persons, have transmitted the disease. But a very crucial experiment was made a short time ago. Mosquitoes which had bitten malarial patients in Italy were sent to London and there allowed to bite Mr. Manson, son of Dr. Manson, who really suggested the mosquito theory of malaria. This gentleman had not lived out of England, and there is no acute malaria in London. He had been a perfectly healthy, strong man. In a few days following the bites of the infected mosquitoes he had a typical attack of malarial fever.

The other experiment, though of a different character, is quite as convincing. In certain regions about Rome, in the Campania, malaria is so prevalent that in the autumn almost every one in the district is attacked, particularly if he is a new-comer. Dr. Sambon and a friend lived in this district from June 1 to September 1, 1900. The test was whether they could live in this exceedingly dangerous climate for the three months without catching malaria, if they used stringent precautions against the bites of mosquitoes. For this purpose the hut in which they lived was thoroughly wired, and they slept with the greatest care under netting. Both of these gentlemen at the end of the period had escaped the disease.

The importance of these studies cannot be overestimated. They explain the relation of malaria to marshy districts, the seasonal incidence of the disease, the nocturnal infection, and many other hitherto obscure problems. More important still, they point out clearly the way by which malaria may be prevented: First, the recognition that any individual with malaria is a source of danger in a community, so that he must be thoroughly treated with quinine;

secondly, the importance of the draining of marshy districts and ponds in which mosquitoes breed; and, thirdly, that even in the most infected regions persons may escape the disease by living in thoroughly protected houses, in this way escaping the bites of mosquitoes.

Venereal Diseases.—These continue to embarrass the social economist and to perplex and distress the profession. The misery and ill-health which they cause are incalculable, and the pity of it is that the cross is not always borne by the offender, but innocent women and children share the penalties. The gonorrhœal infection, so common, and often so little heeded, is a cause of much disease in parts other than those first affected. Syphilis claims its victims in every rank of life, at every age, and in all countries. We now treat it more thoroughly, but all attempts to check its ravages have been fruitless. Physicians have two important duties: the incessant preaching of continence to young men, and scrupulous care, in every case, that the disease may not be a source of infection to others, and that by thorough treatment the patient may be saved from the serious late nervous manifestations. We can also urge that in the interests of public health venereal diseases, like other infections, shall be subject to supervision by the State. The opposition to measures tending to the restriction of these diseases is most natural: on the one hand, from women, who feel that it is an aggravation of a shocking injustice and wrong to their sex; on the other, from those who feel the moral guilt in a legal recognition of the evil. It is appalling to contemplate the frightful train of miseries which a single diseased woman may entail, not alone on her associates, but on scores of the innocent—whose bitter cry should make the opponents of legislation feel that any measures of restriction, any measures of registration, would be preferable to the present disgraceful condition, which makes of some Christian cities open brothels and allows the purest homes to be invaded by the most loathsome of all diseases.

Leprosy.—Since the discovery of the germ of this terrible disease systematic efforts have been made to improve the state of its victims and to promote the study of the conditions under which the disease prevails. The English Leprosy Commission has done good work in calling attention to the widespread prevalence of the disease in India and in the East. In this country leprosy has been introduced into San Fransisco by the Chinese, and into the North-western States by the Norwegians, and there are foci of the disease in the Southern States, particularly Louisiana, and in the province of New Brunswick. The problem has an additional interest since the annexation of Hawaii and the Philippine Islands, in both of which places leprosy prevails extensively. By systematic measures of inspection and the segregation of affected individuals the disease can readily be held in check. It is not likely ever to increase among native Americans, or again gain such a foothold as it had in the Middle Ages.

Puerperal Fever.—Perhaps one of the most striking of all victories of preventive medicine has been the almost total abolition of so-called child-bed fever from the maternity hospitals and from private practice. In many institutions the mortality after child-birth was five or six per cent., indeed sometimes as high as ten per cent., whereas to-day, owing entirely to proper antiseptic precautions, the mortality has fallen to three-tenths to four-tenths per cent. The recognition of the contagiousness of puerperal fever was the most valuable contribution to medical science made by Oliver Wendell Holmes. There had been previous suggestions by several writers, but his essay on the "Contagiousness of Puerperal Fever," published in 1843, was the first strong, clear, logical statement of the case. Semmelweis, a few years later, added the weight of a large practical experience to the side of the contagiousness, but the full recognition of the causes of the disease was not reached until the recent antiseptic views had been put into practical effect.

THE NEW SCHOOL OF MEDICINE

The nineteenth century has witnessed a revolution in the treatment of disease, and the growth of a new school of medicine. The old schools—regular and homœopathic— put their trust in drugs, to give which was the alpha and the omega of their practice. For every symptom there were a score or more of medicines—vile, nauseous compounds in one case; bland, harmless dilutions in the other. The characteristic of the New School is firm faith in a few good, well-tried drugs, little or none in the great mass of medicines still in general use. Imperative drugging—the ordering of medicine in any and every malady—is no longer regarded as the chief function of the doctor. Naturally, when the entire conception of the disease was changed, there came a corresponding change in our therapeutics. In no respect is this more strikingly shown than in our present treatment of fever—say, of the common typhoid fever. During the first quarter of the century the patients were bled, blistered, purged and vomited, and dosed with mercury, antimony, and other compounds to meet special symptoms. During the second quarter the same, with variations in different countries. After 1850 bleeding became less frequent, and the experiments of the Paris and Vienna schools began to shake the belief in the control of fever by drugs. During the last quarter sensible doctors have reached the conclusion that typhoid fever is not a disease to be treated with medicines, but that in a large proportion of all cases diet, nursing and bathing meet the indications. There is active, systematic, careful, watchful treatment, but not with drugs. The public has not yet been fully educated to this point, and medicines have sometimes to be ordered for the sake of their friends, and it must be confessed that there are still in the ranks *antiques* who would insist on a dose of some kind every few hours.

The battle against poly-pharmacy, or the use of a large number of drugs (of the action of which we know little, yet we put them into bodies of the action of which we know less), has not been fought to a finish. There have been two contributing factors on the side of progress—the remarkable growth of the sceptical spirit fostered by Paris, Vienna and Boston physicians, and, above all, the valuable lesson of homœopathy, the infinitesimals of which certainly could not do harm, and quite as certainly could not do good; yet nobody has ever claimed that the mortality among homœopathic practitioners was greater than among those of the regular school. A new school of practitioners has arisen which cares nothing for homœopathy and less for so-called allopathy. It seeks to study, rationally and scientifically, the action of drugs, old and new. It is more concerned that a physician shall know how to apply the few great medicines which all have to use, such as quinine, iron, mercury, iodide of potassium, opium and digitalis, than that he should employ a multiplicity of remedies the action of which is extremely doubtful.

The growth of scientific pharmacology, by which we now have many active principles instead of crude drugs, and the discovery of the art of making medicines palatable, have been of enormous aid in rational practice. There is no limit to the possibility of help from the scientific investigation of the properties and action of drugs. At any day the new chemistry may give to us remedies of extraordinary potency and of as much usefulness as cocaine. There is no reason why we should not even in the vegetable world find for certain diseases specifics of virtue fully equal to that of quinine in the malarial fevers.

One of the most striking characteristics of the modern treatment of disease is the return to what used to be called the natural methods—diet, exercise, bathing and massage. There probably never has been a period in the history of the profession when the value of *diet* in the prevention and the cure of disease was more fully recognized. Dyspepsia, the besetting malady of this country, is largely due to improper diet, imperfectly prepared and too hastily eaten. One of the great lessons to be learned is that the preservation of health depends in great part upon food well cooked and carefully eaten. A common cause of ruined digestion, particularly in young girls, is the eating of sweets between meals and the drinking of the abominations dispensed in the chemists' shops in the form of ice-cream sodas, etc. Another frequent cause of ruined digestion in business men is the hurried meal at the lunch-counter. And a third factor, most important of all, illustrates the old maxim, that more people are killed by over eating and drinking than by the sword. Sensible people have begun to realize that alcoholic excesses lead inevitably to impaired health. A man may take four or five drinks of whiskey a day, or even more, and think perhaps that he transacts his business better with that amount of stimulant; but it only too frequently happens that early in the fifth decade, just as business or political success is assured, Bacchus hands in heavy bills for payment, in the form of serious disease of the arteries or of the liver, or there is a general breakdown. With the introduction of light beer there has been not only less intemperance, but a reduction in the number of cases of organic disease of the heart, liver and stomach caused by alcohol. While temperance in the matter of alcoholic drinks is becoming a characteristic of Americans, intemperance in the quantity of food taken is almost the rule. Adults eat far too much, and physicians are beginning to recognize that the early degenerations, particularly of the arteries and of the kidneys, leading to Bright's disease, which were formerly attributed to alcohol are due in large part to too much food.

Nursing.—Perhaps in no particular does nineteenth-century practice differ from that of the preceding centuries more than in the greater attention which is given to the personal comfort of the patient and to all the accessories comprised in the art of nursing. The physician has in the trained nurse an assistant who carries out his directions with a watchful care, is on the lookout for danger-signals and with accurate notes enables him to estimate the progress of a critical case from hour to hour. The intelligent, devoted women who have adopted the profession of nursing, are not only in their ministrations a public benefaction, but they lighten the anxieties which form so large a part of the load of the busy doctor.

Massage and Hydrotherapy have taken their places as most important measures of relief in many chronic conditions, and the latter has been almost universally adopted as the only safe means of combating the high temperatures of the acute fevers.

Within the past quarter of a century the value of *exercise* in the education of the young has become recognized. The increase in the means of taking wholesome out-of-door exercise is remarkable, and should show in a few years an influence in the reduction of the nervous troubles in young persons.   The prophylactic benefit of systematic exercise, taken in moderation by persons of middle age, is very great.   Golf and the bicycle have in the past few years materially lowered the average incomes which doctors in this country derive from persons under forty.   From the senile contingent—these above this age—the average income has for a time been raised by these exercises, as a large number of persons have been injured by taking up sports which may be vigorously pursued with safety only by those with young arteries.

Of three departures in the art of healing, brief mention may be made.   The use of the extracts of certain organs (or of the organs themselves) in disease is as old as the days of the Romans, but an extraordinary impetus has been given to the subject by the discovery of the curative powers of the extract of the thyroid gland in the diseases known as cretinism and myxœdema.   The brilliancy of the results in these diseases has had no parallel in the history of modern medicine, but it cannot be said that in the use of the extracts of other organs for disease the results have fulfilled the sanguine expectations of many.   There was not, in the first place, the same physiological basis, and practitioners have used these extracts too indiscriminately and without sufficient knowledge of the subject.

Secondly, as I have already mentioned, we possess a sure and certain hope that for many of the acute infections anti-toxins will be found.

A third noteworthy feature in modern treatment has been a return to psychical methods of cure, in which *faith in something is suggested* to the patient.   After all, faith is the great lever of life.   Without it, man can do nothing; with it, even with a fragment, as a grain of mustard-seed, all things are possible to him.   Faith in us, faith in our drugs and methods, is the great stock in trade of the profession. In one pan of the balance, put the pharmacopœias of the world, all the editions from Dioscorides to the last issue of the United States Dispensatory; heap them on the scales as did Euripides his books in the celebrated contest in the "Frogs"; in the other put the simple faith with which from the days of the Pharaohs until now the children of men have swallowed the mixtures these works describe, and the bulky tomes will kick the beam. It is the *aurum potabile*, the touchstone of success in medicine. As Galen says, confidence and hope do more good than physic—"he cures most in whom most are confident." That strange compound of charlatan and philosopher, Paracelsus, encouraged his patients "to have a good faith, a strong imagination, and they shall find the effects" (Burton). While we doctors often overlook or are ignorant of our own faith-cures, we are just a wee bit too sensitive about those performed outside our ranks. We have never had, and cannot expect to have a monopoly in this panacea, which is open to all, free as the sun, and which may make of every one in certain cases, as was the Lacedemonian of Homer's day, "a good physician out of Nature's grace." Faith in the gods or in the saints cures one, faith in little pills another, hypnotic suggestion a third, faith in a plain common doctor a fourth. In all ages the prayer of faith has healed the sick, and the mental attitude of the suppliant seems to be of more consequence than the powers to which the prayer is addressed. The cures in the temples of Æsculapius, the miracles of the saints, the remarkable cures of those noble men, the Jesuit missionaries, in this country, the modern miracles at Lourdes and at St. Anne de Beaupré in Quebec, and the wonder-workings of the so-called Christian Scientists, are often genuine, and must be considered in discussing the foundations of therapeutics. We physicians use the same power every day. If a poor lass, paralyzed apparently, helpless, bed-ridden for years, comes to me, having worn out in mind, body and estate a devoted family; if she in a few weeks or less by faith in me, and faith alone, takes up her bed and walks, the saints of old could not have done more, St. Anne and many others can scarcely to-day do less. We enjoy, I say, no monopoly in the faith business. The faith with which we work, the faith, indeed, which is available to-day in everyday life, has its limitations. It will not raise the dead; it will not put in a new eye in place of a bad one (as it did to an Iroquois Indian boy for one of the Jesuit fathers), nor will it cure cancer or pneumonia, or knit a bone; but, in spite of these nineteenth-century restrictions, such as we find it, faith is a most precious commodity, without which we should be very badly off.

Hypnotism, introduced by Mesmer in the eighteenth century, has had several revivals as a method of treatment during the nineteenth century. The first careful study of it was made by Braid, a Manchester surgeon, who introduced the terms hypnotism, hypnotic, and nervous sleep; but at this time no very great measure of success followed its use in practice, except perhaps in the case of an Anglo-Indian surgeon, James Esdaile, who, prior to the introduction of anæsthesia, had performed two hundred and sixty-one surgical operations upon patients in a state of hypnotic unconsciousness. About 1880 the French physicians, particularly Charcot and Bernheim, took up the study, and since that time hypnotism has been extensively practised. It may be defined as a subjective psychical condition, which Braid called nervous sleep, resembling somnambulism, in which, as Shakespeare says, in the description of Lady Macbeth, the person receives at once the benefit of sleep and does the effects or acts of watching or waking. Therapeutically, the important fact is that the individual's natural susceptibility to suggestion is increased, and this may hold after the condition of hypnosis has passed away. The condition of hypnosis is usually itself induced by suggestion, requesting the subject to close the eyes, to think of sleep, and the operator then repeats two or three times sentences suggesting sleep, and suggesting that the limbs are getting heavy and that he is feeling drowsy. During this state it has been found that the subjects are very susceptible to suggestion. Too much must not be expected of hypnotism, and the claims which have been made for it have been too often grossly exaggerated. It seems, as it has been recently well put, that hypnotism "at best permits of making suggestions more effective for good or bad than can be done upon one in his waking state." It is found to be of very little use in organic disease. It has been helpful in some cases of hysteria, in certain functional spasmodic affections of the nervous system, in the vicious habits of childhood, and in suggesting to the victims of alcohol and drugs that they should get rid of their inordinate desires. It has been used successfully in certain cases for the relief of labour pains, and in surgical operations; but on the whole, while a valuable agent in a few cases, it has scarcely fulfilled the expectations of its advocates. It is a practice not without serious dangers, and should never be performed except in the presence of a third person, while its indiscriminate employment by ignorant persons should be prevented by law.

One mode of faith-healing in modern days, which passes under the remarkable name of Christian Science, is probably nothing more than mental suggestion under another name. "The patient is told to be calm, and is assured that all will go well; that he must try to aid the healer by believing that what is told him is true. The healer then, quietly but firmly, asserts and reiterates that there is no pain, no suffering, that it is disappearing, that relief will come, that the patient is getting well." This is precisely the method which Bernheim used to use with such success with his hypnotic patients at Nancy, iterating and reiterating, in a most wearisome way, that the disease would disappear and the patient would feel better. As has been pointed out by a recent writer (Dr. Harry Marshall), the chief basis for the growth of Christian Science is that which underlies every popular fallacy: "Oliver Wendell Holmes outlined very clearly the factors concerned, showing (a) how easily abundant facts can be collected to prove anything whatsoever; (b) how insufficient 'exalted wisdom, immaculate honesty, and vast general acquirements' are to prevent an individual from having the most primitive ideas upon subjects out of his line of thought; and, finally, demonstrating 'the boundless credulity and excitability of mankind upon subjects connected with medicine.' "

XIV
CHAUVINISM IN MEDICINE

I feel not in myself those common antipathies that I can discover in others: those national repugnances do not touch me, nor do I behold with prejudice the French, Italian, Spaniard, or Dutch: but where I find their actions in balance with my countrymen's, I honour, love, and embrace them in the same degree.   I was born in the eighth climate, but seem for to be framed and constellated unto all: I am no plant that will not prosper out of a garden; all places, all airs, make unto me one country; I am in England, everywhere, and under any meridian.

> SIR THOMAS BROWNE, *Religio Medici.*

All's not offence that indiscretion finds
And dotage terms so.

> SHAKESPEARE, *King Lear*, Act II.

Still in thy right hand carry gentle peace,
To silence envious tongues.

> SHAKESPEARE, *King Henry VIII*, Act III.

XIV

CHAUVINISM[1] IN MEDICINE[2]

A RARE and precious gift is the Art of Detachment, by which a man may so separate himself from a life-long environment as to take a panoramic view of the conditions under which he has lived and moved: it frees him from Plato's den long enough to see the realities as they are, the shadows as they appear. Could a physician attain to such an art he would find in the state of his profession a theme calling as well for the exercise of the highest faculties of description and imagination as for the deepest philosophic insight. With wisdom of the den only and of my fellow-prisoners, such a task is beyond my ambition and my powers, but to emphasize duly the subject that I wish to bring home to your hearts I must first refer to certain distinctive features of our profession:

I. FOUR GREAT FEATURES OF THE GUILD

Its noble ancestry.—Like everything else that is good and durable in this world, modern medicine is a product of the Greek intellect, and had its origin when that wonderful people created positive or rational science, and no small credit is due to the physicians who, as Professor Gomperz remarks (in his brilliant chapter "On the Age of Enlightenment," *Greek Thinkers*, Vol. 1), very early brought to bear the spirit of criticism on the arbitrary and superstitious

[1] Definition: A narrow, illiberal spirit in matters national, provincial, collegiate, or personal.

[2] Canadian Medical Association, Montreal, 1902.

views of the phenomena of life. If science was ever to acquire "steady and accurate habits instead of losing itself in a maze of phantasies, it must be by quiet methodical research." "It is the undying glory of the school of Cos that it introduced this innovation into the domain of its Art, and thus exercised the most beneficial influence on the whole intellectual life of mankind. Fiction to the right! Reality to the left! was the battle cry of this school in the war it was the first to wage against the excesses and defects of the nature philosophy"(Gomperz). The critical sense and sceptical attitude of the Hippocratic school laid the foundations of modern medicine on broad lines, and we owe to it: *first*, the emancipation of medicine from the shackles of priestcraft and of caste; *secondly*, the conception of medicine as an art based on accurate observation, and as a science, an integral part of the science of man and of nature; *thirdly*, the high moral ideals, expressed in that most "memorable of human documents" (Gomperz), the Hippocratic oath; and *fourthly*, the conception and realization of medicine as the profession of a cultivated gentleman.[1] No other profession can boast of the same unbroken continuity of methods and of ideals. We may indeed be justly proud of our apostolic succession. Schools and systems have flourished and gone, schools which have swayed for generations the thought of our guild, and systems that have died before their founders; the philosophies of one age have become the absurdities of the next, and the foolishness of yesterday has become the wisdom of to-morrow; through long ages which

[1] Nowhere in literature do we have such a charming picture illustrating the position of a cultivated physician in society as that given in Plato's *Dialogues* of Eryximachus, himself the son of a physician, Acumenus. In that most brilliant age the physician was the companion and friend, and in intellectual intercourse the peer of its choicest spirits.

were slowly learning what we are hurrying to forget—amid all the changes and chances of twenty-five centuries, the profession has never lacked men who have lived up to these Greek ideals.   They were those of Galen and of Aretæus, of the men of the Alexandrian and Byzantine schools, of the best of the Arabians, of the men of the Renaissance, and they are ours to-day.

A second distinctive feature is the *remarkable solidarity.* Of no other profession is the word universal applicable in the same sense.   The celebrated phrase used of the Catholic Church is in truth much more appropriate when applied to medicine.   It is not the prevalence of disease or the existence everywhere of special groups of men to treat it that betokens this solidarity, but it is the identity throughout the civilized world of our ambitions, our methods and our work.   To wrest from nature the secrets which have perplexed philosophers in all ages, to track to their sources the causes of disease, to correlate the vast stores of knowledge, that they may be quickly available for the prevention and cure of disease—these are our ambitions.   To carefully observe the phenomena of life in all its phases, normal and perverted, to make perfect that most difficult of all arts, the art of observation, to call to aid the science of experimentation, to cultivate the reasoning faculty, so as to be able to know the true from the false—these are our methods.   To prevent disease, to relieve suffering and to heal the sick— this is our work.   The profession in truth is a sort of guild or brotherhood, any member of which can take up his calling in any part of the world and find brethren whose language and methods and whose aims and ways are identical with his own.

Thirdly, *its progressive character.*—Based on science, medicine has followed and partaken of its fortunes, so that in the great awakening which has made the nineteenth memorable among centuries, the profession received a quickening impulse more powerful than at any period in its history. With the sole exception of the mechanical sciences, no other department of human knowledge has undergone so profound a change—a change so profound that we who have grown up in it have but slight appreciation of its momentous character. And not only in what has been actually accomplished in unravelling the causes of disease, in perfecting methods of prevention, and in wholesale relief of suffering, but also in the unloading of old formulæ and in the substitution of the scientific spirit of free inquiry for cast-iron dogmas we see a promise of still greater achievement and of a more glorious future.

And lastly, the profession of medicine is distinguished from all others by its *singular beneficence*. It alone does the work of charity in a Jovian and God-like way, dispensing with free hand truly Promethean gifts. There are those who listen to me who have seen three of the most benign endowments granted to the race since the great Titan stole fire from the heavens. Search the scriptures of human achievement and you cannot find any to equal in beneficence the introduction of Anæsthesia, Sanitation, with all that it includes, and Asepsis—a short half-century's contribution towards the practical solution of the problems of human suffering, regarded as eternal and insoluble. We form almost a monopoly or trust in this business. Nobody else comes into active competition with us, certainly not the other learned professions which continue along the old lines. Every few years sees some new conquest, so that we have ceased to wonder. The work of half a dozen men, headed by Laveran, has made waste places of the earth habitable and the wilderness to blossom as the rose. The work of

Walter Reed and his associates will probably make yellow fever as scarce in the Spanish Main as is typhus fever with us. There seems to be no limit to the possibilities of scientific medicine, and while philanthropists are turning to it as to the hope of humanity, philosophers see, as in some far-off vision, a science from which may come in the prophetic words of the Son of Sirach, "Peace over all the earth."

Never has the outlook for the profession been brighter. Everywhere the physician is better trained and better equipped than he was twenty-five years ago. Disease is understood more thoroughly, studied more carefully and treated more skilfully. The average sum of human suffering has been reduced in a way to make the angels rejoice. Diseases familiar to our fathers and grandfathers have disappeared, the death rate from others is falling to the vanishing point, and public health measures have lessened the sorrows and brightened the lives of millions. The vagaries and whims, lay and medical, may neither have diminished in number nor lessened in their capacity to distress the faint-hearted who do not appreciate that to the end of time people must imagine vain things, but they are dwarfed by comparison with the colossal advance of the past fifty years.

So vast, however, and composite has the profession become, that the physiological separation, in which dependent parts are fitly joined together, tends to become pathological, and while some parts suffer necrosis and degeneration, others, passing the normal limits, become disfiguring and dangerous outgrowths on the body medical. The dangers and evils which threaten harmony among the units, are internal, not external. And yet, in it more than in any other profession, owing to the circumstances of which I have spoken, is complete organic unity possible. Of the many hindrances in the way time would fail me to speak, but there is one aspect of the question to which I would direct your attention in the hope that I may speak a word in season.

Perhaps no sin so easily besets us as a sense of self-satisfied superiority to others. It cannot always be called pride, that master sin, but more often it is an attitude of mind which either leads to bigotry and prejudice or to such a vaunting conceit in the truth of one's own beliefs and positions, that there is no room for tolerance of ways and thoughts which are not as ours are. To avoid some smirch of this vice is beyond human power; we are all dipped in it, some lightly, others deeply grained. Partaking of the nature of uncharitableness, it has not the intensity of envy, hatred and malice, but it shades off in fine degrees from them. It may be a perfectly harmless, even an amusing trait in both nations and individuals, and so well was it depicted by Charelt, Horace Vernet, and others, under the character of an enthusiastic recruit named Chauvin, that the name Chauvinism has become a by-word, expressing a bigoted, intolerant spirit. The significance of the word has been widened, and it may be used as a synonym for a certain type of nationalism, for a narrow provincialism, or for a petty parochialism. It does not express the blatant loudness of Jingoism, which is of the tongue, while Chauvinism is a condition of the mind, an aspect of character much more subtle and dangerous. The one is more apt to be found in the educated classes, while the other is pandemic in the fool multitude—"that numerous piece of monstrosity which, taken asunder, seem men and reasonable creatures of God, but confused together, make but one great beast, and a monstrosity more prodigious than Hydra" (*Religio Medici*). Wherever found, and in whatever form, Chauvinism is a great enemy of progress and of peace and concord among the units. I have not the time, nor if I had, have I the ability to portray this failing in all its varieties; I can but touch upon some of its aspects, national, provincial and parochial.

II. NATIONALISM IN MEDICINE

Nationalism has been the great curse of humanity. In no other shape has the Demon of Ignorance assumed more hideous proportions; to no other obsession do we yield ourselves more readily. For whom do the hosannas ring higher than for the successful butcher of tens of thousands of poor fellows who have been made to pass through the fire to this Moloch of nationalism? A vice of the blood, of the plasm rather, it runs riot in the race, and rages today as of yore in spite of the precepts of religion and the practice of democracy. Nor is there any hope of change; the pulpit is dumb, the press fans the flames, literature panders to it and the people love to have it so. Not that all aspects of nationalism are bad. Breathes there a man with soul so dead that it does not glow at the thought of what the men of his blood have done and suffered to make his country what it is? There is room, plenty of room, for proper pride of land and birth. What I inveigh against is a cursed spirit of intolerance, conceived in distrust and bred in ignorance, that makes the mental attitude perennially antagonistic, even bitterly antagonistic to everything foreign, that subordinates everywhere the race to the nation, forgetting the higher claims of human brotherhood.

While medicine is everywhere tinctured with national characteristics, the wider aspects of the profession, to which I have alluded—our common lineage and the community of interests—should always save us from the more vicious aspects of this sin, if it cannot prevent it altogether. And yet I cannot say, as I wish I could, that we are wholly free from this form of Chauvinism. Can we say, as English,

French, German or American physicians, that our culture
is always cosmopolitan, not national, that our attitude of
mind is always as frankly open and friendly to the French
as to the English, to the American as to the German, and
that we are free at all times and in all places from prejudice,
at all times free from a self-satisfied feeling of superiority
the one over the other? There has been of late years a
closer union of the profession of the different countries
through the International Congress and through the international meetings of the special societies; but this is not
enough, and the hostile attitude has by no means disappeared. Ignorance is at the root. When a man talks
slightingly of the position and work of his profession in any
country, or when a teacher tells you that he fails to find
inspiration in the work of his foreign colleagues, in the
words of the Arabian proverb—he is a fool, shun him!
Full knowledge, which alone disperses the mists of ignorance, can only be obtained by travel or by a thorough
acquaintance with the literature of the different countries.
Personal, first-hand intercourse with men of different lands,
when the mind is young and plastic, is the best vaccination
against the disease. The man who has sat at the feet of
Virchow, or has listened to Traube, or Helmholtz, or Cohn-
heim, can never look with unfriendly eyes at German medicine or German methods. Who ever met with an English
or American pupil of Louis or of Charcot, who did not love
French medicine, if not for its own sake, at least for the
reverence he bore his great master? Let our young men,
particularly those who aspire to teaching positions, go
abroad. They can find at home laboratories and hospitals
as well equipped as any in the world, but they may find
abroad more than they knew they sought—widened sympathies, heightened ideals and something perhaps of a *Welt-*

cultur which will remain through life as the best protection against the vice of nationalism.

Next to a personal knowledge of men, a knowledge of the literature of the profession of different countries will do much to counteract intolerance and Chauvinism. The great works in the department of medicine in which a man is interested, are not so many that he cannot know their contents, though they be in three or four languages. Think of the impetus French medicine gave to the profession in the first half of the last century, of the debt we all owe to German science in the latter half, and of the lesson of the practical application by the English of sanitation and asepsis! It is one of our chief glories and one of the unique features of the profession that, no matter where the work is done in the world, if of any value, it is quickly utilized. Nothing has contributed more to the denationalization of the profession of this continent than, on the one hand, the ready reception of the good men from the old countries who have cast in their lot with us, and, on the other, the influence of our young men who have returned from Europe with sympathies as wide as the profession itself. There is abroad among us a proper spirit of eclecticism, a willingness to take the good wherever found, that augurs well for the future. It helps a man immensely to be a bit of a hero-worshipper, and the stories of the lives of the masters of medicine do much to stimulate our ambition and rouse our sympathies. If the life and work of such men as Bichat and Laënnec will not stir the blood of a young man and make him feel proud of France and of Frenchmen, he must be a dull and muddy mettled rascal. In reading the life of Hunter, of Jenner, who thinks of the nationality which is merged and lost in our interest in the man and in his work? In the halcyon days of the Renaissance there was no nationalism in medicine, but a fine catholic spirit made great leaders like Vesalius, Eustachius, Stensen and others at home in every country in Europe. While this is impossible to-day, a great teacher of any country may have a world-wide audience in our journal literature, which has done so much to make medicine cosmopolitan.

III. PROVINCIALISM IN MEDICINE

While we may congratulate ourselves that the worst aspects of nationalism in medicine are disappearing before the broader culture and the more intimate knowledge brought by ever-increasing intercourse, yet in English-speaking countries conditions have favoured the growth of a very unpleasant subvariety, which may be called provincialism or sectionalism. In one sense the profession of this continent is singularly homogeneous. A young man may be prepared for his medical course in Louisiana and enter McGill College, or he may enter Dalhousie College, Halifax, from the State of Oregon, and in either case he will not feel strange or among strangers so soon as he has got accustomed to his environment. In collegiate life there is a frequent interchange of teachers and professors between all parts of the country. To better his brains the scholar goes freely where he wishes—to Harvard, McGill, Yale, or Johns Hopkins; there are no restrictions. The various medical societies of the two countries are, without exception, open to the members of the profession at large. The President of the Association of American Physicians this year (Dr. James Stewart), is a resident of this city, which gave also last year I believe, presidents to two of the special societies. The chief journals are supported by men of all sections. The text-books and manuals are everywhere in common; there is, in fact, a remarkable homogeneity in the

English-speaking profession, not only on this continent but throughout the world. Naturally, in widely scattered communities sectionalism—a feeling or conviction that the part is greater than the whole—does exist, but it is diminishing, and one great function of the national associations is to foster a spirit of harmony and brotherhood among the scattered units of these broad lands. But we suffer sadly from a provincialism which has gradually enthralled us, and which sprang originally from an attempt to relieve conditions insupportable in themselves. I have praised the unity of the profession of this continent, in so many respects remarkable, and yet in another respect it is the most heterogeneous ever known. Democracy in full circle touches tyranny, and as Milton remarks, the greatest proclaimers of liberty may become its greatest engrossers (or enslavers). The tyranny of labour unions, of trusts, and of an irresponsible press may bear as heavily on the people as autocracy in its worst form. And, strange irony of fate! the democracy of Provincial and State Boards has imposed in a few years a yoke more grievous than that which afflicts our brethren in Great Britain, which took generations to forge.

The delightful freedom of intercourse of which I spoke, while wide and generous, is limited to intellectual and social life, and on the practical side, not only are genial and courteous facilities lacking, but the bars of a rigid provincialism are put up, fencing each State as with a Chinese wall. In the Dominion of Canada there are eight portals of entry to the profession, in the United States almost as many as there are States, in the United Kingdom nineteen, I believe, but in the latter the license of any one of these bodies entitled a man to registration anywhere in the kingdom. Democracy in full circle has reached on this hemisphere a much worse condition than that in which the conservatism of many generations has entangled the profession of Great Britain. Upon the origin and growth of the Provincial and State Boards I do not propose to touch. The ideal has been reached so far as organization is concerned, when the profession elects its own Parliament, to which is committed the control of all matters relating to the license. The recognition, in some form, of this democratic principle, has been one great means of elevating the standard of medical education, and in a majority of the States of the Union it has secured a minimum period of four years of study, and a State Examination for License to Practise. All this is as it should be. But it is high time that the profession realized the anomaly of eight boards in the Dominion and some scores in the United States. One can condone the iniquity in the latter country more readily than in Canada, in which the boards have existed for a longer period, and where there has been a greater uniformity in the medical curriculum. After all these years that a young man, a graduate of Toronto and a registered practitioner in Ontario, cannot practise in the Province of Quebec, his own country, without submitting to vexatious penalties of mind and pocket, or that a graduate from Montreal and a registered practitioner of this province cannot go to Manitoba, his own country again, and take up his life's work without additional payments and penalties, is, I maintain, an outrage; it is provincialism run riot. That this pestiferous condition should exist throughout the various provinces of this Dominion and so many States of the Union, illustrates what I have said of the tyranny of democracy and how great enslavers of liberty its chief proclaimers may be.

That the cure of this vicious state has to be sought in Dominion bills and National examining boards, indicates into what debasing depths of narrow provincialism we have sunk. The solution seems to be so simple, particularly in this country, with its uniformity of methods of teaching and length of curriculum. A generous spirit that will give to local laws a liberal interpretation, that limits its hostility to ignorance and viciousness, that has regard as much or more for the good of the guild as a whole as for the profession of any province—could such a spirit brood over the waters, the raging waves of discord would soon be stilled. With the attitude of mind of the general practitioner in each province rests the solution of the problem. Approach it in a friendly and gracious spirit and the difficulties which seem so hard will melt away. Approach it in a Chauvinistic mood, fully convinced that the superior and unparalleled conditions of your province will be jeopardized by reciprocity or by Federal legislation, and the present antiquated and disgraceful system must await for its removal the awakening of a younger and more intelligent generation.

It would ill become me to pass from this subject—familiar to me from my student days from the interest taken in it by that far-sighted and noble-minded man, Dr. Palmer Howard—it would ill become me, I say, not to pay a tribute of words to Dr. Roddick for the zeal and persistence with which he has laboured to promote union in the compound, comminuted fracture of the profession of this Dominion. My feeling on the subject of international, intercolonial, and interprovincial registration is this—a man who presents evidence of proper training, who is a registered practitioner in his own country and who brings credentials of good standing at the time of departure, should be welcomed as a brother, treated as such in any country, and registered upon payment of the usual fee. The ungenerous treatment of English physicians in Switzerland, France, and Italy, and the chaotic state of internecine warfare existing on this continent, indicate how far a miserable Chauvinism can corrupt the great and gracious ways which should characterize a liberal profession.

Though not germane to the subject, may I be allowed to refer to one other point in connexion with the State Boards—a misunderstanding, I believe, of their functions. The profession asks that the man applying for admission to its ranks shall be of good character and fit to practise the science and art of medicine. The latter is easily ascertained if practical men have the place and the equipment for practical examinations. Many of the boards have not kept pace with the times, and the questions set too often show a lack of appreciation of modern methods. This has, perhaps, been unavoidable since, in the appointment of examiners, it has not always been possible to select experts. The truth is, that however well organized and equipped, the State Boards cannot examine properly in the scientific branches, nor is there need to burden the students with additional examinations in anatomy, physiology and chemistry. The Provincial and State Boards have done a great work for medical education on this continent, which they would crown and extend by doing away at once with all theoretical examinations and limiting the tests for the license to a rigid practical examination in medicine, surgery, and midwifery, in which all minor subjects could be included.

IV. PAROCHIALISM IN MEDICINE

Of the parochial and more personal aspects of Chauvinism I hesitate to speak; all of us, unwittingly as a rule, illustrate its varieties. The conditions of life which round us and bound us, whether in town or country, in college or institution, give to the most liberal a smack of parochialism, just as surely as we catch the tic of tongue of the land in which we live. The dictum put into the mouth of Ulysses, "I am a part of all that I have met," expresses the truth of the influence upon us of the social environment, but it is not the whole truth, since the size of the parish, representing the number of points of contact, is of less moment than the mental fibre of the man. Who has not known lives of the greatest freshness and nobility hampered at every turn and bound in chains the most commonplace and sordid, lives which illustrate the liberty and freedom enjoyed by minds innocent and quiet, in spite of stone walls and iron bars. On the other hand, scan the history of progress in the profession, and men the most illiberal and narrow, reeking of the most pernicious type of Chauvinism, have been among the teachers and practitioners in the large cities and great medical centres; so true is it, that the mind is its own place and in itself can make a man independent of his environment.

There are shades and varieties which are by no means offensive. Many excellent features in a man's character may partake of its nature. What, for example, is more proper than the pride which we feel in our teachers, in the university from which we have graduated, in the hospital at which we have been trained? He is a "poor sort" who is free from such feelings, which only manifest a proper loyalty. But it easily degenerates into a base intolerance which looks with disdain on men of other schools and other ways. The pride, too, may be in inverse proportion to the justness of the claims. There is plenty of room for honest and friendly rivalry between schools and hospitals, only a blind Chauvinism puts a man into a hostile and intolerant attitude of mind at the mention of a name. Alumni and friends should remember that indiscriminate praise of institutions or men is apt to rouse the frame of mind illustrated by the ignorant

Athenian who, so weary of hearing Aristides always called the Just, very gladly took up the oyster shell for his ostracism, and even asked Aristides himself, whom he did not know, to mark it.

A common type of collegiate Chauvinism is manifest in the narrow spirit too often displayed in filling appointments. The professoriate of the profession, the most mobile column of its great army, should be recruited with the most zealous regard to fitness, irrespective of local conditions that are apt to influence the selection. Inbreeding is as hurtful to colleges as to cattle. The interchange of men, particularly of young men, is most stimulating, and the complete emancipation of the chairs which has taken place in most of our universities should extend to the medical schools. Nothing, perhaps, has done more to place German medicine. in the forefront to-day than a peripatetic professoriate, owing allegiance only to the profession at large, regardless of civic, sometimes, indeed, of national limitations and restrictions. We acknowledge the principle in the case of the scientific chairs, and with increasing frequency act upon it, but an attempt to expand it to other chairs may be the signal for the display of rank parochialism.

Another unpleasant manifestation of collegiate Chauvinism is the outcome, perhaps, of the very keen competition which at present exists in scientific circles. Instead of a generous appreciation of the work done in other places, there is a settled hostility and a narrowness of judgment but little in keeping with the true spirit of science. Worse still is the "lock and key" laboratory in which suspicion and distrust reign, and everyone is jealous and fearful lest the other should know of or find out about his work. Thank God! this base and bastard spirit is not much seen, but it is about, and I would earnestly entreat any young man who unwittingly finds himself in a laboratory pervaded with this atmosphere, to get out ere the contagion sinks into his soul.

Chauvinism in the unit, in the general practitioner, is of much more interest and importance. It is amusing to read and hear of the passing of the family physician. There never was a time in our history in which he was so much in evidence, in which he was so prosperous, in which his prospects were so good or his power in the community so potent. The public has even begun to get sentimental over him! He still does the work; the consultants and the specialists do the talking and the writing; and take the fees! By the work, I mean that great mass of routine practice which brings the doctor into every household in the land and makes him, not alone the adviser, but the valued friend. He is the standard by which we are measured. What he is, we are; and the estimate of the profession in the eyes of the public is their estimate of him. A well-trained, sensible doctor is one of the most valuable assets of a community, worth to-day, as in Homer's time, many another man. To make him efficient is our highest ambition as teachers, to save him from evil should be our constant care as a guild. I can only refer here to certain aspects in which he is apt to show a narrow Chauvinism hurtful to himself and to us.

In no single relation of life does the general practitioner show a more illiberal spirit than in the treatment of himself. I do not refer so much to careless habits of living, to lack of routine in work, or to failure to pay due attention to the business side of the profession—sins which so easily beset him—but I would speak of his failure to realize *first*, the need of a lifelong progressive personal training, and *secondly*, the danger lest in the stress of practice he sacrifice that most precious of all possessions, his mental independence. Medicine is a most difficult art to acquire. All the college can do is to teach the student principles, based on facts in science, and give him good methods of work. These simply start him in the right direction, they do not make him a good practitioner—that is his own affair. To master the art requires sustained effort, like the bird's flight which depends on the incessant action of the wings, but this sustained effort is so hard that many give up the struggle in despair. And yet it is only by persistent intelligent study of disease upon a methodical plan of examination that a man gradually learns to correlate his daily lessons with the facts of his previous experience and of that of his fellows, and so acquires clinical wisdom. Nowadays it is really not a hard matter for a well-trained man to keep abreast of the best work of the day. He need not be very scientific so long as he has a true appreciation of the dependence of his art on science, for, in a way, it is true that a good doctor may have practice and no theory, art and no science. To keep up a familiarity with the use of instruments of precision is an all-important help in his art, and I am profoundly convinced that as much space should be given to the clinical laboratory as to the dispensary. One great difficulty is that while waiting for the years to bring the inevitable yoke, a young fellow gets stale and loses that practised familiarity with technique which gives confidence. I wish the older practitioners would remember how important it is to encourage and utilize the young men who settle near them. In every large practice there are a dozen or more cases requiring skilled aid in the diagnosis, and this the general practitioner can have at hand. It is his duty to avail himself of it, and failing to do so he acts in a most illiberal and unjust way to himself and to the profession at large. Not only may the older man, if he has soft arteries in his grey cortex, pick up many points from the young fellow, but there is much clinical wisdom afloat in each parish which is now wasted or dies with the old doctor, because he and the young men have never been on friendly terms.

In the fight which we have to wage incessantly against ignorance and quackery among the masses and follies of all sorts among the classes, *diagnosis*, not *drugging*, is our chief weapon of offence. *Lack of systematic personal training in the methods of the recognition of disease leads to the misapplication of remedies, to long courses of treatment when treatment is useless, and so directly to that lack of confidence in our methods which is apt to place us in the eyes of the public on a level with empirics and quacks.*

Few men live lives of more devoted self-sacrifice than the family physician, but he may become so completely absorbed in work that leisure is unknown; he has scarce time to eat or to sleep, and, as Dr. Drummond remarks in one of his poems, "He's the only man, I know me, don't get no holiday." There is danger in this treadmill life lest he lose more than health and time and rest—his intellectual independence. More than most men he feels the tragedy of isolation—that inner isolation so well expressed in Matthew Arnold's line "We mortal millions live *alone*." Even in populous districts the practice of medicine is a lonely road which winds up-hill all the way and a man may easily go astray and never reach the Delectable Mountains unless he early finds those shepherd guides of whom Bunyan tells, *Knowledge, Experience, Watchful,* and *Sincere*. The circumstances of life mould him into a masterful, self-confident, self-centered man, whose worst faults often partake of his best qualities. The peril is that should he cease to think for himself he becomes a mere automaton, doing a penny-in-the-slot business which places him on a level with the chemist's clerk who can hand out specifics for every ill, from the "pip" to the pox.   The salt of life for him is a judicious scepticism, not the coarse, crude form, but the sober sense of honest doubt expressed in the maxim of the sly old Sicilian Epicharmus, "Be sober and distrustful; these are the sinews of the understanding." A great advantage, too, of a sceptical attitude of mind is, as Green the historian remarks, "One is never very surprised or angry to find that one's opponents are in the right."   It may keep him from self-deception and from falling into that medical slumber into which so many drop, deep as the theological slumber so lashed by Erasmus, in which a man may write letters, debauch himself, get drunk, and even make money—a slumber so deep at times that no torpedo-touch can waken him.

It may keep the practitioner out of the clutches of the arch enemy of his professional independence—the pernicious literature of our camp-followers, a literature increasing in bulk, in meretricious attractiveness, and in impudent audacity.   To modern pharmacy we owe much, and to pharmaceutical methods we shall owe much more in the future, but the profession has no more insidious foe than the large borderland pharmaceutical houses.   No longer an honoured messmate, pharmacy in this form threatens to become a huge parasite, eating the vitals of the body medical.   We all know only too well the bastard literature which floods the mail, every page of which illustrates the truth of the axiom, the greater the ignorance the greater the dogmatism.   Much of it is advertisements of nostrums foisted on the profession by men who trade on the innocent credulity of the regular physician, quite as much as any quack preys on the gullible public.   Even the most respectable houses are not free from this sin of arrogance and of ignorant dogmatism in their literature.   A still more dangerous enemy to the mental virility of the general practitioner, is the "drummer" of the drug house. While many of them are good, sensible fellows, there are others, voluble as Cassio, impudent as Autolycus, and senseless as Caliban, who will tell you glibly of the virtues of extract of the coccygeal gland in promoting pineal metabolism, and are ready to express the most emphatic opinions on questions about which the greatest masters of our art are doubtful. No class of men with which we have to deal illustrates more fully that greatest of ignorance—the ignorance which is the conceit that a man knows what he does not know; but the enthralment of the practitioner by the manufacturing chemist and the revival of a pseudoscientific polypharmacy are too large questions to be dealt with at the end of an address.

But there is a still greater sacrifice which many of us make, heedlessly and thoughtlessly forgetting that "Man does not live by bread alone." One cannot practise medicine alone and practise it early and late, as so many of us have to do, and hope to escape the malign influences of a routine life. The incessant concentration of thought upon one subject, however interesting, tethers a man's mind in a narrow field. The practitioner needs culture as well as learning. The earliest picture we have in literature of a scientific physician, in our sense of the term, is as a cultured Greek gentleman; and I care not whether the young man labours among the beautiful homes on Sherbrooke Street, or in the slums of Caughnawauga, or in some sparsely settled country district, he cannot afford to have learning only. In no profession does culture count for so much as in medicine, and no man needs it more than the general practitioner, working among all sorts and conditions of men, many of whom are influenced quite as much by his general ability, which they can appreciate, as by his learning of which they have no measure. The day has passed for the "practiser of physic" to be like Mr. Robert Levet, Dr. Johnson's friend, "Obscurely wise and coarsely kind." The wider and freer a men's general education the better practitioner is he likely to be, particularly among the higher classes to whom the reassurance and sympathy of a cultivated gentleman of the type of Eryximachus, may mean much more than pills and potions. But what of the men of the type of Mr. Robert Levet, or "Ole Docteur Fiset," whose virtues walk a narrow round, the men who do the hard general practices in the poorer districts of the large cities, in the factory towns and in the widely scattered rough agricultural regions—what, I hear you say, has culture to do with them? Everything! It is the bichloride which may prevent the infection and may keep a man sweet and whole amid the most debasing surroundings. Of very little direct value to him in his practice—though the poor have a pretty keen appreciation of a gentleman—it may serve to prevent the degeneration so apt to overtake the overworked practitioner, whose nature isonly too prone to be subdued like the dyer's hand to what it works in. If a man does not sell his soul, if he does not part with his birthright of independence for a mess of pottage to the Ishmaelites who harass our borders with their clubs and oppress us with their exactions, if he can only keep *free*, the conditions of practice are nowhere incompatible with St. Paul's noble Christian or Aristotle's true gentleman (Sir Thomas Browne).

Whether a man will treat his professional brethren in a gentlemanly way or in a narrow illiberal spirit is partly a matter of temperament, partly a matter of training. If we had only to deal with one another the difficulties would be slight, but it must be confessed that the practice of medicine among our fellow creatures is often a testy and choleric business.   When one has done his best or when a mistake has arisen through lack of special knowledge, but more particularly when, as so often happens, our heart's best sympathies have been engaged, to be misunderstood by the patient and his friends, to have evil motives imputed and to be maligned, is too much for human endurance and justifies a righteous indignation.   Women, our greatest friends and our greatest enemies, are the chief sinners, and while one will exhaust the resources of the language in describing our mistakes and weaknesses, another will laud her pet doctor so indiscriminately that all others come under a sort of oblique condemnation.   "Feminæ sunt medicorum tubæ" is an old and true saying.   It is hard to say whether as a whole we do not suffer just as much from the indiscriminate praise.   But against this evil we are helpless.   Far otherwise, when we do not let the heard word die; not to listen is best, though that is not always possible, but silence is always possible, than which we have no better weapon in our armoury against evil-speaking, lying, and slandering.   The bitterness is when the tale is believed and a brother's good name is involved.   Then begins the worst form of ill-treatment that the practitioner receives—and at his own hands!   He allows the demon of resentment to take possession of his soul, when five minutes' frank conversation might have gained a brother.   In a small or a large community what more joyful than to see the brethren dwelling together in unity.   The bitterness, the rancour, the personal hostility which many of us remember in our younger days has been largely replaced by a better feeling and while the golden rule is not always, as it should be, our code of ethics, we have certainly become more charitable the one towards the other.

To the senior man in our ranks we look for an example, and in the smaller towns and country districts if he would remember that it is his duty to receive and welcome the young fellow who settles near him, that he should be willing to act as his adviser and refuse to regard him as a rival, he may make a good friend and perhaps gain a brother. In speaking of professional harmony, it is hard to avoid the trite and commonplace, but neglecting the stale old chaps whose ways are set and addressing the young, to whom sympathy and encouragement are so dear, and whose way of life means so much to the profession we love, upon them I would urge the practice of St. Augustine, of whom it is told in the *Golden Legend* that "he had these verses written at his table:

> Quisquis amat dictis absentum rodere vitam,
> Hanc mensam indignam noverit esse sibi:

That is to say: Whosoever loves to missay any creature that is absent, it may be said that this table is denied to him at all."

With our History, Traditions, Achievements, and Hopes, there is little room for Chauvinism in medicine. The open mind, the free spirit of science, the ready acceptance of the best from any and every source, the attitude of rational receptiveness rather than of antagonism to new ideas, the liberal and friendly relationship between different nations and different sections of the same nation, the brotherly feeling which should characterize members of the oldest, most beneficent and universal guild that the race has evolved in its upward progress—these should neutralize the tendencies upon which I have so lightly touched.

I began by speaking of the art of detachment as that rare and precious quality demanded of one who wished to take a philosophical view of the profession as a whole.

In another way and in another sense this art may be still more precious. There is possible to each one of us a higher type of intellectual detachment, a sort of separation from the vegetative life of the work-a-day world—always too much with us—which may enable a man to gain a true knowledge of himself and of his relations to his fellows. Once attained, self-deception is impossible, and he may see himself even as he is seen—not always as he would like to be seen—and his own deeds and the deeds of others stand out in their true light. In such an atmosphere pity for himself is so commingled with sympathy and love for others that there is no place left for criticism or for a harsh judgment of his brother. But as Sir Thomas Browne—most liberal of men and most distinguished of general practitioners—so beautifully remarks: "These are Thoughts of things which Thoughts but tenderly touch," and it may be sufficient to remind this audience, made up of practical men, *that the word of action is stronger than the word of speech.*

XV
SOME ASPECTS OF AMERICAN MEDICAL BIBLIOGRAPHY

Without History a man's soul is purblind, seeing only the things which almost touch his eyes.

FULLER, *Holy and Profane State*, 1642.

Every physician will make, and ought to make, observations from his own experience; but he will be able to make a better judgment and juster observations by comparing what he reads and what he sees together. It is neither an affront to any man's understanding, nor a cramp to his genius, to say that both the one and the other may be usefully employed, and happily improved in searching and examining into the opinions and methods of those who lived before him, especially considering that no one is tied up from judging for himself, or obliged to give into the notions of any author, any further than he finds them agreeable to reason, and reducible to practice. No one therefore need fear that his natural sagacity, whatever it is, should be perplexed or misled by reading. For there is as large and fruitful a field for sagacity and good judgment to display themselves in, by distinguishing between one author and another, and sometimes between the several parts and passages in the same author. as is to be found in the greatest extent and variety of practice . . . It has not usually been looked upon as an extraordinary mark of wisdom for a man to think himself too wise to be taught; and yet this seems to be the case of those who rely wholly upon their own experience, and despise all teachers but themselves.

FRIEND, *History of Physic*, Volume I.

SOME ASPECTS OF AMERICAN MEDICAL BIBLIOGRAPHY[1]

I

IN conferring upon me the presidency of this Association, I felt that you wished to pay a compliment to a man who had been much helped by libraries and who knew their value, and I hoped that it was, perhaps, in recognition of the fact that a practical and busy physician may be at the same time a book lover, even a book worm.

You are familiar, of course, with the objects of this Association, but as there are present with us also those who are not members, this is an occasion in which a little missionary work is timely, and I may briefly refer to some of them. An association of the medical libraries of the country, our membership includes both the great libraries, with 50,000–100,000 volumes, and the small collections just started of a few hundred books. The former gain nothing directly from an affiliation with us—they give more than they get, but the blessing that goes with this attitude is not to be despised, and from their representatives we look for guidance and advice. Please understand that in this address I am not talking to the men in charge of them who are familiar with what I shall say, and who are experts where I am only a dabbler; but I wish to catch the inexperienced, those in charge of the small but growing libraries, upon whom I wish to impress some wider aspects of the work. In the recent history of the profession there is nothing more

[1] Association of Medical Librarians, 1902.

encouraging than the increase in the number of medical libraries. The organization of a library means effort, it means union, it means progress. It does good to men who start it, who help with money, with time and with the gifts of books. It does good to the young men, with whom our hopes rest, and a library gradually and insensibly moulds the profession of a town to a better and higher status.

We trust that this Association may be a medium through which men interested in the promotion of the welfare of the profession may do much good in a quiet way. We have to thank some twenty physicians who have kindly joined us in this work and whose subscriptions help to pay the expenses of our exchange; but their names on our list do more—it is an encouragement to know that they are with us, and as they get nothing in return (except the BULLETIN) they should know how much we appreciate their fellowship. We have to thank, in particular, many editors who send us their journals for distribution, and the editors of many Transactions. The liberality with which the work of our Exchange has been aided by the large libraries is beyond all praise. Time and again the Library of the Surgeon-General's Office, the Academy of Medicine of New York, the Boston Medical Library Association, and the College of Physicians' Library of Philadelphia have filled long lists of wants for smaller libraries. The profession is deeply indebted to Drs. Merrill, Chadwick, and Brigham, to Mr. Browne and to Mr. C. P. Fisher for their disinterested labours. In some details our machinery could be better adjusted, but we have had to work with very little money, which means slight clerical help where much is needed, but with an increasing membership we can look forward confidently to a much more complete organization and to a wider field of usefulness.

But this Association may have other ambitions and hopes. We desire to foster among our members and in the profession at large a proper love of books. For its own sake and for the sake of what it brings, medical bibliography is worthy of a closer study than it has received heretofore in this country. The subject presents three aspects, the book itself, the book as a literary record, i.e., its contents, and the book in relation to the author. Strictly speaking, bibliography means the science of everything relating to the book itself, and has nothing to do with its contents. In the words of a recent writer, the bibliographer "has to do with editions and their peculiarities, with places, printers, and dates, with types and illustrations, with sizes and collations, with bindings and owners, with classifications, collections, and catalogues. It is the book as a material object in the world that is his care, not the instruction of which it may be, or may fail to be, the vehicle. Bibliography is the science or the art, or both, of book description."[1]

But there is a larger sense of the word, and I shall discuss some aspects of American medical bibliography in the threefold relationship to which I have referred.

II

The typographical considerations may be passed over with a few words. We have no Aldus or Froben or Stephanus or Elzevir, whose books are sought and prized for themselves, irrespective of their contents. With few exceptions the medical works published here at the end of the eighteenth and the beginning of the nineteenth centuries were poor specimens of the printer's art. Compare a Sydenham first edition of 1682 with Caldwell's Cullen, issued in

[1] Professor Ferguson, *Some Aspects of Bibliography*, Edinburgh, 1900.

Philadelphia more than 100 years later, and the comparison is in favour of the former; and yet there is much of bibliographical interest in early American publications. It would make an instructive exhibit to take a series of surgical books issued in this country from *Jones' Manual* in 1776 to *Kelly's Operative Gynecology;* it would illustrate the progress in the art of book making, and while there would be nothing striking or original, such volumes as *Dorsey's Elements of Surgery* (1813), particularly in the matter of illustrations, would show that there were good book makers at that date. At one of the meetings of the American Medical Association a selection of the works issued during the 117 years of the existence of the house of Lea Brothers would form an instructive exhibition.   There are few medical works in this country the genealogy of which requires any long search. Other than the "Code of Ethics" of the American Medical Association and the "American Pharmacopeia," both of which, by the way, have histories worth tracking, and the "Dispensatory" of Wood and Bache, I know of no works fifty years old which continue to be reprinted.   Compared with the text-books, etc., the journals of the early days were more presentable, and the general appearance of such publications as the *Medical Repository*, of New York, the *Medical Museum*, of Philadelphia, and later the *Medical and Physical Journal*, the *North American Medical and Surgical Journal* and the *Medical Recorder*, not only contrasts favourably with that of European journals of the period, but one gets an impression of capable and scholarly editorial control and a high grade of original contribution.   The *Medical and Physical Journal*, founded in 1820, has a special interest and should be put on the shelves just before the *American Journal of the Medical Sciences*, into which it merged, one of the few great journals of the world, and the one from which one can almost write the progress of American medicine during the past century.

While there is not in American medicine much of pure typographical interest, compensation is offered in one of the most stupendous bibliographical works ever undertaken. The Index-Catalogue of the Library of the Surgeon-General's Office atones for all shortcomings, as in it is furnished to the world a universal medical bibliography from the earliest times. It will ever remain a monument to the Army Medical Department, to the enterprise, energy and care of Dr. Billings, and to the scholarship of his associate, Dr. Robert Fletcher. Ambitious men before Dr. Billings had dreamt of a comprehensive medical bibliography. Conrad Gesner, the learned Swiss naturalist and physician, published his *Bibliotheca Universalis* as early as 1545 and followed it in 1548–9 by a supplement entitled *Pandectarum sive Partitionum universalium Conradi Gesneri, libri* xxi. Book xx, which was to represent the quintessence of the labours of his life and which was to include the medical bibliography, never appeared, owing to his untimely yet happy death—*felix mors Gesneri*, as Caius says, in the touching tribute to his friend.[1] Merklin, von Haller, Ploucquet, Haeser, Young, Forbes, Atkinson and others have dipped into the vast subject, but their efforts are Lilliputian beside the Gargantuan undertaking of the Surgeon-General's Office. One work I cannot pass without a regret and a reference—the unfinished medical bibliography of James Atkinson, London, 1834. If not on your shelves, keep your eyes on the London catalogues for it. It only includes the letters A and B, but it is a unique work by a Thelemite, a true disciple of Rabelais. I need not refer in this audience to the use of the Index-Catalogue in library work; it is also

[1] *Caii Opera,* Jebb's edition.

of incalculable value to any one interested in books. Let me give an everyday illustration. From the library of my friend, the late Dr. Rush Huidekoper, was sent to me a set of very choice old tomes, among which was a handsome folio of the works of Du Laurens, a sixteenth century anatomist and physician. I had never heard of him, but was very much interested in some of his medical dissertations. In a few moments from the Index-Catalogue the whole bibliography of the man was before me, the dates of his birth and death, the source of his biography, and where to look for his portrait. It is impossible to overestimate the boon which this work is to book lovers. One other point— the Index is not used enough by students. Take under the subject of diseases of the heart. Only the other day I referred to a journal article which had a very full bibliography, and I turned to Volume V in the old series, and to the just issued Volume VI of the new series, and there was the literature in full on this subject and in it many articles which the author had overlooked. The entire bibliography might have been omitted with advantage from the paper and simply a reference made to the Index-Catalogue. It would be well in future if writers would bear in mind that on many subjects, particularly those covered by the second series of the Catalogue, the bibliography is very complete, and only supplementary references should be made to the articles which have appeared since the volume of the new series dealing with the subject was printed.

III

The second aspect of a book relates to its contents, which may have an enduring value or which may be of interest only as illustrating a phase in the progress of knowledge, or the importance may relate to the conditions under which the book appeared.

It is sad to think how useless are a majority of the works on our shelves—the old cyclopedias and dictionaries, the files of defunct journals, the endless editions of text-books as dead as the authors. Only a few epoch-making works survive. Editions of the Hippocratic writings appear from time to time, and in the revival of the study of the history of medicine the writings of such masters as Galen and Aretæus reappear, but the interest is scholastic, and amid the multiplicity of studies how can we ask the student to make himself familiar with the ancients? We can, however, approach the consideration of most subjects from an historical standpoint, and the young doctor who thinks that pathology began with Virchow gets about the same erroneous notion as the student who begins the study of American history with the Declaration of Independence.

Now among the colossal mass of rubbish on the shelves there are precious gems which should be polished and well set and in every library put out on view. But let me first mollify the harshness of the expression just used. The other day, thinking in this way, I took from a shelf of old books the first one I touched. It was Currie's *Historical Account of the Climates and Diseases of the United States of America*, published in Philadelphia in 1792. I had possessed it for years, but had never before looked into it. I found the first comprehensive study on climatology and epidemiology made in this country, one which antedates by several years Noah Webster's work on epidemics. With remarkable industry Dr. Currie collected from correspondents in all parts of the country information about the prevalent diseases, and I know of no other work from which we can get a first-hand sketch from the practitioners themselves of the maladies prevalent in the different States.   Then 1 had to look up his possible relationship with James Currie, of Liverpool, the strong advocate of hydrotherapy, the friend and editor of Burns, who had had, I remember, interesting affiliations with Virginia.   At the outbreak of the Revolutionary War he was employed as a clerk at one of the landings on the James River, and suffered not a little for the Tory cause.   His letters, given in his *Life*, which are well worth reading, give a valuable picture of the period. The American Currie's book at least was not rubbish in 1792, but who will read it now?   And yet it is on our shelves for a purpose.   It may not be called for once in five years; it did a good work in its day, and the author lived a life of unselfish devotion to the profession.   As a maker of much which in a few years will be *rubbish* of this kind, let me take back the harsh expression.

But I wish to refer particularly to certain treasures in American bibliography which you should all have on your shelves.   Of course the great libraries have most of them, and yet not all have all of them, but with a little effort they can be picked up.   Take that notable *Discourse upon the Institution of Medical Schools in America*, by John Morgan, M.D., 1765.   From it dates the organization of medical colleges in this country, but there is much more in this scholarly address.   The introduction contains a picture of the state of practice in Philadelphia which is in its way unique, and for the first time in the history of the profession in this country Morgan tried to introduce what he calls the regular mode of practising physic, as apart from the work of the surgeon and apothecary.   What interests us, too, is his plea for the establishment of a medical library. Listen to his appeal: "Perhaps the physicians of Phila-delphia, touched with generous sentiments of regard for the rising generation and the manifest advantages accruing to the College thereby, would spare some useful books or contribute somewhat as a foundation on which we might begin." The biographical fragments in the introduction show the remarkable care with which some of the young colonial physicians sought the best available education. Few to-day, after a protracted apprenticeship, do as did Morgan, spend five years in Europe under the most celebrated masters, but he returned a distinguished Fellow of the Royal Society of London, and a Correspondent of the Royal Academy of Surgery in Paris.

John Jones's *Plain, Practical, Concise, Remarks on the Treatment of Wounds and Fractures, Designed for the Use of Young Military and Naval Surgeons in North America,* 1775, was the *vade mecum* of the young surgeons in the Revolutionary War. As the first separate surgical treatise published in this country it has a distinct bibliographical value, and, when, possible, you should put the three editions together.

Samuel Bard's study on *Angina Suffocativa* (1771), or diphtheria, as it would be now termed, is an American classic of the first rank. It is difficult to get, but it is worth looking for. Get, too, his work on *Midwifery,* 1807, the first published in this country. An enterprising librarian will have all the editions of such a work.

Thomas Bond's *Lecture Introductory to the Study of Clinical Medicine at the Pennsylvania Hospital,* 1766, remained in manuscript until printed in Vol. IV of the *North American Medical Journal,* 1827, a copy of which is not difficult to obtain. It is also republished in Morton's *History of the Pennsylvania Hospital,* and I republished it in the *University Medical Magazine* in 1897.

The works of Rush should be fully represented even in the smaller libraries. His collected writings passed through five editions and are easy to get. Rush "is the father not only of American medicine, but of American medical literature, the type of a great man, many-sided, far-seeing, full of intellect, and genius; abused and vilified, as man hardly ever was before, by his contemporaries, professional and non-professional; misunderstood by his immediate successors, and unappreciated by the present generation, few of whom know anything of his real character." I gladly quote this estimate of Rush by S. D. Gross. Owing to the impression that he was disloyal to Washington, there has arisen of late a certain feeling of antagonism to his name. The truth is he was a strong hater, and, as was common at that period, a bitter partisan. I wish some one would give us the account from contemporary letters, and from the side of Rush. There is an astonishing amount of bibliographical interest in the writings of Rush, and a good story awaits the leisure hours of some capable young physician. His letters are innumerable and scattered in many libraries. I came across one the other day (*Bulletin of the New York Library*, vol. I, No. 8), dated July 27, 1803, in which, replying to an invitation from Horatio Gates, he says pathetically, "A large and expensive family chain me to the pestle and mortar," and in a postscript he adds that as he now confines his labours to his patients, without trying to combat ignorance and error, he is kindly tolerated by his fellow-citizens.

Many early works of great importance are difficult to find, such as Elisha North on *Spotted Typhus* or cerebrospinal fever, 1811. Noah Webster's *History of Epidemics* has a special value, apart from its interest as the most important medical work written in this country by a layman.

The tracts on vaccination by Waterhouse—the American Jenner—should be sought for carefully. Try to have a copy of Nathan Smith's *A Practical Essay on Typhous Fever* (1824) to hand to any young physician who asks for something good and fresh on typhoid fever. There is a long list of important essays which you should have. I cannot begin to name them all, but I may mention, as an example, Jacob Bigelow on *Self-limited Diseases*, 1835, which is a tract every senior student should read, mark, learn and inwardly digest. If not obtainable, his *Nature in Disease*, 1859, contains it and many other essays of value. James Jackson's *Letters to a Young Physician*, 1856, are still worth reading—and worth republishing.

The stories of the great epidemics offer material for careful bibliographical research. Matthew Carey's graphic description of the great epidemic of yellow fever in Philadelphia, while not so lifelike and brilliant as De Foe's great story of the plague in London, has the advantage of the tale of an eye-witness and of a brave man, one of the small band who rose above the panic of those awful days. It is a classic of the first rank. The little book, by the way, had a remarkable sale. The first edition is dated November 13, 1793, the second, November 23, the third, November 30, and the fourth, January 16, 1794. Brockden Brown's *Arthur Mervyn*, while it gives in places a vivid description of this epidemic, is, in comparison, disappointing and lame, not worthy to be placed on the same shelf with Carey's remarkable account.

Even the smaller libraries should have the works of this type. They are not hard to get, if looked for in the right way. Early American works on special subjects should be sought for. The collection of works exhibited in the section on ophthalmology at the meeting of the American Medical Association shows in the most instructive manner the early publications on the subject in this country.

IV

The third aspect of medical bibliography relates to writings which have a value to us from our interest in the author.   After all, the true bibliophile cares not so much for the book as for the man whose life and mind are illustrated in it.   There are men of noble life and high character, every scrap of whose writings should be precious to us, and such men are not rare.   The works are not always of any special value to-day, or even of any intrinsic interest, but they appeal to us through the sympathy and even the affection, stirred in us by the story of the man's life.   It is, I know, a not uncommon feeling—a feeling which pervades No. XXXII of Shakespeare's *Sonnets* and is so beautifully expressed in the concluding line, "Theirs for their style I'll read, his for his love."   Such an attitude I feel personally toward the literary remains of John Morgan, David Ramsay, Daniel Drake, John D. Godman, James Jackson, junr., Elisha Bartlett and others.

In our libraries under John Morgan, to whose remarkable essay I have already referred, there should be also his *Vindication*, which gives the story of the Army Medical Department in the early days of the Revolution.   One of the most famous names in America medicine is David Ramsay, perhaps the most distinguished pupil of Benjamin Rush, a man of high character, full of zeal and ambition and devoted to his profession, yet what he has left in general literature far excels in importance his medical writings. The larger libraries should have his famous *History of the American Revolution*, 1789, his *Life of Washington*, and the *History of South Carolina*, 1809.   The memory of such a man should be cherished among us, and one way—and the best—is to put a complete set of his writings on our shelves.

Another noble soul of the same stamp was John D. Godman, the tragedy of whose life and early death has a pathos unequalled in the annals of the profession of America. Besides his anatomical works, his *Museum of American Natural History* and *The Rambles of a Naturalist* should be among your treasured Americana.

There is a large literature in this group illustrating the excursions of medical men into pure literature. A complete set of the writings of Oliver Wendell Holmes should be in every medical library. His Boylston prize essays on *Neuralgia*, on *Malarial Fever*, and on *Direct Explorations* can be had bound in one volume. One of his writings is inestimable, and will be remembered in the profession as long, I believe, as posterity will cherish his *Chambered Nautilus* or the *Last Leaf*. If you can find the original pamphlet on the *Contagiousness of Puerperal Fever*, a reprint from the *New England Journal of Medicine and Surgery*, 1843, have it bound in crushed levant—'tis worthy of it. The reprint of 1855 is more accessible. Failing either of these, get the journal and cut out and bind the article. Semmelweiss, who gets the credit for introducing asepsis in midwifery, came some years later. Occasionally, a well-known medical writer will dabble in pure literature, and will sometimes, as in the case of Dr. Weir Mitchell, attain a success as remarkable as that which he has had in his profession. Put his writings on the shelves—they illustrate his breadth and his strength. A volume of poems may illustrate some strong man's foible. George B. Wood's epic poem, "First and Last," and the "Eolopoesis" of Jacob Bigelow illustrate the dangers which beset physicians who write poetry.

Biography is a department which you will find a very attractive and most profitable field to cultivate for your

readers. The foreign literature includes several comprehensive encyclopedias, but it is not a department very well
represented in this country. It is true that an enormous
literature exists, chiefly in periodicals, but the sort of
biography to which I refer has a threefold distinction. The
subject is a worthy one, he is dead, and the writer has the
necessary qualifications for the task. We possess three
notable works on American medical biography: James
Thacher, 1828; Stephen W. Williams, 1845, and Samuel D.
Gross, 1861, which remain to-day the chief works of reference to the latter date. Thacher's is a remarkable production and for the period a most ambitious work. It has been
a common tap to which writers have gone for information
on the history of medicine in this country, and the lives of
the prominent physicians to about 1825. It is a rare volume now, but worth its price, and I know of no more
fascinating book, or one more difficult to put down. Even
the printed list of subscribers—a long one, too—is most
interesting. Many of Thacher's best known books come
in the third category, and are of value in a medical library
only so far as they illustrate the remarkable versatility of
the man. His *Practice*, the first American one, you will,
of course, try to get, and you should also have one of the
editions of his *Journal of the Revolutionary War*, through
which he served with pencil, as well as scalpel, in hand. It
is a most graphic account, and of interest to us here since
he describes very fully the campaign in this region, which
led to the surrender of Burgoyne, the treachery of Arnold,
and he was an eye-witness of the tragic end of poor Major
André. You will not find it easy to get a complete set of
his writings.

There are many single volumes for which you will be on
the look out. Caldwell's *Autobiography* is a storehouse of

facts (and fancies!) relating to the University of Pennsylvania, to Rush and to the early days of the Transylvania University and the Cincinnati schools. Pickled, as it is, in vinegar, the work is sure to survive.

Have carefully rebound James Jackson's memoir of his son (1835), and put it in the way of the young men among your readers. Few biographies will do them more good.

For the curious pick up the literature on the Chapman-Pattison quarrel, and anything, in fact, relating to that vivacious and pugnacious Scot, Granville Sharpe Pattison.

There are a few full-blown medical biographies of special interest to us: The life and writings of that remarkable philosopher and physician, Wells, of Charleston. The life of John C. Warren (1860) is full of interest, and in the *Essays* of David Hosack you will get the inner history of the profession in New York during the early years of the last century. In many ways Daniel Drake is the most unique figure in the history of American medicine. Get his *Life*, by Mansfield, and his *Pioneer Life in Kentucky*. He literally made Cincinnati, having "boomed" it in the early days in his celebrated *Picture of Cincinnati*, 1815. He founded nearly everything that is old and good in that city. His monumental work on *The Diseases of the Mississippi Valley* is in every library; pick out from the catalogues every scrap of his writings.

I must bring these "splintery," rambling remarks to a close, but I hope that I may have stirred in you an interest in some of the wider aspects of American medical biobibliography—I mean aspects other than the daily demand upon you for new books, new editions and new journals.

Keep ever in view, each one in this circle, the important fact that a library should be a storehouse of everything relating to his history of the profession of the locality.

Refuse nothing, especially if it is old; letters, manuscripts of all kinds, pictures, everything illustrating the growth as well as the past condition, should be preserved and tabulated. There is usually in each community a man who is fond of work of this sort. Encourage him in every possible way. Think of the legacy left by Dr. Toner, of Washington, rich in materials for the history of the profession during the Revolutionary War! There should be a local pride in collecting the writings and manuscripts of the men who have made a school or a city famous. It is astonishing how much manuscript material is stowed away in old chests and desks. Take, for example, the recent "find" of Dr. Cordell of the letters of the younger Wiesenthal, of Baltimore, describing student life in London about the middle of the eighteenth century. Think of the precious letters of that noble old man, Nathan Smith, full of details about the foundations of the Dartmouth and the Yale Schools of Medicine! Valuable now (too valuable to be in private hands), what will they be 100 or 200 years hence!

What should attract us all is a study of the growth of the American mind in medicine since the starting of the colonies. As in a mirror this story is reflected in the literature of which you are the guardians and collectors—in letters, in manuscripts, in pamphlets, in books, and in journals. In the eight generations which have passed, the men who have striven and struggled—men whose lives are best described in the words of St. Paul, in journeyings often, in perils of water, in perils in the city, in perils in the wilderness, in perils in the sea, in weariness and painfulness, in watchings often, in hunger and thirst, and in fastings—these men, of some of whom I have told you somewhat, have made us what we are. With the irrevocable past into which they have gone lies our future, since our condition is the resultant of forces which, in these generations, have moulded the profession of a new and mighty empire. From the vantage ground of a young century we can trace in the literature how three great streams of influence—English, French and German—have blended into the broad current of American medicine on which we are afloat. Adaptiveness, lucidity and thoroughness may be said to be the characteristics of these Anglican, Gallic and Teutonic influences, and it is no small part of your duty to see that these influences, the combination of which gives to medicine on this continent its distinctively eclectic quality, are maintained and extended.

XVI
THE HOSPITAL AS A COLLEGE

The Hospital is the only proper College in which to rear a true disciple of Aesculapius.

ABERNETHY.

The most essential part of a student's instruction is obtained, as I believe, not in the lecture room, but at the bedside. Nothing seen there is lost; the rhythms of disease are learned by frequent repetition; its unforeseen occurrences stamp themselves indelibly on the memory. Before the student is aware of what he has acquired he has learned the aspects and causes and probable issue of the diseases he has seen with his teacher, and the proper mode of dealing with them, so far as his master knows.

OLIVER WENDELL HOLMES, *Introductory Lecture*, 1867.

XVI

THE HOSPITAL AS A COLLEGE[1]

I

THE last quarter of the last century saw many remarkable changes and reformations, among which in
far-reaching general importance not one is to be compared
with the reform, or rather revolution, in the teaching of
the science and art of medicine. Whether the conscience
of the professors at last awoke, and felt the pricking of
remorse, or whether the change, as is more likely, was only
part of that larger movement toward larger events in the
midst of which we are to-day, need not be here discussed.
The improvement has been in three directions: in demanding of the student a better general education; in lengthening
the period of professional study; and in substituting
laboratories for lecture rooms—that is to say, in the replace-
ment of theoretical by practical teaching. The problem
before us as teachers may be very briefly stated: to give
to our students an education of such a character that
they can become sensible practitioners—the destiny of
seven-eighths of them. Toward this end are all our endowments, our multiplying laboratories, our complicated
curricula, our palatial buildings. In the four years' course
a division is very properly made between the preparatory
or scientific branches and the practical; the former are
taught in the school or college, the latter in the hospital.
Not that there is any essential difference; there may be as

---

[1] Academy of Medicine, New York, 1903.

much science taught in a course of surgery as in a course of embryology. The special growth of the medical school in the past 25 years has been in the direction of the practical teaching of science. Everywhere the lectures have been supplemented or replaced by prolonged practical courses, and instead of a single laboratory devoted to anatomy, there are now laboratories of physiology, or physiological chemistry, of pathology, of pharmacology, and of hygiene. Apart from the more attractive mode of presentation and the more useful character of the knowledge obtained in this way, the student learns to use the instruments of precision, gets a mental training of incalculable value, and perhaps catches some measure of the scientific spirit. The main point is that he has no longer merely theoretical knowledge acquired in a lecture room, but a first-hand practical acquaintance with the things themselves. He not only has dissected the sympathetic system, but he has set up a kymograph and can take a blood pressure observation, he has personally studied the action of digitalis, of chloroform and of ether, he has made his own culture media and he has "plated" organisms. The young fellow who is sent on to us in his third year is nowadays a fairly well trained man and in a position to begin his life's work in those larger laboratories, private and public, which nature fills with her mistakes and experiments.

How can we make the work of the student in the third and fourth year as practical as it is in his first and second? I take it for granted we all feel that it should be. The answer is, take him from the lecture-room, take him from the amphitheatre—put him in the out-patient department —put him in the wards. It is not the systematic lecture, not the amphitheatre clinic, not even the ward class—all of which have their value—in which the reformation is

needed but in the whole relationship of the senior student to
the hospital.   During the first two years, he is thoroughly at
home in the laboratories, domiciled, we may say, with his
place in each one, to which he can go and work quietly under
a tutor's direction and guidance.   To parallel this condition
in the third and fourth years certain reforms are necessary.
First, in the conception of how the art of medicine and
surgery can be taught.   My firm conviction is that we
should start the third year student at once on his road of
life.   Ask any physician of twenty years' standing how he
has become proficient in his art, and he will reply, by constant contact with disease; and he will add that the medicine
he learned in the schools was totally different from the
medicine he learned at the bedside.   The graduate of a
quarter of a century ago went out with little practical
knowledge, which increased only as his practice increased.
In what may be called the natural method of teaching the
student begins with the patient, continues with the patient,
and ends his studies with the patient, using books and lectures as tools, as means to an end.   The student starts, in
fact, as a *practitioner*, as an observer of disordered machines,
with the structure and orderly functions of which he is
perfectly familiar.   Teach him how to observe, give him
plenty of facts to observe, and the lessons will come out of
the facts themselves.   For the junior student in medicine
and surgery it is a safe rule to have no teaching without
a patient for a text, and the best teaching is that taught
by the patient himself.   The whole art of medicine is
in observation, as the old motto goes, but to educate the
eye to see, the ear to hear and the finger to feel takes time,
and to make a beginning, to start a man on the right path, is
all that we can do.   We expect too much of the student
and we try to teach him too much.   Give him good methods

and a proper point of view, and all other things will be added, as his experience grows.

The second, and what is the most important reform, is in the hospital itself. In the interests of the medical student, of the profession, and of the public at large we must ask from the hospital authorities much greater facilities than are at present enjoyed, at least by the students of a majority of the medical schools of this country. The work of the third and fourth year should be taken out of the medical school entirely and transferred to the hospital, which, as Abernethy remarks, is the proper college for the medical student, in his last years at least. An extraordinary difficulty here presents itself. While there are institutions in which the students have all the privileges to be desired, there are others in which they are admitted by side entrances to the amphitheatre of the hospital, while from too many the students are barred as hurtful to the best interests of the patients. The work of an institution in which there is no teaching is rarely first class. There is not that keen interest, nor the thorough study of the cases, nor amid the exigencies of the busy life is the hospital physician able to escape clinical slovenliness unless he teaches and in turn is taught by assistants and students. It is, I think, safe to say that in a hospital with students in the wards the patients are more carefully looked after, their diseases are more fully studied and fewer mistakes made. The larger question, of the extended usefulness of the hospital in promoting the diffusion of medical and surgical knowledge, I cannot here consider.

I envy for our medical students the advantages enjoyed by the nurses, who live in daily contact with the sick, and who have, in this country at least, supplanted the former in the affections of the hospital trustees.

The objection often raised that patients do not like to have students in the wards is entirely fanciful. In my experience it is just the reverse. On this point I can claim to speak with some authority, having served as a hospital physician for more than 25 years, and having taught chiefly in the wards. With the exercise of ordinary discretion, and if one is actuated by kindly feelings towards the patients, there is rarely any difficulty. In the present state of medicine it is very difficult to carry on the work of a first-class hospital without the help of students. We ask far too much of the resident physicians, whose number has not increased in proportion to the enormous increase in the amount of work thrust upon them, and much of the routine work can be perfectly well done by senior students.

II

How, practically, can this be carried into effect? Let us take the third year students first. A class of 100 students may be divided into ten sections, each of which may be called a clinical unit, which should be in charge of one instructor. Let us follow the course of such a unit through the day. On Mondays, Wednesdays, and Fridays at 9 a.m. elementary instruction in physical diagnosis. From 10 to 12 a.m. practical instruction in the out-patient department. This may consist in part in seeing the cases in a routine way, in receiving instruction how to take histories, and in becoming familiar with the ordinary aspect of disease as seen in a medical outclinic. At 12 o'clock a senior teacher could meet four, or even five, of the units, dealing more systematically with special cases. The entire morning, or, where it is customary to have the hospital practice in the afternoon, a large part of the afternoon, two or three hours at least, should be spent in the out-patient department. No short six weeks' course, but each clinical unit throughout the session should as a routine see out-patient practice under skilled direction.   Very soon these students are able to take histories, have learned how to examine the cases, and the out-patient records gradually become of some value.   Of course all of this means abundance of clinical material, proper space in the out-patient department for teaching, sufficient apparatus and young men who are able and willing to undertake the work.

On the alternate days, Tuesdays, Thursdays and Saturdays, the clinical unit (which we are following) is in the surgical out-patient department, seeing minor surgery, learning how to bandage, to give ether, and helping in all the interesting work of a surgical dispensary.   Groups of three or four units should be in charge of a demonstrator of morbid anatomy, who would take them to postmortems, the individual men doing the work, and one day in the week all the units could attend the morbid anatomy demonstration of the professor of pathology.   I take it for granted that the student has got so far that he has finished his pathological histology in his second year, which is the case in the more advanced schools.

Other hours of the day for the third year could be devoted to the teaching of obstetrics, materia medica, therapeutics, hygiene and clinical microscopy.   At the end of the session in a well-conducted school the third-year student is really a very well-informed fellow.   He knows the difference between Pott's disease and Pott's fracture; he can readily feel an enlarged spleen, and he knows the difference between Charcot's crystals and Charcot's joint.

In the fourth yea: I would still maintain the clinical unit of ten men, whose work would be transferred from the out-patient department to the wards.   Each man should be allowed to serve in the medical, and, for as long a period as possible, in the surgical wards. He should be assigned four or five beds. He has had experience enough in his third year to enable him to take the history of the new cases, which would need, of course, supervision or correction by the senior house officer or attending physician. Under the supervision of the house physician he does all of the work connected with his own patients; analysis of the urine, etc., and takes the daily record as dictated by the attending physician. One or two of the clinical units are taken round the wards three or four times in the week by one of the teachers for a couple of hours, the cases commented upon, the students asked questions and the groups made familiar with the progress of the cases. In this way the student gets a familiarity with disease, a practical knowledge of clinical methods and a practical knowledge of how to treat disease. With equal advantage the same plan can be followed in the surgical wards and in the obstetrical and gynæcological departments.

An old method, it is the only method by which medicine and surgery can be taught properly, as it is the identical manner in which the physician is himself taught when he gets into practice. The radical reform needed is in the introduction into this country of the system of clinical clerks and surgical dressers, who should be just as much a part of the machinery of the wards as the nurses or the house physicians.

There is no scarcity of material; on the contrary, there is abundance. Think of the plethora of patients in this city, the large majority of whom are never seen, not to say touched, by a medical student! Think of the hundreds of typhoid fever patients, the daily course of whose disease is never watched or studied by our pupils! Think how few of the hundreds of cases of pneumonia which will enter the hospitals during the next three months, will be seen daily, hourly, in the wards by the fourth year men! And yet it is for this they are in the medical school, just as much as, more indeed, than they are in it to learn the physiology of the liver or the anatomy of the hip-joint.

But as you may ask, how does such a plan work in practice? From a long experience I can answer, admirably! It has been adopted in the Johns Hopkins Medical School, of which the hospital, by the terms of the founder's will, is an essential part. There is nothing special in our material, our wards are not any better than those in other first-class hospitals, but a distinctive feature is that greater provision is made for teaching students and perhaps for the study of disease. Let me tell you in a few words just how the work is conducted. The third year students are taught medicine:

First, in a systematic course of physical diagnosis conducted by Drs. Thayer and Futcher, the Associate Professors of Medicine, in the rooms adjacent to the out-patient department. In the second half of the year, after receiving instruction in history-taking, the students take notes and examine out-patients.

Secondly, three days in the week at the conclusion of the out-patient hours, the entire class meets the teacher in an adjacent room, and the students are taught how to examine and study patients. It is remarkable how many interesting cases can be shown in the course of a year in this way. Each student who takes a case is expected to report upon and "keep track" of it, and is questioned with reference to its progress. The opportunity is taken to teach the student how to look up questions in the literature by setting subjects upon which to report in connexion with the cases they have seen. A class of fifty can be dealt with very conveniently in this manner.

Thirdly, the clinical microscopy class. The clinical laboratory is part of the hospital equipment. It is in charge of a senior assistant, who is one of the resident officers of the hospital. There is room in it for about one hundred students on two floors, each man having his own work-table and locker and a place in which he can have his own specimens and work at odd hours. The course is a systematic one, given throughout the session, from two hours to two hours and a half twice a week, and consists of routine instruction in the methods of examining the blood and secretions, the gastric contents, urine, etc. This can be made a most invaluable course, enabling the student to continue the microscopic work which he has had in his first and second years, and he familiarizes himself with the use of a valuable instrument, which becomes in this way a clinical tool and not a mere toy. The clinical laboratory in the medical school, should be connected with the hospital, of which it is an essential part. Nowadays the microscopical, bacteriological and chemical work of the wards demands skilled labour, and the house physicians as well as the students need the help and supervision of experts in clinical chemistry and bacteriology, who should form part of the resident staff of the institution.

Fourthly, the general medical clinic. One day in the week, in the amphitheatre, a clinic is held for the third and fourth year students and the more interesting cases in the wards are brought before them. As far as possible we present the diseases of the seasons, and in the autumn special attention is given to malarial and typhoid fever, and later in the winter to pneumonia. Committees are appointed to report on every case of pneumonia and the

complications of typhoid fever.   There are no systematic
lectures, but in the physical diagnosis classes there are set
recitations, and in what I call the observation class in the
dispensary held three times a week, general statements are
often made concerning the diseases under consideration.

Fourth Year Ward Work.—The class is divided into three
groups (one in medicine, one in surgery, and one in obstetrics
and gynecology) which serve as clinical clerks and surgical
dressers.   In medicine each student has five or six beds.
He takes notes of the new cases as they come in, does the
urine and blood work and helps the house physician in the
general care of the patients.   From nine to eleven the visit
is made with the clinical clerks, and systematic instruction
is given.   The interesting cases are seen and new cases
are studied, and the students questioned with reference to
the symptoms and nature of the disease and the course of
treatment.   What I wish to emphasize is that this method
of teaching is not a ward-class in which a group of students
is taken into the ward and a case or two demonstrated; it
is *ward-work*, the students themselves taking their share in
the work of the hospital, just as much as the attending
physician, the interne, or the nurse.   Moreover, it is not
an occasional thing.   His work in medicine for the three
months is his major subject and the clinical clerks have
from nine to twelve for their ward-work, and an hour in the
afternoon in which some special questions are dealt with
by the senior assistant or by the house physicians.

The Recitation Class.—As there are no regular lectures,
to be certain that all of the subjects in medicine are brought
before the students in a systematic manner, a recitation
class is held once a week upon subjects set beforehand.

The Weekly Clinic in the amphitheatre, in which the
clinical clerks take leading parts, as they report upon

their cases and read the notes of their cases brought before
the class for consideration.   Certain important aspects of
medicine are constantly kept before this class.   Week after
week the condition of the typhoid fever cases is discussed,
the more interesting cases shown, the complications systematically placed upon the board.   A pneumonia committee deals with all the clinical features of this common
disease, and a list of the cases is kept on the blackboard,
and during a session the students have reports upon fifty
or sixty cases, a large majority of which are seen in the
clinic by all of them, while the clinical clerks have in the
wards an opportunity of studying them daily.

The general impression among the students and the junior
teachers is that the system has worked well.   There are
faults, perhaps more than we see, but I am sure they are
not in the system.   Many of the students are doubtless
not well informed theoretically on some subjects, as personally I have always been opposed to that base and
most pernicious system of educating them with a view to
examinations, but even the dullest learn how to examine
patients, and get familiar with the changing aspects of the
important acute diseases.   The pupil handles a sufficient
number of cases to get a certain measure of technical skill,
and there is ever kept before him the idea that he is not in
the hospital to learn everything that is known but to learn
how to study disease and how to treat it, or rather, how to
treat patients.

III

A third change is in reorganization of the medical school.
This has been accomplished in the first two years by an
extraordinary increase in the laboratory work, which has
necessitated an increase in the teaching force, and indeed an

entirely new conception of how such subjects as physiology, pharmacology and pathology should be taught. A corresponding reformation is needed in the third and fourth years. Control of ample clinical facilities is as essential to-day as large, well-endowed laboratories, and the absence of this causes the clinical to lag behind the scientific education. Speaking for the Department of Medicine, I should say that three or four well-equipped medical clinics of fifty to seventy-five beds each, with out-patient departments under the control of the directors, are required for a school of maximum size, say 800 students. Within the next quarter of a century the larger universities of this country will have their own hospitals in which the problems of nature known as disease will be studied as thoroughly as are those of geology or Sanscrit. But even with present conditions much may be done. There are hundreds of earnest students, thousands of patients, and scores of well-equipped young men willing and anxious to do practical teaching. Too often, as you know full well, "the hungry sheep look up and are not fed;" for the bread of the wards they are given the stones of the lecture-room and amphitheatre. The dissociation of student and patient is a legacy of the pernicious system of theoretical teaching from which we have escaped in the first and second years.

For the third and fourth year students, the hospital is the college; for the juniors, the out-patient department and the clinics; for the seniors, the wards. They should be in the hospital as part of its equipment, as an essential part, without which the work cannot be of the best. They should be in it as the place in which alone they can learn the elements of their art and the lessons which will be of service to them when in practice for themselves. The hospital with students in its dispensaries and wards doubles its usefulness in a community. The stimulus of their presence neutralizes that clinical apathy certain, sooner or later, to beset the man who makes lonely "rounds" with his house-physician. Better work is done for the profession and for the public; the practical education of young men, who carry with them to all parts of the country good methods, extends enormously the work of an institution, and the profession is recruited by men who have been taught to think and to observe for themselves, and who become independent practitioners of the new school of scientific medicine—men whose faith in the possibilities of their art has been strengthened, not weakened, by a knowledge of its limitations. It is no new method which I advocate, but the old method of Boerhaave, of the elder Rutherford of the Edinburgh school, of the older men of this city, and of Boston and of Philadelphia—the men who had been pupils of John Hunter and of Rutherford and of Saunders. It makes of the hospital a college in which, as clinical clerks and surgical dressers, the students slowly learn for themselves, under skilled direction, the phenomena of disease. It is the true method, because it is the natural one, the only one by which a physician grows in clinical wisdom after he begins practice for himself—all others are bastard substitutes.

XVII
ON THE EDUCATIONAL VALUE OF THE MEDICAL SOCIETY

Let us hold fast the profession of our faith without wavering . . . . and let us consider one another, to provoke unto love and to good works: not forsaking the assembling of ourselves together, as the manner of some is.

EPISTLE TO THE HEBREWS, Chapter x.

The want of energy is one of the main reasons why so few persons continue to improve in later years. They have not the will, and do not know the way. They "never try an experiment" or look up a point of interest for themselves; they make no sacrifices for the sake of knowledge; their minds, like their bodies, at a certain age become fixed. Genius has been defined as "the power of taking pains"; but hardly any one keeps up his interest in knowledge throughout a whole life. The troubles of a family, the business of making money, the demands of a profession destroy the elasticity of the mind. The waxen tablet of the memory, which was once capable of receiving "true thoughts and clear impressions," becomes hard and crowded; there is no room for the accumulations of a long life (*Theæt.*, 194 ff.). The student, as years advance, rather makes an exchange of knowledge than adds to his stores.

JOWETT's *Introductions ic Plato.*

XVII

ON THE EDUCATIONAL VALUE OF THE MEDICAL SOCIETY[1]

A S the Autocrat remarks:

> Little of all we value here
> Wakes on the morn of its hundredth year.

All the more reason to honour such occasions as the present in an appropriate manner. The tribute of words
that I gladly bring—and that you may take as expressing
the sentiments of your brethren at large—necessarily
begins with congratulations that your society has passed
into the select group of those that have reached a century
of existence. But congratulations must be mingled with
praise of the band of noble men who, in 1803, made this
gathering possible. It is true they did but follow the lead
of their colleagues of Litchfield County and their own
example when, in 1784, the physicians of this county
organized what is now one of the oldest medical societies
in the land. In the introduction to the volume of *Transactions* of this Society, published in 1788, the following brief
statements are made as to the objects of the organization,
which may be transposed from the parent to the child,
and which I quote in illustration of the character of the
men and as giving in brief the chief uses of a medical

Centennial celebration of the New Haven Medical Association, New
Haven. January 6, 1903.

329

society: "This society was formed on the most liberal and generous principles, and was designed, first, to lay a foundation for that unanimity and friendship which is essential to the dignity and usefulness of the profession; to accomplish which, they resolved, secondly, to meet once in three months; thirdly, that in all cases where counsel is requisite they will assist each other without reserve; fourthly, that all reputable practitioners in the country, who have been in the practice for one year or more, may be admitted members; fifthly, that they will communicate their observations on the air, seasons and climate, with such discoveries as they may make in physic, surgery, botany or chemistry, and deliver faithful histories of the various diseases incident to the inhabitants of this country, with the mode of treatment and event in singular cases; sixthly, to open a correspondence with the medical societies in the neighbouring states and in Europe, for which purpose they have a standing committee of correspondence; seventhly, to appoint a committee for the purpose of examining candidates for the profession, and to give certificates to the deserving." Changed conditions have changed some of these objects, but in the main they hold good to-day.

Some of the paragraphs have suggested to me the subject of my address—the educational value of the medical society. There are many problems and difficulties in the education of a medical student, but they are not more difficult than the question of the continuous education of the general practitioner. Over the one we have some control, over the other, none. The university and the state board make it certain that the one has a minimum, at least, of professional knowledge, but who can be certain of the state of that knowledge of the other in five or ten

years from the date of his graduation? The specialist
may be trusted to take care of himself—the conditions
of his existence demand that he shall be abreast of the
times; but the family doctor, the private in our great
army, the essential factor in the battle, should be carefully
nurtured by the schools and carefully guarded by the
public. Humanly speaking, with him are the issues of
life and death, since upon him falls the grievous responsibility in those terrible emergencies which bring darkness
and despair to so many households. No class of men
needs to call to mind more often the wise comment of
Plato that education is a life-long business. The difficulties
are partly adherent to the subject, partly have to do with
the individual and his weakness. The problems of disease
are more complicated and difficult than any others with
which the trained mind has to grapple; the conditions
in any given case may be unlike those in any other; each
case, indeed, may have its own problem. Law, constantly
looking back, has its forms and procedures, its precedents
and practices. Once grasped, the certainties of divinity
make its study a delight and its practice a pastime; but
who can tell of the uncertainties of medicine as an art?
The science on which it is based is accurate and definite
enough; the physics of a man's circulation are the physics
of the waterworks of the town in which he lives, but once
out of gear, you cannot apply the same rules for the repair
of the one as of the other. Variability is the law of life,
and as no two faces are the same, so no two bodies are alike,
and no two individuals react alike and behave alike under
the abnormal conditions which we know as disease. This is
the fundamental difficulty in the education of the physician,
and one which he may never grasp, or he takes it so tenderly
that it hurts instead of boldly accepting the axiom of

Bishop Butler, more true of medicine than of any other profession: "Probability is the guide of life." Surrounded by people who demand certainty, and not philosopher enough to agree with Locke that "*Probability supplies the defect of our knowledge and guides us when that fails and is always conversant about things of which we have no certainty*," the practitioner too often gets into a habit of mind which resents the thought that opinion, not full knowledge, must be his stay and prop. There is no discredit, though there is at times much discomfort, in this everlasting *perhaps* with which we have to preface so much connected with the practice of our art. It is, as I said, inherent in the subject. Take in illustration an experience of last week. I saw a patient with Dr. Bolgiano who presented marked pulsation to the left of the sternum in the second, third and fourth interspaces, visible even before the night-dress was removed, a palpable impulse over the area of pulsation, flatness on percussion, accentuated heart sounds and a soft systolic bruit. When to this were added paralysis of the left recurrent laryngeal nerve, smallness of the radial pulse on the left side, and tracheal tugging, there is not one of you who would not make, under such circumstances, the diagnosis of aneurism of the aorta. Few of us, indeed, would put in the *perhaps*, or think of it as a probability with such a combination of physical signs, and yet the associate conditions which had been present—a small primary tumour of the left lobe of the thyroid, with secondary nodules in the lymph glands of the neck and involvement of the mediastinum and metastases in the brain with optic neuritis—left no question that the tumour causing the remarkable intrathoracic combination was not aneurismal but malignant. Listen to the appropriate comment of the Father of Medicine, who twenty-five centuries ago had not only grasped the fundamental conception of our art as one based on observation, but had laboured also through a long life to give to the profession which he loved the saving health of science—listen, I say, to the words of his famous aphorism: *"Experience is fallacious and judgment difficult!"*

But the more serious problem relates to the education of the practitioner after he has left the schools. The foundation may not have been laid upon which to erect an intellectual structure, and too often the man starts with a total misconception of the prolonged struggle necessary to keep the education he has, to say nothing of bettering the instruction of the schools. As the practice of medicine is not a business and can never be one,[1] the education of the heart—the moral side of the man—must keep pace with the education of the head. Our fellow creatures cannot be dealt with as man deals in corn and coal; "the human heart by which we live" must control our professional relations. After all, the personal equation has most to do with success or failure in medicine, and in the trials of life the fire which strengthens and tempers the metal of one may soften and ruin another. In his philosophy

---

[1] In every age there have been Elijahs ready to give up in despair at the progress of commercialism in the profession. Garth says in 1699 (*Dispensary*)—

How sickening Physick hangs her pensive head
And what was once a Science, now's a Trade.

Of medicine, many are of the opinion expressed by one of Akenside's disputants at Tom's Coffee House, that the ancients endeavoured to make it a science and failed, and the moderns to make it a trade and have succeeded. To-day the cry is louder than ever, and in truth there are grounds for alarm; but, on the other hand, we can say to these Elijahs that there are many more than 7,000 left who have not bowed the knee to this Baal, but who practise *caute caste et probe.*

of life the young doctor will find Rabbi Ben Ezra[1] a better guide, with his stimulating

> Then, welcome each rebuff
> That turns earth's smoothness rough,
> Each sting that bids nor sit nor stand but go!

than Omar, whose fatalism, so seductive in Fitzgerald's verses, leaves little scope for human effort.

For better or worse, there are few occupations of a more satisfying character than the practice of medicine, if a man can but once get *orientirt* and bring to it the philosophy of honest work, the philosophy which insists that we are here, not to get all we can out of the life about us, but to see how much we can add to it. The discontent and grumblings which one hears have their source in the man more often than in his environment. In the nature of the material in which we labour and of which, by the way, we are partakers, there is much that could be improved, but, as Mrs. Poyser remarks, we must accept men as the Lord made them, and not expect too much. But let me say this of the public: it is rarely responsible for the failures in the profession. Occasionally a man of superlative merit is neglected, but it is because he lacks that most essential gift, the knowledge how to use his gifts. The failure in 99 per cent. of the cases is in the man himself; he has not started right, the poor chap has not had the choice of his parents, or his education has been faulty, or he has fallen away to the worship of strange gods, Baal or Ashtoreth, or worse still, Bacchus. But after all the killing vice of the young doctor is intellectual laziness. He may have worked hard at college, but the years of probation have

[1] See Browning's poem. A good little edition has just been issued (with an introduction by William Adams Slade), which I commend to young graduates.

been his ruin. Without specific subjects upon which to work, he gets the newspaper or the novel habit, and fritters his energies upon useless literature. There is no greater test of a man's strength than to make him mark time in the "stand and wait" years. Habits of systematic reading are rare, and are becoming more rare, and five or ten years from his license, as practice begins to grow, may find the young doctor knowing less than he did when he started and without fixed educational purpose in life.

Now here is where the medical society may step in and prove his salvation. The doctor's post-graduate education comes from patients, from books and journals, and from societies, which should be supplemented every five or six years by a return to a post-graduate school to get rid of an almost inevitable slovenliness in methods of work. Of his chief teachers, his patients, I cannot here speak. Each case has its lesson—a lesson that may be, but is not always, learnt, for clinical wisdom is not the equivalent of experience. A man who has seen 500 cases of pneumonia may not have the understanding of the disease which comes with an intelligent study of a score of cases, so different are knowledge and wisdom, which, as the poet truly says, "far from being one have ofttimes no connexion." Nor can I speak of his books and journals, but on such an occasion as the present it seems appropriate to say a few words on the *educational value of the medical society.*

The first, and in some respects the most important, function is that mentioned by the wise founders of your parent society—to lay a foundation for that unity and friendship which is essential to the dignity and usefulness of the profession. Unity and friendship! How we all long for them, but how difficult to attain! Strife seems rather to be the very life of the practitioner, whose warfare is incessant against disease and against ignorance and prejudice, and, sad to have to admit, he too often lets his angry passions rise against his professional brother. The quarrels of doctors make a pretty chapter in the history of medicine. Each generation seems to have had its own. The Coans and the Cnidians, the Arabians and the Galenists, the humoralists and the solidists, the Brunonians and the Broussaisians, the homœopaths and the regulars, have, in different centuries, rent the robe of Æsculapius. But these larger quarrels are becoming less and less intense, and in the last century no new one of moment sprang up, while it is easy to predict that in the present century, when science has fully leavened the dough of homœpathy, the great breach of our day will be healed. But in too many towns and smaller communities miserable frictions prevail, and bickerings and jealousies mar the dignity and usefulness of the profession. So far as my observation goes, the fault lies with the older men. The young fellow, if handled aright and made to feel that he is welcomed and not regarded as an intruder to be shunned, is only too ready to hold out the hand of fellowship. The society comes in here as professional cement. The meetings in a friendly social way lead to a free and open discussion of differences in a spirit that refuses to recognize differences of opinion on the non-essentials of life as a cause of personal animosity or ill-feeling. An attitude of mind habitually friendly, more particularly to the young man, even though you feel him to be the David to whom your kingdom may fall, a little of the old-fashioned courtesy which makes a man shrink from wounding the feelings of a brother practitioner—in honour preferring one another; with such a spirit abroad in the society and among its older men, there is no room for envy, hatred, malice or any uncharitableness. It is the confounded tales of patients that so often set us by the ears, but if a man makes it a rule never under any circumstances to believe a story told by a patient to the detriment of a fellow-practitioner—even if he knows it to be true!—though the measure he metes may not be measured to him again, he will have the satisfaction of knowing that he has closed the ears of his soul to ninety-nine lies, and to have missed the hundredth truth will not hurt him. Most of the quarrels of doctors are about non-essential, miserable trifles and annoyances—the pin pricks of practice—which would sometimes try the patience of Job, but the good-fellowship and friendly intercourse of the medical society should reduce these to a minimum.

The well-conducted medical society should represent a clearing house, in which every physician of the district would receive his intellectual rating, and in which he could find out his professional assets and liabilities. We doctors do not "take stock" often enough, and are very apt to carry on our shelves stale, out-of-date goods. The society helps to keep a man "up to the times," and enables him to refurnish his mental shop with the latest wares. Rightly used, it may be a touchstone to which he can bring his experiences to the test and save him from falling into the rut of a few sequences. It keeps his mind open and receptive, and counteracts that tendency to premature senility which is apt to overtake a man who lives in a routine. Upon one or two specially valuable features of the society I may dwell for a moment or two.

In a city association the demonstration of instructive specimens in morbid anatomy should form a special feature of the work. After all has been done, many cases of great obscurity in our daily rounds remain obscure, and as post-mortems are few and far between, the private practitioner

is at a great disadvantage, since his mistakes in diagnosis
are less often corrected than are those of hospital physicians.
No more instructive work is possible than carefully demonstrated specimens illustrating disturbance of function and
explanatory of the clinical symptoms. It is hard in this
country to have the student see enough morbid anatomy,
the aspects of which have such an important bearing upon
the mental attitude of the growing doctor. For the crass
therapeutic credulity, so widespread to-day, and upon which
our manufacturing chemists wax fat, there is no more
potent antidote than the healthy scepticism bred of long
study in the post-mortem room. The new pathology, so
fascinating and so time-absorbing, tends, I fear, to grow
away from the old morbid anatomy, a training in which
is of such incalculable advantage to the physician. It is a
subject which one must learn in the medical school, but
the time assigned is rarely sufficient to give the student
a proper grasp of the subject. The younger men should be
encouraged to make the exhibition of specimens part of the
routine work of each meeting. Something may be learned
from the most ordinary case if it is presented with the
special object of illustrating the relation of disturbed
function to altered structure. Of still greater educational
value is the clinical side of the society. No meeting should
be arranged without the presentation of patients, particularly those illustrating rare and unusual forms of
disease. Many diseases of the skin and of the joints, a
host of nervous affections, and many of the more remarkable
of general maladies, as myxœdema, cretinism, achon-
droplasia, etc., are seen so rarely and yet are so distinctive, requiring only to be seen to be recognized, that it is
incumbent upon members to use the society to show such
cases. A clinical evening devoted to these rarer affections

is of very great help in diffusing valuable knowledge. The importance of a clinical demonstration was never better illustrated than at the International Congress in London in 1881, when Dr. Ord and others presented one morning at the Clinical Museum a group of cases of myxœdema. There were men from all parts of the world, and the general recognition of the disease outside of England dates from that meeting. The physiognomy of disease is learned slowly, and yet there are a great many affections which can be recognized, sometimes at a glance, more often by careful inspection, without any history. The society should be a school in which the scholars teach each other, and there is no better way than by the demonstration of the more unusual cases that happen to fall in your way. I have gone over my history cards of private patients brought or sent to me by last-year physicians, in which the disease was not diagnosed though recognizable *de visu*. Gout, pseudo-hypertrophic muscular paralysis, hysterical lordosis, spondylitis deformans, preataxic tabes (myosis, ptosis, etc.), Graves' disease, Parkinson's disease, anorexia nervosa, Raynaud's disease, pernicious anæmia, spastic diplegia, spastic hemiplegia and cyanosis of chronic emphysema were on the list. Some of these are rare diseases, but at an active society in the course of a few years every one of them could be demonstrated.

The presentation of the histories of cases may be made very instructive, but this is often a cause of much weariness and dissatisfaction. A brief oral statement of the special features of a case is much to be preferred to a long, written account. The protocol or daily record of a long case should never be given in full. The salient points should be brought out, particularly the relation the case bears to the known features of the disease and to diagnosis and treatment. The volume of the *Transactions of the New Haven County Medical Society*, 1788, contains many admirably reported cases. I select one for special comment, as it is, so far as I know, the first case on record of a most remarkable disease, to which much attention has been paid of late—the hypertrophic stenosis of the pylorus in children (see full discussion in the *Lancet* of December 20, 1902). Dr. Hezekiah Beardsley reports a *Case of Schirrhus of the Pylorus of an Infant*. Every feature of the disease as we know it now is noted—the constant puking, the leanness, the wizened, old look of the child are well described, and the diagnosis was made four months before death! The post-mortem showed a dilated and hypertrophied stomach and "the pylorus was invested with a hard, compact substance or schirrosity which so completely obstructed the passage into the duodenum, as to admit with the greatest difficulty the finest fluid." If other men had been as accurate and careful as Dr. Beardsley, and if other societies had followed the good example set so early by the New Haven County Medical Association, not only would this rare disease have been recognized, but by the accumulation of accurate observations many another disease would have yielded its secret. But it illustrates the old story—there is no more difficult art to acquire than the art of observation, and for some men it is quite as difficult to record an observation in brief and plain language.

In no way can a society better help in the education of its members than in maintaining for them a good library, and I am glad to know that this is one of your functions. It is most gratifying to note the growing interest in this work in all parts of the country. In the last number of the *Bulletin* of the Association of Medical Librarians there is a list of twenty-five societies with medical libraries.

An attractive reading-room, with the important weekly journals, and with shelves stocked with the new books in different departments, becomes an educational centre in which the young man can keep up his training and to which the older practitioner can go for advice when he is in despair and for reassurance when he is in doubt. The self-sacrifice necessary to establish and maintain such a library does good to the men who take part in it; harmony is promoted, and, in the words of your fathers, the dignity and usefulness of the profession are maintained.

Why is it that a large majority of all practitioners are not members of a medical society? Dr. Simmons estimates that there are 77,000 physicians in the United States who do not belong to any medical society whatever! In part this is due to apathy of the officers and failure to present an attractive programme, but more often the fault is in the men. Perhaps given over wholly to commercialism a doctor feels it a waste of time to join a society, and so it is if he is in the profession only for the money he can get out of patients without regard to the sacred obligation to put himself in the best possible position to do the best that is known for them. More frequently, I fear, the "dollar-doctor" is a regular frequenter of the society, knowing full well how suicidal in the long run is isolation from the general body of the profession. The man who knows it all and gets nothing from the society reminds one of that little dried-up miniature of humanity, the prematurely senile infant, whose tabetic marasmus has added old age to infancy. Why should he go to the society and hear Dr. Jones on the gastric relations of neurasthenia when he can get it all so much better in the works of Einhorn or Ewald? He is weary of seeing appendices, and there are no new pelvic viscera for demonstration. It is a waste of time, he says, and he feels better at home, and perhaps that is the best place for a man who has reached this stage of intellectual stagnation.

Greater sympathy must be felt for the man who has started all right and has worked hard at the societies, but as the rolling years have brought ever-increasing demands on his time, the evening hours find him worn out yet not able to rest, much less to snatch a little diversion or instruction in the company of his fellows whom he loves so well. Of all men in the profession the forty-visit-a-day man is the most to be pitied. Not always an automaton, he may sometimes by economy of words and extraordinary energy do his work well, but too often he is the one above all others who needs the refreshment of mind and recreation that is to be had in a well-conducted society. Too often he is lost beyond all recall, and, like Ephraim joined to his idols, we may leave him alone. Many good men are ruined by success in practice, and need to pray the prayer of the Litany against the evils of prosperity. It is only too true, as you know well, that a most successful—as the term goes—doctor may practise with a clinical slovenliness that makes it impossible for that kind old friend, Dame Nature, to cover his mistakes. A well-conducted society may be of the greatest help in stimulating the practitioner to keep up habits of scientific study. It seems a shocking thing to say, but you all know it to be a fact that many, very many men in large practice never use a stethoscope, and as for a microscope, they have long forgotten what a leucocyte or a tube cast looks like. This in some cases may be fortunate, as imperfect or half knowledge might only lead to mistakes, but the secret of this neglect of means of incalculable help is the fact that he has not attained the full and enduring knowledge which should have been given to him in the medical school. It is astonishing with how little outside aid a large practice may be conducted, but it is not astonishing that in it cruel and unpardonable mistakes are made. At whose door so often lies the responsibility for death in cases of empyema but at that of the busy doctor, who has not time to make routine examinations, or who is "so driven" that the urine of his scarlet fever or puerperal patients is not examined until the storm has broken?

But I hear it sometimes said you cannot expect the general practitioner, particularly in country districts, to use the microscope and stethoscope—these are refinements of diagnosis. They are not! They are the essential means which can be used and should be used by every intelligent practitioner. In our miserable, antiquated system of teaching we send our graduates out wholly unprepared to make a rational diagnosis, but a man who is in earnest —and, thank heaven! most of the young men to-day in the profession are in earnest—can supply the defects in his education by careful study of his cases, and can supplement the deficiency by a post-graduate course. A room fitted as a small laboratory, with the necessary chemicals and a microscope, will prove a better investment in the long run than a static machine or a new-fangled air-pressure spray apparatus.

It is not in the local society only that a man can get encouragement in his day's work and a betterment of mind and methods. Every practitioner should feel a pride in belonging to his state society, and should attend the meetings whenever possible, and gradually learn to know his colleagues, and here let me direct your attention to an important movement on the part of the American Medical Association, which has for its object the organization of the profession throughout the entire country. This can be accomplished only by a uniformity in the organization of the state societies, and by making the county society the unit through which members are admitted to the state and national bodies. Those of you interested will find very instructive information on this subject in the *Journal* of the association in a series of papers by Dr. Simmons, the editor, which have been reprinted in pamphlet form. As now managed, with active sections conducted by good men from all parts of the country, the meeting of the National Association is in itself a sort of brief post-graduate course. Those of you at the receptive age who attended the Saratoga meeting last June must have been impressed with the educational value of such a gathering. The Annual Museum was itself an important education in certain lines, and the papers and discussions in the various sections were of the greatest possible value, But I need say no more to this audience on the subject of medical societies; you of New England have not "forsaken the gathering of yourselves together as the manner of some is," but have been an example to the whole country.

In the dedication of his *Holy War*, Thomas Fuller has some very happy and characteristic remarks on the bounden duty of a man to better his heritage of birth or fortune, and what the father found glass and made crystal, he urges the son to find crystal and make pearl. Your heritage has been most exceptional, and, I believe, from all that I know of the profession in this city and State, that could your fathers return they would say that of their crystal you had made pearl. One cannot read their history as told by Bronson, or as sketched by your distinguished citizen, my colleague, Dr. Welch, without a glow of admiration for their lofty ideals, their steadfastness and devotion, and for their faith in the profession which they loved. The times have changed, conditions of practice have altered and are altering rapidly, but when such a celebration takes us back to your origin in simpler days and ways, we find that the ideals which inspired them are ours to-day— ideals which are ever old, yet always fresh and new, and we can truly say in Kipling's words:

The men bulk big on the old trail, our own trail, the out trail,
They're God's own guides on the Long Trail, the trail that is always new.

XVIII
THE MASTER-WORD IN MEDICINE

If any one is desirous of carrying out in detail the Platonic education of after-life, some such counsels as the following may be offered to him: That he shall choose the branch of knowledge to which his own mind most distinctly inclines, and in which he takes the greatest delight, either one which seems to connect with his own daily employment, or, perhaps, furnishes the greatest contrast to it. He may study from the speculative side the profession or business in which he is practically engaged. He may make Homer, Dante, Shakespeare, Plato, Bacon the friends and companions of his life. He may find opportunities of hearing the living voice of a great teacher. He may select for inquiry some point of history, or some unexplained phenomenon of nature. An hour a day passed in such scientific or literary pursuits will furnish as many facts as the memory can retain, and will give him "a pleasure not to be repented of" (*Timæus*, 59 D). Only let him beware of being the slave of crotchets, or of running after a Will o' the Wisp in his ignorance, or in his vanity of attributing to himself the gifts of a poet, or assuming the air of a philosopher. He should know the limits of his own powers. Better to build up the mind by slow additions, to creep on quietly from one thing to another, to gain insensibly new powers and new interests in knowledge, than to form vast schemes which are never destined to be realized.

JOWETT, *Introductions to Plato.*

> Contend, my soul, for moments and for hours;
> Each is with service pregnant, each reclaimed
> Is like a Kingdom conquered, where to reign.

ROBERT LOUIS STEVENSON.

In the case of our habits we are only masters of the beginning, their growth by gradual stages being imperceptible, like the growth of disease.

ARISTOTLE, *Ethics.*

XVIII

THE MASTER-WORD IN MEDICINE[1]

I

BEFORE proceeding to the pleasing duty of addressing the undergraduates, as a native of this province and as an old student of this school, I must say a few words on the momentous changes inaugurated with this session, the most important, perhaps, which have taken place in the history of the profession in Ontario. The splendid laboratories which we saw opened this afternoon, a witness to the appreciation by the authorities of the needs of science in medicine, make possible the highest standards of education in the subjects upon which our Art is based. They may do more. A liberal policy, with a due regard to the truth that the greatness of a school lies in brains not bricks, should build up a great scientific centre which will bring renown to this city and to our country. The men in charge of the departments are of the right stamp. See to it that you treat them in the right way by giving skilled assistance enough to ensure that the vitality of men who could work for the world is not sapped by the routine of teaching. One regret will, I know, be in the minds of many of my younger hearers. The removal of the department of anatomy and physiology from the biological laboratory of the university breaks a connexion which has had an important influence on medicine in this city. To Professor Ramsay Wright is due much of the inspiration which has made possible these

[1] University of Toronto, 1903.

fine new laboratories. For years he has encouraged in every way the cultivation of the scientific branches of medicine and has unselfishly devoted much time to promoting the best interests of the Medical Faculty. And in passing let me pay a tribute to the ability and zeal with which Dr. A. B. Macallum has won for himself a world-wide reputation by intricate studies which have carried the name of this University to every nook and corner of the globe where the science of physiology is cultivated. How much you owe to him in connexion with the new buildings I need scarcely mention in this audience.

But the other event which we celebrate is of much greater importance. When the money is forthcoming it is an easy matter to join stone to stone in a stately edifice, but it is hard to find the market in which to buy the precious cement which can unite into an harmonious body the professors of medicine of two rival medical schools in the same city. That this has been accomplished so satisfactorily is a tribute to the good sense of the leaders of the two faculties, and tells of their recognition of the needs of the profession in the province. Is it too much to look forward to the absorption or affiliation of the Kingston and London schools into the Provincial University? The day has passed in which the small school without full endowment can live a life beneficial to the students, to the profession or to the public. I know well of the sacrifice of time and money which is freely made by the teachers of those schools; and they will not misunderstand my motives when I urge them to commit suicide, at least so far as to change their organizations into clinical schools in affiliation with the central university, as part, perhaps, of a widespread affiliation of the hospitals of the province. A school of the first rank in the world, such as this must become, should have ample clinical faculties

under its own control. It is as much a necessity that the
professors of medicine and surgery, etc., should have large
hospital services under their control throughout the year,
as it is that professors of pathology and physiology should
have laboratories such as those in which we here meet.   It
should be an easy matter to arrange between the provincial
authorities and the trustees of the Toronto General Hospital
to replace the present antiquated system of multiple small
services by modern well-equipped clinics—three in medicine
and three in surgery to begin with.   The increased efficiency of the service would be a substantial *quid pro quo*, but
there would have to be a self-denying ordinance on the part
of many of the attending physicians.   With the large number of students in the combined school no one hospital can
furnish in practical medicine, surgery and the specialties a
training in the art an equivalent of that which the student
will have in the science in the new laboratories.   An affiliation should be sought with every other hospital in the city
and province of fifty beds and over, in each of which two
or three extra-mural teachers could be recognized, who
would recieve for three or more months a number of students proportionate to the beds in the hospital.   I need
not mention names.   We all know men in Ottawa, Kingston, London, Hamilton, Guelph and Chatham, who could
take charge of small groups of the senior students and make
of them good practical doctors.   I merely throw out the
suggestion.   There are difficulties in the way; but is there
anything worth struggling for in this life which does not
bristle with them?

Students of Medicine: May this day be to each of you,
as it was to me when I entered this school thirty-five years
ago, the beginning of a happy life in a happy calling.   Not
one of you has come here with such a feeling of relief as that

which I experienced at an escape from conic sections and logarithms and from Hooker and Pearson. The dry bones became clothed with interest, and I felt that I had at last got to work. Of the greater advantages with which you start I shall not speak. Why waste my words on what you cannot understand. To those of us only who taught and studied in the dingy old building which stood near here is it given to feel the full change which the years have wrought, a change which my old teachers, whom I see here to-day— Dr. Richardson, Dr. Ogden, Dr. Thorburn and Dr. Oldright —must find hard to realize. One looks about in vain for some accustomed object on which to rest the eye in its backward glance—all, all are gone, the old familiar places. Even the landscape has altered, and the sense of loneliness and regret, the sort of homesickness one experiences on such occasions, is relieved by a feeling of thankfulness that at least some of the old familiar faces have been spared to see this day. To me at least the memory of those happy days is a perpetual benediction, and I look back upon the two years I spent at this school with the greatest delight. There were many things that might have been improved—and we can say the same of every medical school of that period—but I seem to have got much more out of it than our distinguished philosopher friend, J. Beattie Crozier, whose picture of the period seems hardly drawn. But after all, as someone has remarked, instruction is often the least part of an education, and, as I recall them, our teachers in their life and doctrine set forth a true and lively word to the great enlightenment of our darkness. They stand out in the background of my memory as a group of men whose influence and example were most helpful. In William R. Beaumont and Edward Mulberry Hodder, we had before us the highest type of the cultivated English surgeon. In Henry H. Wright we saw the incarnation of faithful devotion to duty—too faithful, we thought, as we trudged up to the eight o'clock lecture in the morning. In W. T. Aikins, a practical surgeon of remarkable skill and an ideal teacher for the general practitioner. How we wondered and delighted in the anatomical demonstrations of Dr. Richardson, whose infective enthusiasm did much to make anatomy the favourite subject among the students. I had the double advantage of attending the last course of Dr. Ogden and the first of Dr. Thorburn on materia medica and therapeutics. And Dr. Oldright had just begun his career of unselfish devotion to the cause of hygiene.

To one of my teachers I must pay in passing the tribute of filial affection. There are men here to-day who feel as I do about Dr. James Bovell—that he was of those finer spirits, not uncommon in life, touched to finer issues only in a suitable environment. Would the Paul of evolution have been Thomas Henry Huxley had the Senate elected the young naturalist to a chair in this university in 1851? Only men of a certain metal rise superior to their surroundings, and while Dr. Bovell had that all-important combination of boundless ambition with energy and industry, he had that fatal fault of diffuseness, in which even genius is strangled. With a quadrilateral mind, which he kept spinning like a teetotum, one side was never kept uppermost for long at a time. Caught in a storm which shook the scientific world with the publication of the *Origin of Species*, instead of sailing before the wind, even were it with bare poles, he put about and sought a harbour of refuge in writing a work on Natural Theology, which you will find on the shelves of second-hand book shops in a company made respectable at least by the presence of Paley. He was an omnivorous reader and transmutor, he could talk pleasantly, even at times transcendentally, upon anything in the science of the day, from protoplasm to evolution; but he lacked concentration and that scientific accuracy which only comes with a long training (sometimes, indeed, never comes,) and which is the ballast of the boat. But the bent of his mind was devotional, and early swept into the Tractarian movement, he became an advanced Churchman, a good Anglican Catholic. As he chaffingly remarked one day to his friend, the Rev. Mr. Darling, he was like the waterman in *Pilgrim's Progress*, rowing one way towards Rome, but looking steadfastly in the other direction towards Lambeth. His *Steps to the Altar* and his *Lectures on the Advent* attest the earnestness of his convictions; and later in life, following the example of Linacre, he took orders and became another illustration of what Cotton Mather calls the angelic conjunction of medicine with divinity. Then, how well I recall the keen love with which he would engage in metaphysical discussions, and the ardour with which he studied Kant, Hamilton, Reed, and Mill. At that day, to the Rev. Prof. Bevan was intrusted the rare privilege of directing the minds of the thinking youths at the Provincial University into proper philosophical channels. It was rumoured that the hungry sheep looked up and were not fed. I thought so at least, for certain of them, led by T. Wesley Mills, came over daily after Dr. Bovell's four o'clock lecture to reason high and long with him.

> On Providence, Foreknowledge, Will and Fate,
> Fixed Fate, Freewill, Foreknowledge absolute.

Yet withal, his main business in life was as a physician, much sought after for his skill in diagnosis, and much beloved for his loving heart. He had been brought up in the very best practical schools. A pupil of Bright and of Addison, a warm personal friend of Stokes and of Graves, he maintained loyally the traditions of Guy's, and taught us to reverence his great masters. As a teacher he had grasped the fundamental truth announced by John Hunter of the unity of physiological and pathological processes, and, as became the occupant of the chair of the Institutes of Medicine, he would discourse on pathological processes in lectures on physiology, and illustrate the physiology of bioplasm in lectures on the pathology of tumours to the bewilderment of the students. When in September, 1870, he wrote to me that he did not intend to return from the West Indies I felt that I had lost a father and a friend; but in Robert Palmer Howard, of Montreal, I found a noble step-father, and to these two men, and to my first teacher, the Rev. W. A. Johnson, of Weston, I owe my success in life—if success means getting what you want and being satisfied with it.

II

Of the value of an introductory lecture I am not altogether certain. I do not remember to have derived any enduring benefit from the many that I have been called upon to hear, or from the not a few that I have inflicted in my day. On the whole, I am in favour of abolishing the old custom, but as this is a very special occasion, with special addresses, I consider myself most happy to have been selected for this part of the programme. To the audience at large I fear that what I have to say will appear trite and commonplace, but bear with me, since, indeed, to most of you how good soever the word, the season is long past in which it could be spoken to your edification. As I glance from face to face the most striking single peculiarity is the extraordinary diversity that exists among you. Alike in

that you are men and white, you are unlike in your features, very unlike in your minds and in your mental training, and your teachers will mourn the singular inequalities
in your capacities. And so it is sad to think will be your
careers; for one success, for another failure; one will tread
the primrose path to the great bonfire, another the straight
and narrow way to renown; some of the best of you will be
striken early on the road, and will join that noble band of
youthful martyrs who loved not their lives to the death;
others, perhaps the most brilliant among you, like my old
friend and comrade, Dick Zimmerman (how he would have
rejoiced to see this day!), the Fates will overtake and whirl
to destruction just as success seems assured. When the
iniquity of oblivion has blindly scattered her poppy over
us, some of you will be the trusted counsellors of this community, and the heads of the departments of this Faculty;
while for the large majority of you, let us hope, is reserved
the happiest and most useful lot given to man—to
become vigorous, whole-souled, intelligent, general practitioners.

It seems a bounden duty on such an occasion to be honest
and frank, so I propose to tell you the secret of life as I have
seen the game played, and as I have tried to play it myself.
You remember in one of the Jungle Stories that when
Mowgli wished to be avenged on the villagers he could only
get the help of Hathi and his sons by sending them the
master-word. This I propose to give you in the hope, yes,
in the full assurance, that some of you at least will lay hold
upon it to your profit. Though a little one, the master-
word looms large in meaning. It is the open sesame to
every portal, the great equalizer in the world, the true philosopher's stone, which transmutes all the base metal of humanity into gold. The stupid man among you it will make

bright, the bright man brilliant, and the brilliant student steady. With the magic word in your heart all things are possible, and without it all study is vanity and vexation. The miracles of life are with it; the blind see by touch, the deaf hear with eyes, the dumb speak with fingers. To the youth it brings hope, to the middle-aged confidence, to the aged repose. True balm of hurt minds, in its presence the heart of the sorrowful is lightened and consoled. It is directly responsible for all advances in medicine during the past twenty-five centuries. Laying hold upon it Hippocrates made observation and science the warp and woof of our art. Galen so read its meaning that fifteen centuries stopped thinking, and slept until awakened by the *De Fabrica* of Vesalius, which is the very incarnation of the master-word. With its inspiration Harvey gave an impulse to a larger circulation than he wot of, an impulse which we feel to-day. Hunter sounded all its heights and depths, and stands out in our history as one of the great exemplars of its virtue. With it Virchow smote the rock, and the waters of progress gushed out; while in the hands of Pasteur it proved a very talisman to open to us a new heaven in medicine and a new earth in surgery. Not only has it been the touchstone of progress, but it is the measure of success in every-day life. Not a man before you but is beholden to it for his position here, while he who addresses you has that honour directly in consequence of having had it graven on his heart when he was as you are to-day. And the master-word is *Work*, a little one, as I have said, but fraught with momentous sequences if you can but write it on the tablets of your hearts, and bind it upon your foreheads. But there is a serious difficulty in getting you to understand the paramount importance of the work-habit as part of your organization. You are not far from the

Tom Sawyer stage with its philosophy "that work consists of whatever a body is obliged to do, and that play consists of whatever a body is not obliged to do."

A great many hard things may be said of the work-habit: For most of us it means a hard battle; the few take to it naturally; the many prefer idleness and never learn to love labour. Listen to this: "Look at one of your industrious fellows for a moment, I beseech you," says Robert Louis Stevenson. "He sows hurry and reaps indigestion; he puts a vast deal of activity out to interest, and receives a large measure of nervous derangement in return. Either he absents himself entirely from all fellowship, and lives a recluse in a garret, with carpet slippers and a leaden inkpot, or he comes among people swiftly and bitterly, in a contraction of his whole nervous system, to discharge some temper before he returns to work. I do not care how much or how well he works, this fellow is an evil feature in other people's lives." These are the sentiments of an overworked, dejected man; let me quote the motto of his saner moments: "To travel hopefully is better than to arrive, and the true success is in labour." If you wish to learn of the miseries of scholars in order to avoid them, read Part I, Section 2, Member 3, Subsection XV, of that immortal work, the *Anatomy of Melancholy*; but I am here to warn you against these evils, and to entreat you to form good habits in your student days.

At the outset appreciate clearly the aims and objects each one of you should have in view—a knowledge of disease and its cure, and a knowledge of yourself. The one special education, will make you a practitioner of medicine; the other, an inner education, may make you a truly good man, four square and without a flaw. The one is extrinsic and is largely accomplished by teacher and tutor, by text and by tongue; the other is intrinsic and is the mental salvation to be wrought out by each one for himself. The first may be had without the second; any one of you may become an active practitioner, without ever having had sense enough to realize that through life you have been a fool; or you may have the second without the first, and, without knowing much of the art, you may have the endowments of head and heart that make the little you do possess go very far in the community. With what I hope to infect you is a desire to have a due proportion of each.

So far as your professional education is concerned, what I shall say may make for each one of you an easy path easier. The multiplicity of the subjects to be studied is a difficulty, and it is hard for teacher and student to get a due sense of proportion in the work. We are in a transition stage in our methods of teaching, and have not everywhere got away from the idea of the examination as the "be-all and end-all;" so that the student has constantly before his eyes the magical letters of the degree he seeks. And this is well, perhaps, if you will remember that having, in the old phrase, commenced Bachelor of Medicine, you have only reached a point from which you can begin a life-long process of education.

So many and varied are the aspects presented by this theme that I can only lay stress upon a few of the more essential. The very first step towards success in any occupation is to become interested in it. Locke put this in a very happy way when he said, give a pupil "a relish of knowledge" and you put life into his work. And there is nothing more certain than that you cannot study well if you are not interested in your profession. Your presence here is a warrant that in some way you have become attracted to the study of medicine, but the speculative possibilities so warmly cherished at the outset are apt to cool when in contact with the stern realities of the class-room. Most of you have already experienced the all-absorbing attraction of the scientific branches, and nowadays the practical method of presentation has given a zest which was usually lacking in the old theoretical teaching. The life has become more serious in consequence, and medical students have put away many of the childish tricks with which we used to keep up their bad name. Compare the picture of the "sawbones" of 1842, as given in the recent biography of Sir Henry Acland, with the representatives to-day, and it is evident a great revolution has been effected, and very largely by the salutary influences of improved methods of education. It is possible now to fill out a day with practical work, varied enough to prevent monotony, and so arranged that the knowledge is picked out by the student himself, and not thrust into him, willy-nilly, at the point of the tongue. He exercises his wits and is no longer a passive Strasbourg goose, tied up and stuffed to repletion.

How can you take the greatest possible advantage of your capacities with the least possible strain? By cultivating system. I say cultivating advisedly, since some of you will find the acquisition of systematic habits very hard. There are minds congenitally systematic; others have a life-long fight against an inherited tendency to diffuseness and carelessness in work. A few brilliant fellows try to dispense with it altogether, but they are a burden to their brethren and a sore trial to their intimates. I have heard it remarked that order is the badge of an ordinary mind. So it may be, but as practitioners of medicine we have to be thankful to get into that useful class. Let me entreat those of you who are here for the first time to lay to heart what I say on this matter. Forget all else, but take away this counsel of a man who has had to fight a hard battle, and not always a successful one, for the little order he has had in his life; take away with you a profound conviction of the value of system in your work.   I appeal to the freshmen especially, because you to-day make a beginning, and your future career depends very much upon the habits you will form during this session.   To follow the routine of the classes is easy enough, but to take routine into every part of your daily life is a hard task.   Some of you will start out joyfully as did Christian and Hopeful, and for many days will journey safely towards the Delectable Mountains, dreaming of them and not thinking of disaster until you find yourselves in the strong captivity of Doubt and under the grinding tyranny of Despair.   You have been overconfident.   Begin again and more cautiously.   No student escapes wholly from these perils and trials; be not disheartened, expect them.   Let each hour of the day have its allotted duty, and cultivate that power of concentration which grows with its exercise, so that the attention neither flags nor wavers, but settles with a bull-dog tenacity on the subject before you.   Constant repetition makes a good habit fit easily in your mind, and by the end of the session you may have gained that most precious of all knowledge— the power to work.   Do not underestimate the difficulty you will have in wringing from your reluctant selves the stern determination to exact the uttermost minute on your schedule.   Do not get too interested in one study at the expense of another, but so map out your day that due allowance is given to each.   Only in this way can the average student get the best that he can out of his capacities.   And it is worth all the pains and trouble he can possibly take for the ultimate gain—if he can reach his doctorate with system so ingrained that it has become an integral part of his being. The artistic sense of perfection in work is another much-to-be-desired quality to be cultivated. No matter how trifling the matter on hand, do it with a feeling that it demands the best that is in you, and when done look it over with a critical eye, not sparing a strict judgment of yourself. This it is that makes anatomy a student's touchstone. Take the man who does his "part" to perfection, who has got out all there is in it, who labours over the tags of connective tissue and who demonstrates Meckel's ganglion in his part—this is the fellow in after years who is apt in emergencies, who saves a leg badly smashed in a railway accident, or fights out to the finish, never knowing when he is beaten, in a case of typhoid fever.

Learn to love the freedom of the student life, only too quickly to pass away; the absence of the coarser cares of after days, the joy in comradeship, the delight in new work, the happiness in knowing that you are making progress. Once only can you enjoy these pleasures. The seclusion of the student life is not always good for a man, particularly for those of you who will afterwards engage in general practice, since you will miss that facility of intercourse upon which often the doctor's success depends. On the other hand sequestration is essential for those of you with high ambitions proportionate to your capacity. It was for such that St. Chrysostom gave his famous counsel, "Depart from the highways and transplant thyself into some enclosed ground, for it is hard for a tree that stands by the wayside to keep its fruit till it be ripe."

Has work no dangers connected with it? What of this bogie of overwork of which we hear so much? There are dangers, but they may readily be avoided with a little care. I can only mention two, one physical, one mental. The very best students are often not the strongest. Ill-health, the bridle of Theages, as Plato called it in the case of one of his friends whose mind had thriven at the expense of his body, may have been the diverting influence towards books or the profession.   Among the good men who have studied with me there stands out in my remembrance many a young Lycidas, "dead ere his prime," sacrificed to carelessness in habits of living and neglect of ordinary sanitary laws.   Medical students are much exposed to infection of all sorts, to combat which the body must be kept in first-class condition.   Grosseteste, the great Bishop of Lincoln, remarked that there were three things necessary for temporal salvation—food, sleep and a cheerful disposition.   Add to these suitable exercise and you have the means by which good health may be maintained.   Not that health is to be a matter of perpetual solicitation, but habits which favour the *corpus sanum* foster the *mens sana*, in which the joy of living and the joy of working are blended in one harmony. Let me read you a quotation from old Burton, the great authority on *morbi eruditorum*.   There are "many reasons why students dote more often than others.   The first is their negligence; other men look to their tools, a painter will wash his pencils, a smith will look to his hammer, anvil, forge; a husbandman will mend his plough-irons, and grind his hatchet, if it be dull; a falconer or huntsman will have an especial care of his hawks, hounds, horses, dogs, etc.; a musician will string and unstring his lute, etc.; only scholars neglect that instrument, their brain and spirits (I mean) which they daily use."[1]

Much study is not only believed to be a weariness of the flesh, but also an active cause of ill-health of mind, in all grades and phases.   I deny that work, legitimate work,

[1] Quotation mainly from *Marsilius Ficinus*.

has anything to do with this. It is that foul fiend Worry who is responsible for a large majority of the cases. The more carefully one looks into the causes of nervous breakdown in students, the less important is work *per se* as a factor. There are a few cases of genuine overwork, but they are not common. Of the causes of worry in the student life there are three of prime importance to which I may briefly refer.

An anticipatory attitude of mind, a perpetual forecasting, disturbs the even tenor of his way and leads to disaster. Years ago a sentence in one of Carlyle's essays made a lasting impression on me: "Our duty is not to *see* what lies dimly at a distance, but to *do* what lies clearly at hand." I have long maintained that the best motto for a student is, "Take no thought for the morrow." Let the day's work suffice; live for it, regardless of what the future has in store, believing that to-morrow should take thought for the things of itself. There is no such safeguard against the morbid apprehensions about the future, the dread of examinations and the doubt of the ultimate success. Nor is there any risk that such an attitude may breed carelessness. On the contrary, the absorption in the duty of the hour is in itself the best guarantee of ultimate success. "He that observeth the wind shall not sow, and he that regardeth the clouds shall not reap," which means you cannot work profitably with your mind set upon the future.

Another potent cause of worry is an idolatry by which many of you will be sore let and hindered. The mistress of your studies should be the heavenly Aphrooite, the motherless daughter of Uranus. Give her your whole heart, and she will be your protectress and friend. A jealous creature, brooking no second, if she finds you trifling and coquetting with her rival, the younger, earthly Aphrodite, daughter of

Zeus and Dione, she will whistle you off and let you down
the wind to be a prey, perhaps to the examiners, certainly
to the worm regret.   In plainer language, put your affections in cold storage for a few years, and you will take them
out ripened, perhaps a bit mellow, but certainly less subject
to those frequent changes which perplex so many young
men.   Only a grand passion, an all-absorbing devotion to
the elder goddess can save the man with a congenital tendency to philandering, the flighty Lydgate who sports with
Celia and Dorothea, and upon whom the judgment ultimately falls in a basil-plant of a wife like Rosamond.

And thirdly, one and all of you will have to face the ordeal of every student in this generation who sooner or later
tries to mix the waters of science with the oil of faith.   You
can have a great deal of both if you only keep them separate.   The worry comes from the attempt at mixture.
As general practitioners you will need all the faith you can
carry, and while it may not always be of the conventional
pattern, when expressed in your lives rather than on your
lips, the variety is not a bad one from the standpoint of St.
James; and may help to counteract the common scandal
alluded to in the celebrated diary of that gossipy old pastor-
doctor, the Rev. John Ward: "One told the Bishop of
Gloucester that he imagined physicians of all other men the
most competent judges of all other affairs of religion—and
his reason was because they were wholly unconcerned with
it."

III

Professional work of any sort tends to narrow the mind,
to limit the point of view and to put a hall-mark on a man
of a most unmistakable kind.   On the one hand are the
intense, ardent natures, absorbed in their studies and

quickly losing interest in everything but their profession, while other faculties and interests "fust" unsued. On the other hand are the bovine brethren, who think of nothing but the treadmill and the corn. From very different causes, the one from concentration, the other from apathy, both are apt to neglect those outside studies that widen the sympathies and help a man to get the best there is out of life. Like art, medicine is an exacting mistress, and in the pursuit of one of the scientific branches, sometimes, too, in practice, not a portion of a man's spirit may be left free for other distractions, but this does not often happen. On account of the intimate personal nature of his work, the medical man, perhaps more than any other man, needs that higher education of which Plato speaks,—"that education in virtue from youth upwards, which enables a man eagerly to pursue the ideal perfection." It is not for all, nor can all attain to it, but there is comfort and help in the pursuit, even though the end is never reached. For a large majority the daily round and the common task furnish more than enough to satisfy their heart's desire, and there seems no room left for anything else. Like the good, easy man whom Milton scores in the *Areopagitica*, whose religion was a "traffic so entangled that of all mysteries he could not skill to keep a stock going upon that trade" and handed it over with all the locks and keys to "a divine of note and estimation," so it is with many of us in the matter of this higher education. No longer intrinsic, wrought in us and ingrained, it has become, in Milton's phrase, a "dividual movable," handed over nowadays to the daily press or to the haphazard instruction of the pulpit, the platform or the magazines. Like a good many other things, it comes in a better and more enduring form if not too consciously sought. The all-important thing is to get a relish for the good company of the race in a daily intercourse with some of the great minds of all ages.   Now, in the spring-time of life, pick your intimates among them, and begin a systematic cultivation of their works.   Many of you will need a strong leaven to raise you above the dough in which it will be your lot to labour.   Uncongenial surroundings, an ever-present dissonance between the aspirations within and the actualities without, the oppressive discords of human society, the bitter tragedies of life, the *lacrymae rerum*, beside the hidden springs of which we sit in sad despair—all these tend to foster in some natures a cynicism quite foreign to our vocation, and to which this inner education offers the best antidote.   Personal contact with men of high purpose and character will help a man to make a start—to have the desire, at least, but in its fulness this culture—for that word best expresses it—has to be wrought out by each one for himself.   Start at once a bed-side library and spend the last half hour of the day in communion with the saints of humanity.   There are great lessons to be learned from Job and from David, from Isaiah and St. Paul.   Taught by Shakespeare you may take your intellectual and moral measure with singular precision.   Learn to love Epictetus and Marcus Aurelius.   Should you be so fortunate as to be born a Platonist, Jowett will introduce you to the great master through whom alone we can think in certain levels, and whose perpetual modernness startles and delights. Montaigne will teach you moderation in all things, and to be "sealed of his tribe" is a special privilege.   We have in the profession only a few great literary heroes of the first rank, the friendship and counsel of two of whom you cannot too earnestly seek.   Sir Thomas Browne's *Religio Medici* should be your pocket companion, while from the Breakfast Table Series of Oliver Wendell Holmes you can glean a philosophy of life peculiarly suited to the needs of a physician.   There are at least a dozen or more works which would be helpful in getting wisdom in life which only comes to those who earnestly seek it.[1]

A conscientious pursuit of Plato's ideal perfection may teach you the three great lessons of life.   *You may learn to consume your own smoke.*   The atmosphere is darkened by the murmurings and whimperings of men and women over the non-essentials, the trifles that are inevitably incident to the hurly burly of the day's routine.   Things cannot always go your way.   Learn to accept in silence the minor aggravations, cultivate the gift of taciturnity and consume your own smoke with an extra draught of hard work, so that those about you may not be annoyed with the dust and soot of your complaints.   More than any other the practitioner of medicine may illustrate the second great lesson, *that we are here not to get all we can out of life for ourselves, but to try to make the lives of others happier.*   This is the essence of that oft-repeated admonition of Christ, "He that findeth his life shall lose it, and he that loseth his life for my sake shall find it," on which hard saying if the children of this generation would only lay hold, there would be less misery and discontent in the world.   It is not possible for anyone to have better opportunities to live this lesson than you will enjoy.   The practice of medicine is an art, not a trade; a calling, not a business; a calling in which your heart will be exercised equally with your head.   Often the best part of your work will have nothing to do with potions and powders, but with the exercise of an influence of the strong upon the weak, of the righteous upon the wicked, of the wise upon the foolish.   To you, as the trusted

[1] Note p. 452 "Bedside Library for Medical Students."

family counsellor, the father will come with his anxieties, the mother with her hidden grief, the daughter with her trials, and the son with his follies.   Fully one-third of the work you do will be entered in other books than yours. Courage and cheerfulness will not only carry you over the rough places of life, but will enable you to bring comfort and help to the weak-hearted and will console you in the sad hours when, like Uncle Toby, you have "to whistle that you may not weep."

And the third lesson you may learn is the hardest of all— that *the law of the higher life is only fulfilled by love, i.e. charity.*   Many a physician whose daily work is a daily round of beneficence will say hard things and think hard thoughts of a colleague.   No sin will so easily beset you as uncharitableness towards your brother practitioner.   So strong is the personal element in the practice of medicine, and so many are the wagging tongues in every parish, that evil-speaking, lying, and slandering find a shining mark in the lapses and mistakes which are inevitable in our work. There is no reason for discord and disagreement, and the only way to avoid trouble is to have two plain rules.   From the day you begin practice never under any circumstances listen to a tale told to the detriment of a brother practitioner.   And when any dispute or trouble does arise, go frankly, ere sunset, and talk the matter over, in which way you may gain a brother and a friend.   Very easy to carry out, you may think!   Far from it; there is no harder battle to fight.   Theoretically there seems to be no difficulty, but when the concrete wound is rankling, and after Mrs. Jones has rubbed in the cayenne pepper by declaring that Dr. J. told her in confidence of your shocking bungling, your attitude of mind is that you would rather see him in purgatory than make advances towards reconciliation.   Wait until the day of your trial comes and then remember my words.

And in closing, may I say a few words to the younger practitioners in the audience whose activities will wax not wane with the growing years of the century which opens so auspiciously for this school, for this city, and for our country. You enter a noble heritage, made so by no efforts of your own, but by the generations of men who have unselfishly sought to do the best they could for suffering mankind. Much has been done, much remains to do; a way has been opened, and to the possibilities in the scientific development of medicine there seems to be no limit. Except in its application, as general practitioners, you will not have much to do with this. Yours is a higher and more sacred duty. Think not to light a light to shine before men that they may see your good works; contrariwise, you belong to the great army of quiet workers, physicians and priests, sisters and nurses, all over the world, the members of which strive not neither do they cry, nor are their voices heard in the streets, but to them is given the ministry of consolation in sorrow, need, and sickness. Like the ideal wife of whom Plutarch speaks, the best doctor is often the one of whom the public hears the least; but nowadays, in the fierce light that beats upon the hearth, it is increasingly difficult to lead the secluded life in which our best work is done. To you the silent workers of the ranks, in villages and country districts, in the slums of our large cities, in the mining camps and factory towns, in the homes of the rich, and in the hovels of the poor, to you is given the harder task of illustrating with your lives the Hippocratic standards of Learning, of Sagacity, of Humanity, and of Probity. Of learning, that you may apply in your practice the best that is known in our art, and that with the increase in your knowledge there may be an increase in that priceless endowment of sagacity, so that to all, everywhere, skilled succour may come in the hour of need.   Of a humanity, that will show in your daily life tenderness and consideration to the weak, infinite pity to the suffering, and broad charity to all.   Of a probity, that will make you under all circumstances true to yourselves, true to your high calling, and true to your fellow man.

XIX
THE FIXED PERIOD

"'Tho' much is taken, much abides."
(*Ulysses.*)

TENNYSON

XIX

THE FIXED PERIOD[1]

A S this is the last public function at which I shall
appear as a member of the University, I very gladly
embrace the opportunity which it offers to express the
mingled feelings of gratitude and sorrow which are naturally
in my mind—gratitude to you all for sixteen years of
exceptionally happy life, sorrow that I am to belong to you
no more. Neither stricken deeply in years, nor damaged
seriously by illness, you may well wonder at the motives
that have induced me to give up a position of such influence
and importance, to part from colleagues so congenial, from
associates and students so devoted, and to leave a country
in which I have so many warm friends, and in which I have
been appreciated at so much more than my real worth.
It is best that you stay in the wonder-stage. Who can
understand another man's motives? Does he always
understand his own? This much I may say in explanation
—not in palliation. After years of hard work, at the very
time when a man's energies begin to flag, and when he feels
the need of more leisure, the conditions and surroundings
that have made him what he is and that have moulded his
character and abilities into something useful in the community—these very circumstances ensure an ever increasing
demand upon them; and when the call of the East comes,
which in one form or another is heard by all of us, and which
grows louder as we grow older, the call may come like the
summons to Elijah, and not alone the ploughing of the day,

[1] Johns Hopkins University, Feb. 22, 1905.

but the work of a life, friends, relatives, even father and mother, are left to take up new work in a new field. Or, happier far, if the call comes, as it did to Puran Das in Kipling's story, not to new labours, but to a life "private, unactive, calm, contemplative."

There are several problems in university life suggested by my departure. It may be asked in the first place, whether metabolism is sufficiently active in the professoriate body, is there change enough? May not the loss of a professor bring stimulating benefits to a university? We have not here lost very many—this is not a university that men care to leave—but in looking over its history I do not see that the departure of any one has proved a serious blow. It is strange of how slight value is the unit in a great system. A man may have built up a department and have gained a certain following, local or general; nay, more, he may have had a special value for his mental and moral qualities, and his fission may leave a scar, even an aching scar, but it is not for long. Those of us accustomed to the process know that the organism as a whole feels it about as much as a big polyzoon when a colony breaks off, or a hive of bees after a swarm—'tis not indeed always a calamity, oftentimes it is a relief. Of course upon a few the sense of personal loss falls heavily; in a majority of us the faculty of getting attached to those with whom we work is strongly developed, and some will realize the bitterness of the lines:—

> Alas! that all we loved of him should be
> But for our grief as if it had not been.

But to the professor himself these partings belong to the life he has chosen. Like the hero in one of Matthew Arnold's poems, he knows that his heart was not framed to

be 'long loved.'   Change is the very marrow of his existence—a new set of students every year, a new set of assistants, a new set of associates every few years to replace
those called off to other fields; in any active department
there is no constancy, no stability in the human surroundings.   And in this there is an element of sadness.   A man
comes into one's life for a few years, and you become
attached to him, interested in his work and in his welfare,
and perhaps you grow to love him, as a son, and then off
he goes !—leaving you with a bruised heart.

The question may be asked—whether as professors we do
not stay too long in one place.   It passes my persimmon to
tell how some good men—even lovable and righteous men
in other respects—have the hardihood to stay in the same
position for twenty-five years!   To a man of active mind
too long attachment to one college is apt to breed self-satisfaction, to narrow his outlook, to foster a local spirit, and
to promote senility.   Much of the phenomenal success of
this institution has been due to the concentration of a group
of light-horse intellectuals, without local ties, whose operations were not restricted, whose allegiance indeed was not
always national, yet who were willing to serve faithfully in
whatever field of action they were placed.   And this should
be the attitude of a vigilant professoriate.   As St. Paul
perferred an evangelist without attachments, as more free
for the work, so in the general interests of higher education
a University President should cherish a proper nomadic
spirit in the members of his faculties, even though it be on
occasions a seeming detriment.   A well-organized College
Trust could arrange a rotation of teachers which would be
most stimulating all along the line.   We are apt to grow
stale and thin mentally if kept too long in the same pasture.
Transferred to fresh fields, amid new surroundings and

other colleagues, a man gets a fillip which may last for several years. Interchange of teachers, national and international, will prove most helpful. How bracing the Turnbull lectures have been, for example. It would be an excellent work for the University Association which met here recently to arrange this interchange of instructors. Even to 'swap' College Presidents now and then might be good for the exchequer. We have an excellent illustration of the value of the plan in the transfer this year from Jena of Prof. Keutgen to give the lectures on History. An international university clearing-house might be organized to facilitate the work. How delightful it would be to have a return to the mediaeval practice when the professor roamed Europe at his sweet will, or to the halcyon era of the old Greek teachers—of which Empedocles sings:—

> What days were those Parmenides!
> When we were young, when we could number friends
> In all the Italian cities like ourselves;
> When with elated hearts we joined your train
> Ye Sun-born Virgins on the road of truth.

It is more particularly upon the younger men that I would urge the advantages of an early devotion to a peripatetic philosophy of life. Just so soon as you have your second teeth think of a change; get away from the nurse, cut the apron strings of your old teachers, seek new ties in a fresh environment, if possible where you can have a certain measure of freedom and independence. Only do not wait for a fully equipped billet almost as good as that of your master. A small one, poorly appointed, with many students and few opportunities for research, may be just what is needed to bring out the genius—latent and perhaps unrecognized—that will enable you in an unfavourable posi-

tion to do well what another could not do at all, even in the
most helpful surroundings. There are two appalling
diseases which only a feline restlessness of mind and body
may head off in young men in the academic career. There
is a remarkable bodily condition, known as infantilism, in
which adolescence does not come at the appointed time, or
is deferred until the twentieth year or later, and is then
incomplete, so that the childish mind and the childish form
and features remain. The mental counterpart is even more
common among us. Intellectual infantilism is a well recognized disease, and just as imperfect nutrition may cause
failure of the marvellous changes which accompany puberty
in the body, so the mind too long fed on the same diet in
one place may be rendered rickety or even infantile. Worse
than this may happen. A rare, but still more extraordinary,
bodily state is that of progeria, in which, as though touched
with the wand of some malign fairy, the child does not
remain infantile, but skips adolescence, maturity and manhood, and passes at once to senility, looking at eleven or
twelve years like a miniature Tithonus "marred and wasted,"
wrinkled and stunted, a little old man among his toys. It
takes great care on the part of any one to live the mental
life corresponding to the phases through which his body
passes. How few minds reach puberty, how few come to
adolescence, how fewer attain maturity! It is really tragic
—this wide-spread prevalence of mental infantilism due to
careless habits of intellectual feeding. Progeria is an awful
malady in a college. Few Faculties escape without an
instance or two, and there are certain diets which cause it
just as surely as there are waters in some of the Swiss valleys
that produce cretinism. I have known an entire faculty
attacked. The progeric himself is a nice enough fellow to
look at and to play with, but he is sterile, with the mental

horizon narrowed, and quite incapable of assimilating the new thoughts of his day and generation.

As in the case of many other diseases, it is more readily prevented than cured, and, taken early, change of air and diet may do much to antagonize a tendency, inherited or acquired. Early stages may be relieved by a prolonged stay at the University Baths of Berlin or Leipzic, or if at the proper time a young man is transferred from an American or Anglican to a Gallic or Teutonic diet. Through no fault of the men, but of the system, due to the unfortunate idea on the part of the denominations that in each one of the States they should have their own educational institutions, collegiate infantilism is far too prevalent, against which the freer air and better diet of the fully equipped State Universities is proving a rapid, as it is the rational, antidote.

Nor would I limit this desire for change to the teachers. The student of the technical school should begin his *wander-jahre* early, not postponing them until he has taken his M.D. or Ph.D. A residence of four years in the one school is apt to breed prejudice and to promote mental astigmatism which the after years may never be able to correct. One great difficulty is the lack of harmony in the curricula of the schools, but this time will correct and, once initiated and encouraged, the better students will take a year, or even two years, in schools other than those at which they intend to graduate.

I am going to be very bold and touch upon another question of some delicacy, but of infinite importance in university life: one that has not been settled in this country. I refer to a fixed period for the teacher, either of time of service or of age. Except in some proprietary schools, I do not know of any institutions in which there is a time limit of, say, twenty years' service, as in some of the London hospitals, or in which a man is engaged for a term of years. Usually the appointment is *ad vitam aut culpam*, as the old phrase reads. It is a very serious matter in our young universities to have all of the professors growing old at the same time. In some places, only an epidemic, a time limit, or an age limit can save the situation. I have two fixed ideas well known to my friends, harmless obsessions with which I sometimes bore them, but which have a direct bearing on this important problem. The first is the comparative uselessness of men above forty years of age. This may seem shocking, and yet read aright the world's history bears out the statement. Take the sum of human achievement in action, in science, in art, in literature—subtract the work of the men above forty, and while we should miss great treasures, even priceless treasures, we would practically be where we are to-day. It is difficult to name a great and far-reaching conquest of the mind which has not been given to the world by a man on whose back the sun was still shining. The effective, moving, vitalizing work of the world is done between the ages of twenty-five and forty—these fifteen golden years of plenty, the anabolic or constructive period, in which there is always a balance in the mental bank and the credit is still good. In the science and art of medicine young or comparatively young men have made every advance of the first rank. Vesalius, Harvey, Hunter, Bichat, Laennec, Virchow, Lister, Koch—the green years were yet upon their heads when their epoch-making studies were made. To modify an old saying, a man is sane morally at thirty, rich mentally at forty, wise spiritually at fifty—or never. The young men should be encouraged and afforded every possible chance to show what is in them. If there is one thing more than another upon which the professors of this university are to be congratulated it is this very sympathy and fellowship with their junior associates, upon whom really in many departments, in mine certainly, has fallen the brunt of the work. And herein lies the chief value of the teacher who has passed his climacteric and is no longer a productive factor, he can play the man midwife as Socrates did to Theaetetus, and determine whether the thoughts which the young men are bringing to the light are false idols or true and noble births.

My second fixed idea is the uselessness of men above sixty years of age, and the incalculable benefit it would be in commercial, political and in professional life if, as a matter of course, men stopped work at this age. In his *Biathanatos* Donne tells us that by the laws of certain wise states sexagenarii were precipitated from a bridge, and in Rome men of that age were not admitted to the suffrage and they were called *Depontani* because the way to the senate was *per pontem*, and they from age were not permitted to come thither. In that charming novel, *The Fixed Period*, Anthony Trollope discusses the practical advantages in modern life of a return to this ancient usage, and the plot hinges upon the admirable scheme of a college into which at sixty men retired for a year of contemplation before a peaceful departure by chloroform. That incalculable benefits might follow such a scheme is apparent to any one who, like myself, is nearing the limit, and who has made a careful study of the calamities which may befall men during the seventh and eighth decades. Still more when he contemplates the many evils which they perpetuate unconsciously, and with impunity. As it can be maintained that all the great advances have come from men under forty, so the history of the world shows that a very large proportion of the evils may be traced to the sexagenarians—nearly all the great mistakes politically and socially, all of the worst poems, most of the bad pictures, a majority of the bad novels, not a few of the bad sermons and speeches. It is not to be denied that occasionally there is a sexagenarian whose mind, as Cicero remarks, stands out of reach of the body's decay. Such a one has learned the secret of Hermippus, that ancient Roman who feeling that the silver cord was loosening cut himself clear from all companions of his own age and betook himself to the company of young men, mingling with their games and studies, and so lived to the age of 153, *puerorum halitu refocillatus et educatus.* And there is truth in the story, since it is only those who live with the young who maintain a fresh outlook on the new problems of the world. The teacher's life should have three periods, study until twenty-five, investigation until forty, profession until sixty, at which age I would have him retired on a double allowance. Whether Anthony Trollope's suggestion of a college and chloroform should be carried out or not I have become a little dubious, as my own time is getting so short. (I may say for the benefit of the public that with a woman I would advise an entirely different plan, since, after sixty her influence on her sex may be most helpful, particularly if aided by those charming accessories, a cap and a fichu.)

II

Such an occasion as the present affords an opportunity to say a few words on the work which the Johns Hopkins foundations have done and may do for medicine. The hospital was organized at a most favourable period, when the profession had at last awakened to its responsibilities, the leading universities had begun to take medical education seriously, and to the public at large had come a glimmering sense of the importance of the scientific investigation of disease and of the advantages of well trained doctors in a community. It would have been an easy matter to have made colossal mistakes with these great organizations. There are instances in which larger bequests have been sterile from the start; but in the history of educational institutions it is hard to name one more prolific than the Johns Hopkins University. Not simply a seed farm, it has been a veritable nursery from which the whole country has been furnished with cuttings, grafts, slips, seedlings, etc. It would be superfluous in this audience to refer to the great work which the Trustees and Mr. Gilman did in twenty-five years—their praise is in all the colleges. But I must pay a tribute to the wise men who planned the hospital, who refused to establish an institution on the old lines—a great city charity for the sick poor, but gave it vital organic connexion with a University. I do not know who was directly reponsible for the provision in Mr. Hopkins' will that the hospital should form part of the Medical School, and that it should be an institution for the study as well as for the cure of disease. Perhaps the founder himself may be credited with the idea, but I have always felt that Francis T. King was largely responsible, as he had strong and sensible convictions on the subject, and devoted the last years of his useful life putting them into execution. As first President of the Hospital Board he naturally did much to shape the policy of the institution, and it is a pleasure to recall the zeal and sympathy with which he was always ready to co-operate. It is sad that in so few years all of the members of the original Board have passed away, the last, Mr. Corner—faithful and interested to the end— only a few weeks ago. They did a great work for this city, and their names should be held in everlasting remembrance. Judge Dobbin and James Carey Thomas, in particular, the members of the staff in the early days remember with gratitude for their untiring devotion to the medical school side of the problems which confronted us.   To John S. Billings, so long the skilled adviser of the Board, we all turned for advice and counsel, and his influence was deeper and stronger than was always apparent.   For the admirable plan of preliminary medical study, and for the shaping of the scientific work before the hospital was opened for patients, we are indebted to Newell Martin, Ira Remsen and W. H. Welch.   The present excellent plan of study leading to medicine, in which the classics, science and literature are fully represented, is the outcome of their labours.

About this time sixteen years ago Mr. King, Dr. Billings, Dr. Welch and myself had many conferences with reference to the opening of the hospital.   I had been appointed January 1st, but had not yet left Philadelphia.   As so often happens the last steps in a great organization are the most troublesome, and after some delay the whole matter was intrusted to Mr. Gilman, who became acting director, and in a few months everything was ready, and on May 7 the hospital was opened.   I look back with peculiar pleasure to my association with Mr. Gilman.   It was both an education and a revelation.   I had never before been brought into close contact with a man who loved difficulties just for the pleasure of making them disappear.   But I am not going to speak of those happy days lest it should forestall the story I have written of the inner history of the first period of the hospital.

At the date of the organization of the hospital the two great problems before the profession of this country were, how to give to students a proper education, in other words how to give them the culture, the science and the art commensurate with the dignity of a learned profession; and,

secondly, how to make this great and rich country a contributor to the science of medicine.

The conditions under which the medical school opened in
1893 were unique in the history of American medicine. It
would have been an easy matter, following the lead of the
better schools, to have an entrance examination which
guaranteed that a man had an ordinary education, but
Miss Garett's splendid gift enabled us to say, no! we do not
want a large number of half-educated students; we prefer a
select group trained in the sciences preliminary to medicine,
and in the languages which will be most useful for a modern
physician. It was an experiment, and we did not expect
more than twenty five or thirty students each year for eight
or ten years at least. As is so often the case, the country
was better prepared than we thought to meet our conditions,
and the number of admissions to the school has risen until
we have about reached our capacity. Our example in
demanding the preliminary arts or science course for admission to the school has been followed by Harvard, and is to be
adopted at Columbia. It is not a necessary measure in all
the schools, but there has been everywhere a very salutary
increase in the stringency of the entrance examinations.
Before we took up the work great reforms in the scientific
teaching in medicine had already begun in this country.
Everywhere laboratory work had replaced to some extent
the lecture, and practical courses in physiology, pathology
and pharmacology had been organized. We must not forget
however that to Newell Martin, the first professor of physiology in this university, is due the introduction of practical
classes in biology and physiology. The rapid growth of the
school necessitated the erection of a separate building for
physiology, pharmacology and physiological chemistry,
and in these departments and in anatomy the equipment is

as complete as is required. Of the needs in pathology, hygiene and experimental pathology this is not the occasion to speak. It is sufficient to say that for instruction in the sciences, upon which the practice of the art is based, the school is in first class condition.

Indeed the rapidity with which the scientific instruction in our medical schools has been brought to a high level is one of the most remarkable educational features of the past twenty years. Even in small unendowed colleges admirable courses are given in bacteriology and pathology, and sometimes in the more difficult subject of practical physiology. But the demand and the necessity for these special courses has taxed to the utmost the resources of the private schools. The expense of the new method of teaching is so great that the entire class fees are absorbed by the laboratories. The consequence is that the old proprietary colleges are no longer profitable ventures, certainly not in the north, and fortunately they are being forced into closer affiliation with the universities, as it is not an easy matter to get proper endowments for private corporations.

The great difficulty is in the third part of the education of the student: viz., his art. In the old days when a lad was apprenticed to a general practitioner, he had good opportunities to pick up the essentials of a rough and ready art, and the system produced many self-reliant, resourceful men. Then with the multiplication of the medical schools and increasing rivalry between them came the two year course, which for half a century lay like a blight on the medical profession, retarding its progress, filling its ranks with half-educated men, and pandering directly to all sorts of quackery, humbuggery and fraud among the public. The awakening came about thirty years ago, and now there is scarcely a school in the country which has not a four years course, and all are trying to get clear of the old shackles and teach rational medicine in a rational way. But there are extraordinary difficulties in teaching the medical student his Art. It is not hard, for example, to teach him all about the disease pneumonia, how it prevails in the winter and spring, how fatal it always has been, all about the germ. all about the change which the disease causes in the lungs and in the heart—he may become learned, deeply learned, on the subject—but put him beside a case, and he may not know which lung is involved, and he does not know how to find out, and if he did find out, he might be in doubt whether to put an ice-bag or a poultice on the affected side, whether to bleed or to give opium, whether to give a dose of medicine every hour or none at all, and he may not have the faintest notion whether the signs look ominous or favourable. So also with other aspects of the art of the general practitioner. A student may know all about the bones of the wrist, in fact he may carry a set in his pocket and know every facet and knob and nodule on them, he may have dissected a score of arms, and yet when he is called to see Mrs. Jones who has fallen on the ice and broken her wrist, he may not know a Colles' from a Pott's fracture, and as for setting it *secundum artem*, he may not have the faintest notion, never having seen a case. Or he may be called to preside at one of those awful domestic tragedies—the sudden emergency, some terrible accident of birth or of childhood, that requires skill, technical skill, courage—the courage of full knowledge, and if he has not been in the obstetrical wards, if he has not been trained practically, if he has not had the opportunities that are the rights of every medical student, he may fail at the critical moment, a life, two lives, may be lost, sacrificed to ignorance, often to helpless, involuntary ignorance. By far the greatest work of the Johns Hopkins Hospital has been the demonstration to the profession of the United States and to the public of this country of how medical students should be instructed in their art.   I place it first because it was the most needed lesson, I place it first because it has done the most good as a stimulating example, and I place it first because never before in the history of this country have medical students lived and worked in a hospital as part of its machinery, as an essential part of the work of the wards.   In saying this, Heaven forbid that I should obliquely disparage the good and faithful work of my colleagues elsewhere.   But the amphitheatre clinic, the ward and dispensary classes, are but bastard substitutes for a system which makes the medical student himself help in the work of the hospital as part of its human machinery. He does not see the pneumonia case in the amphitheatre from the benches, but he follows it day by day, hour by hour; he has his time so arranged that he can follow it; he sees and studies similar cases and the disease itself becomes his chief teacher, and he knows its phases and variations as depicted in the living; he learns under skilled direction when to act and when to refrain, he learns insensibly principles of practice and he possibly escapes a "nickel-in-the-slot" attitude of mind which has been the curse of the physician in the treatment of disease.   And the same with the other branches of his art; he gets a first hand knowledge which, if he has any sense, may make him wise unto the salvation of his fellows.   And all this has come about through the wise provision that the hospital was to be part of the medical school, and it has become for the senior students, as it should be, their college.   Moreover they are not in it upon sufferance and admitted through side-doors, but they are welcomed as important aids without which the work could not be done efficiently.   The whole question of the practical education of the medical student is one in which the public is vitally interested. Sane, intelligent physicians and surgeons with culture, science, and art, are worth much in a community, and they are worth paying for in rich endowments of our medical schools and hospitals. Personally, there is nothing in life in which I take greater pride than in my connexion with the organization of the medical clinic of the Johns Hopkins Hospital and with the introduction of the old-fashioned methods of practical instruction. I desire no other epitaph—no hurry about it, I may say—than the statement that I taught medical students in the wards, as I regard this as by far the most useful and important work I have been called upon to do.

The second great problem is a much more difficult one, surrounded as it is with obstacles inextricably connected with the growth and expansion of a comparatively new country. For years the United States had been the largest borrower in the scientific market of the world, and more particularly in the sciences relating to medicine. To get the best that the world offered, our young men had to go abroad; only here and there was a laboratory of physiology or pathology, and then equipped as a rule for teaching. The change in twenty years has been remarkable. There is scarcely to-day a department of scientific medicine which is not represented in our larger cities by men who are working as investigators, and American scientific medicine is taking its rightful place in the world's work. Nothing shows this more plainly than the establishment within a few years of journals devoted to scientific subjects; and the active participation of this school as a leader is well illustrated by the important publications which have been started by its members. The Hospital Trustees early appreciated the value of these scientific publications, and the Bulletin and the Reports have done much to spread the reputation of the Hospital as a medical centre throughout the world. But let us understand clearly that only a beginning has been made.   For one worker in pathology—a man, I mean, who is devoting his life to the study of the causes of diseases— there are twenty-five at least in Germany, and for one in this country there are a dozen laboratories of the first class in any one of the more important sciences cognate to medicine. It is not alone that the money is lacking; the men are not always at hand.   When the right man is available he quickly puts American science into the forefront.   Let me give you an illustration.   Anatomy is a fundamental branch in medicine.   There is no school, even amid sylvan glades, without its dissecting room; but it has been a great difficulty to get the higher anatomy represented in American univer- sities.   Plenty of men have always been available to teach the subject to medical students, but when it came to ques- tions of morphology and embryology and the really scientific study of the innumerable problems connected with them, it was only here and there and not in a thorough manner that the subjects were approached.   And the young men had to go abroad to see a completely equipped, modern working anatomical institute.   There is to-day connected with this university a school of anatomy of which any land might be proud, and the work of Dr. Mall demonstrates what can be done when the man fits his environment.

It is a hopeful sign to see special schools established for the study of disease such as the Rockefeller Institute in New York, the McCormick Institute in Chicago and the Phipps Institute in Philadelphia.   They will give a great impetus in the higher lines of work in which the country has hereto- fore been so weak.   But it makes one green with envy to see how much our German brethren are able to do.   Take, for example, the saddest chapter in the history of disease—

insanity, the greatest curse of civilized life. Much has been done in the United States for the care of the insane, much in places for the study of the disease, and I may say that the good work which has been inaugurated in this line at the Sheppard Hospital is attracting attention everywhere; but what a bagatelle it seems in comparison with the modern development of the subject in Germany, with its great psychopathic clinics connected with each university, where early and doubtful cases are skilfully studied and skilfully treated. The new department for insanity connected with the University of Munich has cost nearly half a million of dollars! Of the four new departments for which one side of the hospital grounds lies vacant, and which will be built within the next twenty-five years, one should be a model psychopathic clinic to which the acute and curable cases may be sent. The second, a clinic for the diseases of children. Much has been done with our out-patient department under Dr. Booker, who has helped to clarify one of the dark problems in infant mortality, but we need a building with fine wards and laboratories in which may be done work of a character as notable and worldwide as that done in Dr. Kelly's division for the diseases of women.[1] The third great department for which a separate building must be provided is that of Syphilis and Dermatology. Already no small share of the reputation of this hospital has come from the good work in these specialities by the late Dr. Brown, by Dr. Gilchrist, and by Dr. Hugh Young; and lastly, for diseases of the eye, ear, and throat, a large separate clinic is needed, which will give to these all-important subjects the equipment they deserve.

[1] It is most gratifying to know that the Harriet Lane Johnston Hospital for children will be associated with the Johns Hopkins Hospital, and will meet the requirements of which I have spoken.

For how much to be thankful have we who have shared in the initiation of the work of these two great institutions. We have been blessed with two remarkable Presidents, whose active sympathies have been a stimulus in every department, and whose good sense has minimized the loss of energy through friction between the various parts of the machine—a loss from which colleges are very prone to suffer. A noteworthy feature is that in so motley a collection from all parts of the country the men should have fitted into each other's lives so smoothly and peacefully, so that the good fellowship and harmony in the faculties has been delightful. And we have been singularly blessed in our relationship with the citizens, who have not only learned to appreciate the enormous benefits which these great trusts confer upon the city and the state, but they have come forward in a noble way to make possible a new era in the life of the university. And we of the medical faculty have to feel very grateful to the profession, to whose influence and support much of the success of the hospital and the medical school is due; and not only to the physicians of the city and of the state, who have dealt so truly with us, but to the profession of the entire country, and more particularly to that of the Southern States, whose confidence we have enjoyed in such a practical way. Upon a maintenance of this confidence the future rests. The character of the work of the past sixteen years is the best guarantee of its permanence.

What has been accomplished is only an earnest of what shall be done in the future. Upon our heels a fresh perfection must tread, born of us, fated to excel us. We have but served and have but seen a beginning. Personally I feel deeply grateful to have been permitted to join in this noble work and to have been united in it with men of such high and human ideals.

XX
THE STUDENT LIFE

"Take therefore no thought for the morrow: for the morrow shall take thought for the things of itself."

SERMON ON THE MOUNT.

XX

THE STUDENT LIFE[1]

I

EXCEPT it be a lover, no one is more interesting as an object of study than a student. Shakespeare might have made him a fourth in his immortal group. The lunatic with his fixed idea, the poet with his fine frenzy, the lover with his frantic idolatry, and the student aflame with the desire for knowledge are of "imagination all compact." To an absorbing passion, a whole-souled devotion, must be joined an enduring energy, if the student is to become a devotee of the grey-eyed goddess to whose law his services are bound. Like the quest of the Holy Grail, the quest of Minerva is not for all. For the one, the pure life; for the other, what Milton calls "a strong propensity of nature." Here again the student often resembles the poet—he is born, not made. While the resultant of two moulding forces, the accidental, external conditions, and the hidden germinal energies, which produce in each one of us national, family, and individual traits, the true student possesses in some measure a divine spark which sets at naught their laws. Like the Snark, he defies definition, but there are three unmistakable signs by which you may recognize the genuine article from a Boojum—an absorbing desire to know the truth, an unswerving steadfastness in its pursuit, and an open, honest heart, free from suspicion, guile, and jealousy.

At the outset do not be worried about this big question —Truth. It is a very simple matter if each one of you

[1] A farewell address to American and Canadian medical students 1905.

starts with the desire to get as much as possible. No
human being is constituted to know the truth, the whole
truth, and nothing but the truth; and even the best of men
must be content with fragments, with partial glimpses,
never the full fruition. In this unsatisfied quest the
attitude of mind, the desire, the thirst—a thirst that from
the soul must rise!—the fervent longing, are the be-all
and the end-all. What is the student but a lover courting
a fickle mistress who ever eludes his grasp? In this very
elusiveness is brought out his second great characteristic
—steadfastness of purpose. Unless from the start the
limitations incident to our frail human faculties are frankly
accepted, nothing but disappointment awaits you. The
truth is the best you can get with your best endeavour,
the best that the best men accept—with this you must
learn to be satisfied, retaining at the same time with due
humility an earnest desire for an ever larger portion. Only
by keeping the mind plastic and receptive does the student
escape perdition. It is not, as Charles Lamb remarks,
that some people do not know what to do with truth when
it is offered to them, but the tragic fate is to reach, after
years of patient search, a condition of mind-blindness in
which the truth is not recognized, though it stares you in
the face. This can never happen to a man who has followed
step by step the growth of a truth, and who knows the painful phases of its evolution. It is one of the great tragedies
of life that every truth has to struggle to acceptance against
honest but mind-blind students. Harvey knew his contemporaries well, and for twelve successive years demonstrated the circulation of the blood before daring to publish
the facts on which the truth was based.[1]   Only steadfast-

[1] "These views, as usual, pleased some more, others less; some chid
and calumniated me, and laid it to me as a crime that I had dared to

ness of purpose and humility enable the student to shift his
position to meet the new conditions in which new truths are
born, or old ones modified beyond recognition. And,
thirdly, the honest heart will keep him in touch with his
fellow students, and furnish that sense of comradeship without which he travels an arid waste alone.   I say advisedly
an honest *heart*—the honest head is prone to be cold and
stern, given to judgment, not mercy, and not always able
to entertain that true charity which, while it thinketh no
evil, is anxious to put the best possible interpretation upon
the motives of a fellow worker.   It will foster, too, an
attitude of generous, friendly rivalry untinged by the green
peril, jealousy, that is the best preventive of the growth
of a bastard scientific spirit, loving seclusion and working
in a lock-and-key laboratory, as timorous of light as is a
thief.

You have all become brothers in a great society, not
apprentices, since that implies a master, and nothing should
be further from the attitude of the teacher than much that
is meant in that word, used though it be in another sense,
particularly by our French brethren in a most delightful
way, signifying a bond of intellectual filiation.   A fraternal
attitude is not easy to cultivate—the chasm between the
chair and the bench is difficult to bridge.   Two things have
helped to put up a cantilever across the gulf.   The successful
teacher is no longer on a height, pumping knowledge at
high pressure into passive receptacles.   The new methods
have changed all this.   He is no longer *Sir Oracle*, perhaps
unconsciously by his very manner antagonizing minds to
whose level he cannot possibly descend, but he is a senior

---

depart from the precepts and opinions of all Anatomists.'—*De Motu
Cordis*, chap. i.

student anxious to help his juniors.   When a simple, earnest spirit animates a college, there is no appreciable interval between the teacher and the taught—both are in the same class, the one a little more advanced than the other.   So animated, the student feels that he has joined a family whose honour is his honour, whose welfare is his own, and whose interests should be his first consideration.

The hardest conviction to get into the mind of a beginner is that the education upon which he is engaged is not a college course, not a medical course, but a life course, for which the work of a few years under teachers is but a preparation.   Whether you will falter and fail in the race or whether you will be faithful to the end depends on the training before the start, and on your staying powers, points upon which I need not enlarge.   You can all become good students, a few may become great students, and now and again one of you will be found who does easily and well what others cannot do at all, or very badly, which is John Ferriar's excellent definition of a genius.

In the hurry and bustle of a business world, which is the life of this continent, it is not easy to train first-class students.   Under present conditions it is hard to get the needful seclusion, on which account it is that our educational market is so full of wayside fruit.   I have always been much impressed by the advice of St. Chrysostom: "Depart from the highway and transplant thyself in some enclosed ground, for it is hard for a tree which stands by the wayside to keep her fruit till it be ripe."   The dilettante is abroad in the land, the man who is always venturing on tasks for which he is imperfectly equipped, a habit of mind fostered by the multiplicity of subjects of the curriculum; and while many things are studied, few are studied thoroughly.   Men will not take time to get to the heart of a matter.   After all, concentration is the price the modern student pays for success. Thoroughness is the most difficult habit to acquire, but it is the pearl of great price, worth all the worry and trouble of the search. The dilettante lives an easy, butterfly life, knowing nothing of the toil and labour with which the treasures of knowledge are dug out of the past, or wrung by patient research in the laboratories. Take, for example, the early history of this country—how easy for the student of the one type to get a smattering, even a fairly full acquaintance with the events of the French and Spanish settlements. Put an original document before him, and it might as well be Arabic. What we need is the other type, the man who knows the records, who, with a broad outlook and drilled in what may be called the embryology of history, has yet a powerful vision for the minutiae of life. It is these kitchen and backstair men who are to be encouraged, the men who know the subject in hand in all possible relationships. Concentration has its drawbacks. It is possible to become so absorbed in the problem of the "enclitic δε," or the structure of the flagella of the Trichomonas, or of the toes of the prehistoric horse, that the student loses the sense of proportion in his work, and even wastes a lifetime in researches which are valueless because not in touch with current knowledge. You remember poor Casaubon, in *Middlemarch*, whose painful scholarship was lost on this account. The best preventive to this is to get denationalized early. The true student is a citizen of the world, the allegiance of whose soul, at any rate, is too precious to be restricted to a single country. The great minds, the great works transcend all limitations of time, of language, and of race, and the scholar can never feel initiated into the company of the elect until he can approach all of life's problems from the cosmopolitan standpoint. I care not in what sub·

ject he may work, the full knowledge cannot be reached without drawing on supplies from lands other than his own —French, English, German, American, Japanese, Russian, Italian—there must be no discrimination by the loyal student, who should willingly draw from any and every source with an open mind and a stern resolve to render unto all their dues.   I care not on what stream of knowledge he may embark, follow up its course, and the rivulets that feed it flow from many lands.   If the work is to be effective he must keep in touch with scholars in other countries.   How often has it happened that years of precious time have been given to a problem already solved or shown to be insoluble, because of the ignorance of what had been done elsewhere. And it is not only book knowledge and journal knowledge, but a knowledge of men that is needed.   The student will, if possible, see the men in other lands.   Travel not only widens the vision and gives certainties in place of vague surmises, but the personal contact with foreign workers enables him to appreciate better the failings or successes in his own line of work, perhaps to look with more charitable eyes on the work of some brother whose limitations and opportunities have been more restricted than his own.   Or, in contact with a mastermind, he may take fire, and the glow of the enthusiasm may be the inspiration of his life. Concentration must then be associated with large views on the relation of the problem, and a knowledge of its status elsewhere; otherwise it may land him in the slough of a specialism so narrow that it has depth and no breadth, or he may be led to make what he believes to be important discoveries, but which have long been current coin in other lands.   It is sad to think that the day of the great polymathic student is at an end; that we may, perhaps, never again see a Scaliger, a Haller, or a Humboldt—men who

took the whole field of knowledge for their domain and
viewed it as from a pinnacle. And yet a great specializing
generalist may arise, who can tell? Some twentieth-cen-
tury Aristotle may be now tugging at his bottle, as little
dreaming as are his parents or his friends of a conquest of
the mind, beside which the wonderful victories of the
Stagirite will look pale. The value of a really great student
to the country is equal to half a dozen grain elevators or a
new transcontinental railway. He is a commodity singularly fickle and variable, and not to be grown to order. So
far as his advent is concerned there is no telling when or
where he may arise. The conditions seem to be present
even under the most unlikely externals. Some of the
greatest students this country has produced have come from
small villages and country places. It is impossible to predict from a study of the environment, which a "strong propensity of nature," to quote Milton's phrase again, will
easily bend or break.

The student must be allowed full freedom in his work,
undisturbed by the utilitarian spirit of the Philistine, who
cries, *Cui bono?* and distrusts pure science. The present
remarkable position in applied science and in industrial
trades of all sorts has been made possible by men who did
pioneer work in chemistry, in physics, in biology, and in
physiology, without a thought in their researches of any
practical application. The members of this higher group
of productive students are rarely understood by the common
spirits, who appreciate as little their unselfish devotion as
their unworldly neglect of the practical side of the problems.

Everywhere now the medical student is welcomed as
an honoured member of the guild. There was a time, I
confess, and it is within the memory of some of us, when,
like Falstaff, he was given to "taverns and sack and wine

and metheglins, and to drinkings and swearings and star-
ings, pribbles and prabbles"; but all that has changed
with the curriculum, and the "Meds" now roar you as
gently as the "Theologs." On account of the peculiar
character of the subject-matter of your studies, what
I have said upon the general life and mental attitude of the
student applies with tenfold force to you. Man, with all
his mental and bodily anomalies and diseases—the machine
in order, the machine in disorder, and the business yours
to put it to rights. Through all the phases of its career
this most complicated mechanism of this wonderful world
will be the subject of our study and of your care—the
naked, new-born infant, the artless child, the lad and the
lassie just aware of the tree of knowledge overhead, the
strong man in the pride of life, the woman with the benediction of maternity on her brow, and the aged, peaceful
in the contemplation of the past. Almost everything has
been renewed in the science and in the art of medicine, but
all through the long centuries there has been no variableness
or shadow of change in the essential features of the life
which is our contemplation and our care. The sick love-
child of Israel's sweet singer, the plague-striken hopes of
the great Athenian statesman, Elpenor bereft of his
beloved Artemidora, and "Tully's daughter mourned so
tenderly," are not of any age or any race—they are here
with us to-day, with the Hamlets, the Ophelias, and the
Lears. Amid an eternal heritage of sorrow and suffering
our work is laid, and this eternal note of sadness would be
insupportable if the daily tragedies were not relieved by
the spectacle of the heroism and devotion displayed by the
actors. Nothing will sustain you more potently than the
power to recognize in your humdrum routine, as perhaps
it may be thought, the true poetry of life—the poetry of

the commonplace, of the ordinary man, of the plain, toil-
worn woman, with their loves and their joys, their sorrows
and their griefs. The comedy, too, of life will be spread
before you, and nobody laughs more often than the doctor at
the pranks Puck plays upon the Titanias and the Bottoms
among his patients. The humorous side is really almost
as frequently turned towards him as the tragic. Lift up
one hand to heaven and thank your stars if they have
given you the proper sense to enable you to appreciate the
inconceivably droll situations in which we catch our fellow
creatures. Unhappily, this is one of the free gifts of the
gods, unevenly distributed, not bestowed on all, or on all in
equal portions. In undue measure it is not without risk,
and in any case in the doctor it is better appreciated by
the eye than expressed on the tongue. Hilarity and good
humour, a breezy cheerfulness, a nature "sloping toward
the southern side," as Lowell has it, help enormously both
in the study and in the practice of medicine. To many of
a sombre and sour disposition it is hard to maintain good
spirits amid the trials and tribulations of the day, and yet
it is an unpardonable mistake to go about among patients
with a long face.

Divide your attentions equally between books and men.
The strength of the student of books is to sit still—two or
three hours at a stretch—eating the heart out of a subject
with pencil and notebook in hand, determined to master
the details and intricacies, focussing all your energies on its
difficulties. Get accustomed to test all sorts of book
problems and statements for yourself, and take as little as
possible on trust. The Hunterian "Do not think, but try"
attitude of mind is the important one to cultivate. The
question came up one day, when discussing the grooves
left on the nails after fever, how long it took for the nail to

grow out, from root to edge. A majority of the class had
no further interest; a few looked it up in books; two men
marked their nails at the root with nitrate of silver, and a
few months later had positive knowledge on the subject.
They showed the proper spirit. The little points that come
up in your reading try to test for yourselves. With one
fundamental difficulty many of you will have to contend
from the outset—a lack of proper preparation for really
hard study. No one can have watched successive groups
of young men pass through the special schools without
profoundly regretting the haphazard, fragmentary character
of their preliminary education. It does seem too bad that
we cannot have a student in his eighteenth year sufficiently
grounded in the humanities and in the sciences preliminary
to medicine—but this is an educational problem upon which
only a Milton or a Locke could discourse with profit. With
pertinacity you can overcome the preliminary defects and
once thoroughly interested, the work in books becomes a
pastime. A serious drawback in the student life is the
selfconsciousness, bred of too close devotion to books. A
man gets shy, "dysopic," as old Timothy Bright calls it,
and shuns the looks of men, and blushes like a girl.

The strength of a student of men is to travel—to study
men, their habits, character, mode of life, their behaviour
under varied conditions, their vices, virtues, and peculiarities. Begin with a careful observation of your fellow
students and of your teachers; then, every patient you see is
a lesson in much more than the malady from which he
suffers. Mix as much as you possibly can with the outside
world, and learn its ways. Cultivated systematically, the
student societies, the students' union, the gymnasium, and
the outside social circle will enable you to conquer the
diffidence so apt to go with bookishness and which may

prove a very serious drawback in after-life. I cannot too strongly impress upon the earnest and attentive men among you the necessity of overcoming this unfortunate failing in your student days. It is not easy for every one to reach a happy medium, and the distinction between a proper self-confidence and "cheek," particularly in junior students, is not always to be made. The latter is met with chiefly among the student pilgrims who, in travelling down the Delectable Mountains, have gone astray and have passed to the left hand, where lieth the country of Conceit, the country in which you remember the brisk lad Ignorance met Christian.

I wish we could encourage on this continent among our best students the habit of wandering. I do not know that we are quite prepared for it, as there is still great diversity in the curricula, even among the leading schools, but it is undoubtedly a great advantage to study under different teachers, as the mental horizon is widened and the sympathies enlarged. The practice would do much to lessen that narrow "I am of Paul and I am of Apollos" spirit which is hostile to the best interests of the profession.

There is much that I would like to say on the question of work, but I can spare only a few moments for a word or two. Who will venture to settle upon so simple a matter as the best time for work? One will tell us there is no best time; all are equally good; and truly, all times are the same to a man whose soul is absorbed in some great problem. The other day I asked Edward Martin, the well-known story-writer, what time he found best for work. "Not in the evening, and never between meals!" was his answer, which may appeal to some of my hearers. One works best at night; another, in the morning; a majority of the students of the past favour the latter. Erasmus, the great exemplar, says, "Never work at night; it dulls the brain and hurts the health." One day, going with George Ross through Bedlam, Dr. Savage, at that time the physician in charge, remarked upon two great groups of patients—those who were depressed in the morning and those who were cheerful, and he suggested that the spirits rose and fell with the bodily temperature—those with very low morning temperatures were depressed, and vice versâ. This, I believe, expresses a truth which may explain the extraordinary difference in the habits of students in this matter of the time at which the best work can be done. Outside of the asylum there are also the two great types, the student-lark who loves to see the sun rise, who comes to breakfast with a cheerful morning face, never so "fit" as at 6 a.m. We all know the type. What a contrast to the student-owl with his saturnine morning face, thoroughly unhappy, cheated by the wretched breakfast bell of the two best hours of the day for sleep, no appetite, and permeated with an unspeakable hostility to his *vis-à-vis*, whose morning garrulity and good humour are equally offensive. Only gradually, as the day wears on and his temperature rises, does he become endurable to himself and to others. But see him really awake at 10 p.m. while our blithe lark is in hopeless coma over his books, from which it is hard to rouse him sufficiently to get his boots off for bed, our lean owl-friend, Saturn no longer in the ascendant, with bright eyes and cheery face, is ready for four hours of anything you wish—deep study, or

> Heart-affluence in discursive talk,

and by 2 a.m. he will undertake to unsphere the spirit of Plato. In neither a virtue, in neither a fault we must recognize these two types of students, differently constituted, owing possibly—though I have but little evidence for the belief—to thermal peculiarities.

II

In the days of probation the student's life may be lived by each one of you in its fullness and in its joys, but the difficulties arise in the break which follows departure from college and the entrance upon new duties.   Much will now depend on the attitude of mind which has been encouraged. If the work has been for your degree, if the diploma has been its sole aim and object, you will rejoice in a freedom from exacting and possibly unpleasant studies, and with your books you will throw away all thoughts of further systematic work.   On the other hand, with good habits of observation you may have got deep enough into the subject to feel that there is still much to be learned, and if you have had ground into you the lesson that the collegiate period is only the beginning of the student life, there is a hope that you may enter upon the useful career of the *student-practitioner*.   Five years, at least, of trial await the man after parting from his teachers, and entering upon an independent course—years upon which his future depends, and from which his horoscope may be cast with certainty.   It is all the same whether he settles in a country village or goes on with hospital and laboratory work; whether he takes a prolonged trip abroad; or whether he settles down in practice with a father or a friend—these five waiting years fix his fate so far as the student life is concerned.   Without any strong natural propensity to study, he may feel such a relief after graduation that the effort to take to books is beyond his mental strength, and a weekly journal with an occasional textbook furnish pabulum enough, at least to

keep his mind hibernating.   But ten years later he is dead
mentally, past any possible hope of galvanizing into life as
a student, fit to do a routine practice, often a capable,
resourceful man, but without any deep convictions, and
probably more interested in stocks or in horses than in
diagnosis or therapeutics.   But this is not always the fate
of the student who finishes his work on Commencement
Day.   There are men full of zeal in practice who give good
service to their fellow creatures, who have not the capacity
or the energy to keep up with the times.   While they have
lost interest in science, they are loyal members of the profession, and apreciate their responsibilities as such.   That
fateful first lustrum ruins some of our most likely material.
Nothing is more trying to the soldier than inaction, to mark
time while the battle is raging all about him; and waiting
for practice is a serious strain under which many yield.   In
the cities it is not so hard to keep up: there is work in the
dispensaries and colleges, and the stimulus of the medical
societies; but in smaller towns and in the country it takes
a strong man to live through the years of waiting without
some deterioration.   I wish the custom of taking junior
men as partners and assistants would grow on this continent.
It has become a necessity, and no man in large general practice can do his work efficiently without skilled help.   How
incalculably better for the seniors, how beneficial to the
patients, how helpful in every way if each one of you, for
the first five or ten years, was associated with an older practitioner, doing his night work, his laboratory work, his
chores of all sorts.   You would, in this way, escape the
chilling and killing isolation of the early years, and amid
congenial surroundings you could, in time, develop into
that flower of our calling—the cultivated general practitioner.   May this be the destiny of a large majority of you!

Have no higher ambition! You cannot reach any better position in a community; the family doctor is the man behind the gun, who does our effective work. That his life is hard and exacting; that he is underpaid and overworked; that he has but little time for study and less for recreation —these are the blows that may give finer temper to his steel, and bring out the nobler elements in his character. What lot or portion has the general practitioner in the student life? Not, perhaps, the fruitful heritage of Judah or Benjamin but he may make of it the goodly portion of Ephraim. A man with powers of observation, well trained in the wards, and with the strong natural propensity to which I have so often referred, may live the ideal student life, and even reach the higher levels of scholarship. Adams, of Banchory (a little Aberdeenshire village), was not only a good practitioner and a skilful operator, but he was an excellent naturalist. This is by no means an unusual or remarkable combination, but Adams became, in addition, one of the great scholars of the profession. He had a perfect passion for the classics, and amid a very exacting practice found time to read "almost every Greek work which has come down to us from antiquity, except the ecclesiastical writers." He translated the works of Paulus Aegineta, the works of Hippocrates, and the works of Aretaeus, all of which are in the Sydenham Society's publications, monuments of the patient skill and erudition of a Scottish village doctor, an incentive to every one of us to make better use of our precious time.

Given the sacred hunger and proper preliminary training the student-practitioner requires at least three things with which to stimulate and maintain his education, a notebook, a library, and a quinquennial braindusting. I wish I had time to speak of the value of note-taking. You can do nothing as a student in practice without it. Carry a small notebook which will fit into your waistcoat pocket, and never ask a new patient a question without notebook and pencil in hand. After the examination of a pneumonia case two minutes will suffice to record the essentials in the daily progress. Routine and system when once made a habit, facilitate work, and the busier you are the more time you will have to make observations after examining a patient. Jot a comment at the end of the notes: "clear case," "case illustrating obscurity of symptoms," "error in diagnosis," etc. The making of observations, may become the exercise of a jackdaw trick, like the craze which so many of us have to collect articles of all sorts. The study of the cases, the relation they bear to each other and to the cases in litera-ture—here comes in the difficulty. Begin early to make a threefold category—clear cases, doubtful cases, mistakes. And learn to play the game fair, no self-deception, no shrinking from the truth; mercy and consideration for the other man, but none for yourself, upon whom you have to keep an incessant watch. You remember Lincoln's famous *mot* about the impossibility of fooling all of the people all the time. It does not hold good for the individual who can fool himself to his heart's content all of the time. If necessary, be cruel; use the knife and the cautery to cure the intumes-cence and moral necrosis which you will feel in the posterior parietal region, in Gall and Spurzheim's centre of self-esteem, where you will find a sore spot after you have made a mistake in diagnosis. It is only by getting your cases grouped in this way that you can make any real progress in your post-collegiate education; only in this way can you gain wisdom with experience. It is a common error to think that the more a doctor sees the greater his experience and the more he knows. No one ever drew a more skilful

distinction than Cowper in his oft-quoted lines, which I am
never tired of repeating in a medical audience:

> Knowledge and wisdom, far from being one,
> Have oft-times no connexion.   Knowledge dwells
> In heads replete with thoughts of other men;
> Wisdom in minds attentive to their own.
> Knowledge is proud that he has learned so much;
> Wisdom is humble that he knows no more.

What we call sense or wisdom is knowledge, ready for use,
made effective, and bears the same relation to knowledge
itself that bread does to wheat.   The full knowledge of the
parts of a steam engine and the theory of its action may be
possessed by a man who could not be trusted to pull the
lever to its throttle.   It is only by collecting data and using
them that you can get sense.   One of the most delightful
sayings of antiquity is the remark of Heraclitus upon his
predecessors—that they had much knowledge but no sense
—which indicates that the noble old Ephesian had a keen
appreciation of their difference; and the distinction, too, is
well drawn by Tennyson in the oft-quoted line:

> Knowledge comes but wisdom lingers.

Of the three well-stocked rooms which it should be the
ambition of every young doctor to have in his house, the
library, the laboratory, and the nursery—books, balances,
and bairns—as he may not achieve all three, I would urge
him to start at any rate with the books and the balances.
A good weekly and a good monthly journal to begin with,
and read them.   Then, for a systematic course of study,
supplement your college textbooks with the larger systems
—Allbutt or Nothnagel—a system of surgery, and, as your
practice increases, make a habit of buying a few special
monographs every year.   Read with two objects: first, to
acquaint yourself with the current knowledge on the

subject and the steps by which it has been reached; and secondly, and more important, read to understand and analyse your cases.   To this line of work we should direct the attention of the student before he leaves the medical school, pointing in specific cases just where the best articles are to be found, sending him to the Index Catalogue—that marvellous storehouse, every page of which is interesting and the very titles instructive.   Early learn to appreciate the differences between the descriptions of disease and the manifestations of that disease in an individual—the difference between the composite portrait and one of the component pictures.   By exercise of a little judgment you can collect at moderate cost a good working library.   Try, in the waiting years, to get a clear idea of the history of medicine.   Read Foster's *Lectures on the History of Physiology* and Baas's *History of Medicine*.   Get the "Masters of Medicine" Series, and subscribe to the *Library and Historical Journal*.[1]

Every day do some reading or work apart from your profession.   I fully realize, no one more so, how absorbing is the profession of medicine; how applicable to it is what Michelangelo says: "There are sciences which demand the whole of a man, without leaving the least portion of his spirit free for other distractions"; but you will be a better man and not a worse practitioner for an avocation.   I care not what it may be; gardening or farming, literature or history or bibliography, any one of which will bring you into contact with books.   (I wish that time permitted me to speak of the other two rooms which are really of equal importance with the library, but which are more difficult to equip, though of co-ordinate value in the education of the head, the heart, and the hand.)   The third essential

[1] Brooklyn.   Price $2 per annum.

for the practitioner as a student is the quinquennial brain-dusting, and this will often seem to him the hardest task to carry out. Every fifth year, back to the hospital, back to the laboratory, for renovation, rehabilitation, rejuvenation, reintegration, resuscitation, etc. Do not forget to take the notebooks with you, or the sheets, in three separate bundles, to work over. From the very start begin to save for the trip. Deny yourself all luxuries for it; shut up the room you meant for the nursery—have the definite determination to get your education thoroughly well started; if you are successful you may, perhaps, have enough saved at the end of three years to spend six weeks in special study; or in five years you may be able to spend six months. Hearken not to the voice of old "Dr. Hayseed," who tells you it will ruin your prospects, and that he "never heard of such a thing" as a young man, not yet five years in practice, taking three months' holiday. To him it seems preposterous. Watch him wince when you say it is a speculation in the only gold mine in which the physician should invest—*Grey Cortex!* What about the wife and babies, if you have them? Leave them! Heavy as are your responsibilities to those nearest and dearest, they are outweighed by the responsibilities to yourself, to the profession, and to the public. Like Isaphaena, the story of whose husband—ardent, earnest soul, peace to his ashes!—I have told in the little sketch of *An Alabama Student*, your wife will be glad to bear her share in the sacrifice you make.

With good health and good habits the end of the second lustrum should find you thoroughly established—all three rooms well furnished, a good stable, a good garden, no mining stock, but a life insurance, and, perhaps, a mortgage or two on neighbouring farms. Year by year you have

dealt honestly with yourself; you have put faithfully the
notes of each case into their proper places, and you will be
gratified to find that, though the doubtful cases and mistakes still make a rather formidable pile, it has grown
relatively smaller. You literally "own" the country-
side, as the expression is. All the serious and dubious
cases come to you, and you have been so honest in the
frank acknowledgment of your own mistakes, and so charitable in the contemplation of theirs, that neighbouring
doctors, old and young, are glad to seek your advice. The
work, which has been very heavy, is now lightened by
a good assistant, one of your own students, who becomes
in a year or so your partner. This is not an overdrawn
picture, and it is one which may be seen in many places
except, I am sorry to say, in the particular as to the partner.
This is the type of man we need in the country districts
and the smaller towns. He is not a whit too good to look
after the sick, not a whit too highly educated—impossible!
And with an optimistic temperament and a good digestion
he is the very best product of our profession, and may do
more to stop quackery and humbuggery, inside and outside
of the ranks, than could a dozen prosecuting county
attorneys. Nay, more! such a doctor may be a daily benediction in the community—a strong, sensible, whole-souled
man, often living a life of great self-denial, and always of
tender sympathy, worried neither by the vagaries of the
well nor by the testy waywardness of the sick, and to him,
if to any, may come (even when he knows it not) the true
spiritual blessing—that "blessing which maketh rich and
addeth no sorrow."

The danger in such a man's life comes with prosperity.
He is safe in the hard-working day, when he is climbing
the hill, but once success is reached, with it come the

temptations to which many succumb.   Politics has been
the ruin of many country doctors, and often of the very
best, of just such a good fellow as he of whom I have been
speaking.   He is popular; he has a little money; and he,
if anybody, can save the seat for the party!   When the
committee leaves you, take the offer under consideration,
and if in the ten or twelve years you have kept on intimate
terms with those friends of your student days, Montaigne
and Plutarch, you will know what answer to return.   If
you live in a large town, resist the temptation to open a
sanatorium.   It is not the work for a general practitioner,
and there are risks that you may sacrifice your independence
and much else besides.   And, thirdly, resist the temptation
to move into a larger place.   In a good agricultural district,
or in a small town, if you handle your resources aright,
taking good care of your education, of your habits, and of
your money, and devoting part of your energies to the
support of the societies, etc., you may reach a position in
the community of which any man may be proud.   There
are country practitioners among my friends with whom
I would rather change places than with any in our ranks,
men whose stability of character and devotion to duty make
one proud of the profession.

Curiously enough, the student-practitioner may find
studiousness to be a stumbling-block in his career.   A
bookish man may never succeed; deep-versed in books,
he may not be able to use his knowledge to practical effect;
or, more likely, his failure is not because he has studied
books much, but because he has not studied men more.
He has never got over that shyness, that diffidence, against
which I have warned you.   I have known instances in
which this malady was incurable; in others I have known
a cure effected not by the public, but by the man's profes-

sional brethren, who, appreciating his work, have insisted
upon utilizing his mental treasures. It is very hard to
carry student habits into a large city practice; only zeal,
a fiery passion, keeps the flame alive, smothered as it is so
apt to be by the dust and ashes of the daily routine. A
man may be a good student who reads only the book of
nature. Such a one[1] I remember in the early days of my
residence in Montreal—a man whose devotion to patients
and whose kindness and skill quickly brought him an enormous practice. Reading in his carriage and by lamplight
at Lucina's bedside, he was able to keep well informed;
but he had an insatiable desire to know the true inwardness
of a disease, and it was in this way I came into contact with
him. Hard pushed day and night, yet he was never too
busy to spend a couple of hours with me searching for data
which had not been forthcoming during life, or helping to
unravel the mysteries of a new disease, such as pernicious
anaemia.

III

The *student-specialist* has to walk warily, as with two
advantages there are two great dangers against which he
has constantly to be on guard. In the bewildering complexity of modern medicine it is a relief to limit the work
of a life to a comparatively narrow field which can be
thoroughly tilled. To many men there is a feeling of great
satisfaction in the mastery of a small department, particularly one in which technical skill is required. How much
we have benefited from this concentration of effort in
dermatology, laryngology, ophthalmology, and in gynecology! Then, as a rule, the specialist is a free man, with
leisure or, at any rate, with some leisure; not the slave of

[1] The late John Bell.

the public, with the incessant demands upon him of the general practitioner. He may live a more rational life, and has time to cultivate his mind, and he is able to devote himself to public interests and to the welfare of his professional brethren, on whose suffrages he so largely depends. How much we are indebted in the larger cities to the disinterested labours of this favoured class the records of our libraries and medical societies bear witness. The dangers do not come to the strong man in a speciality, but to the weak brother who seeks in it an easier field in which specious garrulity and mechanical dexterity may take the place of solid knowledge. All goes well when the man is larger than his speciality and controls it, but when the speciality runs away with the man there is disaster, and a topsy-turvy condition which, in every branch, has done incalculable injury. Next to the danger from small men is the serious risk of the loss of perspective in prolonged and concentrated effort in a narrow field. Against this there is but one safeguard—the cultivation of the sciences upon which the speciality is based. The student-specialist may have a wide vision—no student wider—if he gets away from the mechanical side of the art, and keeps in touch with the physiology and pathology upon which his art depends. More than any other of us, he needs the lessons of the laboratory, and wide contact with men in other departments may serve to correct the inevitable tendency to a narrow and perverted vision, in which the life of the ant-hill is mistaken for the world at large.

Of the *student-teacher* every faculty affords examples in varying degrees. It goes without saying that no man can teach successfully who is not at the same time a student. Routine, killing routine, saps the vitality of many who start with high aims, and who, for years, strive with all

their energies against the degeneration which it is so prone
to entail. In the smaller schools isolation the absence of
congenial spirits working at the same subject, favours stagnation, and after a few years the fires of early enthusiasm
no longer glow in the perfunctory lectures. In many
teachers the ever-increasing demands of practice leave
less and less time for study, and a first-class man may lose
touch with his subject through no fault of his own, but
through an entanglement in outside affairs which he deeply
regrets yet cannot control. To his five natural senses the
student-teacher must add two more—the sense of responsibility and the sense of proportion. Most of us start with
a highly developed sense of the importance of the work,
and with a desire to live up to the responsibilities entrusted
to us. Punctuality, the class first, always and at all times;
the best that a man has in him, nothing less; the best the
profession has on the subject, nothing less; fresh energies
and enthusiasm in dealing with dry details; animated,
unselfish devotion to all alike; tender consideration for
his assistants—these are some of the fruits of a keen sense
of responsibility in a good teacher. The sense of proportion
is not so easy to acquire, and much depends on the training
and on the natural disposition. There are men who never
possess it; to others it seems to come naturally. In the
most careful ones it needs constant cultivation—*nothing
over-much* should be the motto of every teacher. In my
early days I came under the influence of an ideal student-
teacher, the late Palmer Howard, of Montreal. If you
ask what manner of man he was, read Matthew Arnold's
noble tribute to his father in his well-known poem, *Rugby
Chapel*. When young, Dr. Howard had chosen a path—
"path to a clear-purposed goal," and he pursued it with
unswerving devotion. With him the study and the teach-

ing of medicine were an absorbing passion, the ardour of
which neither the incessant and ever-increasing demands
upon his time nor the growing years could quench.   When
I first, as a senior student, came into intimate contact with
him in the summer of 1871, the problem of tuberculosis
was under discussion, stirred up by the epoch-making work
of Villemin and the radical views of Niemeyer.   Every
lung lesion at the Montreal General Hospital had to be
shown to him, and I got my first-hand introduction to
Laennec, to Graves, and to Stokes, and became familiar
with their works.   No matter what the hour, and it usually
was after 10 p.m., I was welcome with my bag, and if Wilks
and Moxon, Virchow, or Rokitanski gave us no help, there
were the Transactions of the Pathological Society and the
big *Dictionnaire* of Dechambre.   An ideal teacher because
a student, ever alert to the new problems, an indomitable
energy enabled him in the midst of an exacting practice
to maintain an ardent enthusiasm, still to keep bright the
fires which he had lighted in his youth.   Since those days
I have seen many teachers, and I have had many colleagues,
but I have never known one in whom was more happily
combined a stern sense of duty with the mental freshness
of youth.

But as I speak, from out the memory of the past there
rises before me a shadowy group, a long line of students
whom I have taught and loved, and who have died prematurely—mentally, morally, or bodily.   To the successful we are willing and anxious to bring the tribute of praise,
but none so poor to give recognition to the failures.   From
one cause or another, perhaps because when not absorbed
in the present, my thoughts are chiefly in the past, I have
cherished the memory of many young men whom I have
loved and lost.   *Io victis:* let us sometimes sing of the vap-

quished. Let us sometimes think of those who have fallen
in the battle of life, who have striven and failed, who have
failed even without the strife. How many have I lost
from the student band by mental death, and from so many
causes—some stillborn from college, others dead within
the first year of infantile marasmus, while mental rickets,
teething, tabes, and fits have carried off many of the most
promising minds! Due to improper feeding within the
first five fateful years, scurvy and rickets head the mental
mortality bills of students. To the teacher-nurse it is a
sore disappointment to find at the end of ten years so few
minds with the full stature, of which the early days gave
promise. Still, so widespread is mental death that we
scarcely comment upon it in our friends. The real tragedy
is the moral death which, in different forms, overtakes
so many good fellows who fall away from the pure, honourable, and righteous service of Minerva into the idolatry
of Bacchus, of Venus, or of Circe. Against the background
of the past these tragedies stand out, lurid and dark, and
as the names and faces of my old boys recur (some of them
my special pride), I shudder to think of the blighted hopes
and wrecked lives, and I force my memory back to those
happy days when they were as you are now, joyous and free
from care, and I think of them on the benches, in the
laboratories, and in the wards—and there I leave them.
Less painful to dwell upon, though associated with a more
poignant grief, is the fate of those whom physical death
has snatched away in the bud or blossom of the student
life. These are among the tender memories of the teacher's
life, of which he does not often care to speak, feeling with
Longfellow that the surest pledge of their remembrance
is "the silent homage of thoughts unspoken." As I look
back it seems now as if the best of us had died, that the

brightest and the keenest had been taken and the more commonplace among us had been spared. An old mother, a devoted sister, a loving brother, in some cases a broken-hearted wife, still pay the tribute of tears for the untimely ending of their high hopes, and in loving remembrance I would mingle mine with theirs. What a loss to our profession have been the deaths of such true disciples as Zimmerman, of Toronto; of Jack Cline and of R. L. MacDonnell, of Montreal; of Fred Packard and of Kirkbride, of Philadelphia; of Livingood, of Lazear, of Oppenheimer, and of Oechsner, in Baltimore—cut off with their leaves still in the green, to the inconsolable grief of their friends!

To each one of you the practice of medicine will be very much as you make it—to one a worry, a care, a perpetual annoyance; to another, a daily joy and a life of as much happiness and usefulness as can well fall to the lot of man. In the student spirit you can best fulfil the high mission of our noble calling—in his *humility*, conscious of weakness, while seeking strength; in his *confidence*, knowing the power, while recognizing the limitations of his art; in his *pride* in the glorious heritage from which the greatest gifts to man have been derived; and in his sure and certain hope that the future holds for us richer blessings than the past.

XXI
UNITY, PEACE, AND CONCORD

"In necessariis unitas, in non-necessariis libertas, in omnibus caritas."

"Life is too short to waste,
   In critic peep or cynic bark,
Quarrel or reprimand:
   'Twill soon be dark;
Up! Mind thine own aim, and
   God speed the mark!"

EMERSON.

XXI
UNITY, PEACE, AND CONCORD[1]

O N this occasion I have had no difficulty in selecting a subject on which to address you. Surely the hour is not for the head but for the heart, out of the abundance of which I may be able to express, however feebly, my gratitude for the many kindnesses I have received from the profession of this country during the past twenty-one years, and from you, my dear colleagues of this state and city, during the sixteen years I have dwelt among you. Truly I can say that I have lived my life in our beloved profession —perhaps too much! but whatever success I have had has come directly through it, and my devotion is only natural. Few men have had more from their colleagues than has fallen to my lot. As an untried young man my appointment at McGill College came directly through friends in the faculty who had confidence in me as a student. In the ten happy years I lived in Montreal I saw little of any save physicians and students, among whom I was satisfied to work—and to play. In Philadelphia the hospitals and the societies absorbed the greater part of my time, and I lived the peaceful life of a student with students. An ever-widening circle of friends in the profession brought me into closer contact with the public, but I have never departed from my ambition to be first of all a servant of my brethren, willing and anxious to do anything in my power to help them. Of my life here you all know. I have studied to be quiet and

[1] A farewell address to the Medical Profession of the United States, delivered before the Medical and Chirurgical Faculty of the State of Maryland, 1905.

to do my own business and to walk honestly toward them that are without; and one of my chief pleasures has been to work among you as a friend, sharing actively in your manifold labours. But when to the sessions of sweet, silent thought I summon up the past, not what I have done but the many things I have left undone, the opportunities I have neglected, the battles I have shirked, the precious hours I have wasted—these rise up in judgment.

A notable period it has been in our history through which we have lived, a period of reconstruction and renovation, a true renaissance, not only an extraordinary revival of learning, but a complete transformation in our educational methods; and I take pride in the thought that, in Philadelphia and in Baltimore, I have had the good fortune to be closely associated with men who have been zealous in the promotion of great reforms, the full value of which we are too close to the events to appreciate. On the far-reaching influence of these changes time will not permit us to dwell. I propose to consider another aspect of our work of equal importance, neither scientific nor educational, but what may be called humanistic, as it deals with our mutual relations and with the public.

Nothing in life is more glaring than the contrast between possibilities and actualities, between the ideal and the real. By the ordinary mortal, idealists are regarded as vague dreamers, striving after the impossible; but in the history of the world how often have they gradually moulded to their will conditions the most adverse and hopeless! They alone furnish the *Geist* that finally animates the entire body and makes possible reforms and even revolutions. Imponderable, impalpable, more often part of the moral than of the intellectual equipment, are the subtle qualities so hard to define, yet so potent in everyday life,

by which these fervent souls keep alive in us the reality of
the ideal.   Even in a lost cause, with aspirations utterly
futile, they refuse to acknowledge defeat, and, still nursing
an unconquerable hope, send up the prayer of faith in face
of a scoffing world.   Most characteristic of aspirations of
this class is the petition of the Litany in which we pray
that to the nations may be given 'unity, peace, and concord.'   Century after century from the altars of Christen-
dom this most beautiful of all prayers has risen from lips
of men and women, from the loyal souls who have refused
to recognize its hopelessness, with the war-drums ever
sounding in their ears.   The desire for unity, the wish for
peace, the longing for concord, deeply implanted in the
human heart, have stirred the most powerful emotions of
the race, and have been responsible for some of its noblest
actions.   It is but a sentiment, you may say: but is not
the world ruled by feeling and by passion?   What but a
strong sentiment baptized this nation in blood; and what
but sentiment, the deep-rooted affection for country which
is so firmly implanted in the hearts of all Americans, gives
to these states to-day unity, peace, and concord?   As
with the nations at large, so with the nation in particular;
as with people, so with individuals; and as with our profession, so with its members, this fine old prayer for unity,
peace, and concord, if in our hearts as well as on our lips,
may help us to realize its aspirations.   What some of its
lessons may be to us will be the subject of my address.

UNITY

Medicine is the only world-wide profession, following
everywhere the same methods, actuated by the same ambitions, and pursuing the same ends.   This homogeneity,
its most characteristic feature, is not shared by the law,

and not by the Church, certainly not in the same degree. While in antiquity the law rivals medicine, there is not in it that extraordinary solidarity which makes the physician at home in any country, in any place where two or three sons of men are gathered together. Similar in its high aims and in the devotion of its officers, the Christian Church, widespread as it is, and saturated with the humanitarian instincts of its Founder, yet lacks that catholicity—*urbi et orbi*—which enables the physician to practise the same art amid the same surroundings in every country of the earth. There is a unity, too, in its aims—the prevention of diseases by discovering their causes, and the cure and relief of sickness and suffering. In a little more than a century a united profession, working in many lands, has done more for the race than has ever before been accomplished by any other body of men. So great have been these gifts that we have almost lost our appreciation of them. Vaccination, sanitation, anaesthesia, antiseptic surgery, the new science of bacteriology, and the new art in therapeutics have effected a revolution in our civilization to which can be compared only the extraordinary progress in the mechanical arts. Over the latter there is this supreme advantage, it is domestic—a bedroom revolution which sooner or later touches each one of us, if not in person, in those near and dear—a revolution which for the first time in the history of poor, suffering humanity brings us appreciably closer to that promised day when the former things should pass away, when there should be no more unnecessary death, when sorrow and crying should be no more, and there should not be any more pain.

One often hears as a reproach that more has been done in the prevention than in the cure of disease. It is true; but this second part of our labours has also made enormous

progress.   We recognize to-day the limitations of the art;
we know better the diseases curable by medicine, and
those which yield to exercise and fresh air; we have learned
to realize the intricacy of the processes of disease, and have
refused to deceive ourselves with half-knowledge, preferring
to wait for the day instead of groping blindly in the dark
or losing our way in the twilight.   The list of diseases which
we can positively cure is an ever-increasing one, the number
of diseases the course of which we can modify favourably
is a growing one, the number of incurable diseases (which is
large and which will probably always be large) is diminishing—so that in this second point we may feel that not
only is the work already done of the greatest importance,
but that we are on the right path, and year by year as we
know disease better we shall be able to treat it more successfully.   The united efforts of countless workers in many
lands have won these greatest victories of science.   Only
by ceaseless co-operation and the intelligent appreciation
by all of the results obtained in each department has the
present remarkable position been reached.   Within a week
or ten days a great discovery in any part of the world is
known everywhere, and, while in a certain sense we speak
of German, French, English, and American medicine, the
differences are trifling in comparison with the general similarity.   The special workers know each other and are familiar with each other's studies in a way that is truly remarkable.   And the knowledge gained by the one, or the special
technic he may devise, or the instrument he may invent is
at the immediate disposal of all.   A new lifesaving operation of the first class devised by a surgeon in Breslau
would be performed here the following week.   A discovery
in practical medicine is common property with the next
issue of the weekly journals.

A powerful stimulus in promoting this wide organic unity is our great international gatherings—not so much the International Congress of the profession, which has proved rather an unwieldy body, but of the special societies which are rapidly denationalizing science. In nearly every civilized country medical men have united in great associations which look after their interests and promote scientific work. It should be a source of special pride to American physicians to feel that the national association of this country—the American Medical Association—has become one of the largest and most influential bodies of the kind in the world. We cannot be too grateful to men who have controlled its course during the past ten years. The reorganization so efficiently carried out has necessitated a readjustment of the machinery of the state societies, and it is satisfactory to know that this meeting of our state society, the first held under the new conditions, has proved so satisfactory. But in the whole scheme of readjustment nothing commands our sympathy and co-operation more than the making of the county societies the materials out of which the state and national associations are built. It is not easy at first to work out such a scheme in full detail, and I would ask of the members of this body not only their co-operation, but an expectant consideration, if the plan at first does not work as smoothly as could be desired. On the county members I would urge the support of a plan conceived on broad national lines—on you its success depends, and to you its benefits will chiefly come.

Linked together by the strong bonds of community of interests, the profession of medicine forms a remarkable world-unit in the progressive evolution of which there is a fuller hope for humanity than in any other direction.

Concentration, fusion, and consolidation are welding together various subunits in each nation. Much has been done, much remains to do; and to three desiderata I may refer briefly.

In this country reciprocity between the state licensing boards remains one of the most urgent local needs. Given similar requirements, and examinations practically of the same character, with evidence of good character, the state board should be given power to register a man on payment of the usual fee. It is preposterous to restrict in his own country, as is now done, a physician's liberty. Take a case in point: A few months ago a man who is registered in three states, an able, capable practitioner of twenty years' standing, a hard student in his profession, a physician who has had charge of some of the most important lives of this country, had to undergo another examination for licence. What an anomaly! What a reflection on a united profession! I would urge you all most strongly to support the movement now in progress to place reciprocity on a proper basis. International reciprocity is another question of equal importance, but surrounded with greater difficulties; and, though a long way off, it will come within this century.

The second urgent need is a consolidation of many of our medical schools. Within the past twenty-five years conditions have so changed that the tax on the men in charge of the unendowed schools has become ever more burdensome. In the old days of a faculty with seven professors, a school with 300 students was a good property, paying large salaries, but the introduction of laboratory and practical teaching has so increased the expenses that very little is now left for distribution at the end of the year. The students' fees have not increased proportionately, and only the self-sacrifice and devotion of men who ungrudgingly give their time, and often their means, save a hopeless situation. A fusion of the schools is the natural solution of the problem. Take a concrete example: A union of three of the medical schools of this city would enable the scientific departments to be consolidated at an enormous saving of expense and with a corresponding increase in efficiency. Anatomy, physiology, pathology, physiological chemistry, bacteriology, and pharmacology could be taught in separately organized departments which the funds of the united school could support liberally. Such a school could appeal to the public for aid to build and endow suitable laboratories. The clinical work could be carried on at the separate hospitals, which would afford unequalled facilities for the scientific study of disease. Not only in this city, but in Richmond, in Nashville, in Columbus, in Indianapolis, and in many cities a "merger" is needed. Even the larger schools of the larger cities could "pool" their scientific interests to the great advantage of the profession.

And the third desideratum is the recognition by our homoeopathic brethren that the door is open. It is too late in this day of scientific medicine to prattle of such antique nonsense as is indicated in the "pathies." We have long got past the stage when any "system" can satisfy a rational practitioner, long past the time when a difference of belief in the action of drugs—the most uncertain element in our art!—should be allowed to separate men with the same noble traditions, the same hopes, the same aims and ambitions. It is not as if our homoeopathic brothers are asleep; far from it, they are awake—many of them at any rate—to the importance of the scientific study of disease, and all of them must realize the anomaly of their position.

It is distressing to think that so many good men live isolated, in a measure, from the great body of the profession.
The original grievous mistake was ours—to quarrel with
our brothers over infinitesimals was a most unwise and
stupid thing to do.   That we quarrel with them now is
solely on account of the old Shibboleth under which they
practise.   Homoeopathy is as inconsistent with the new
medicine as is the old-fashioned polypharmacy, to the
destruction of which it contributed so much.   The rent in
the robe of Aesculapius, wider in this country than elsewhere, could be repaired by mutual concessions—on the one
hand by the abandonment of special designations, and on
the other by an intelligent toleration of therapeutic vagaries
which in all ages have beset the profession, but which have
been mere flies on the wheels of progress.

PEACE

Many seek peace, few ensue it actively, and among these
few we, alas! are not often to be found.   In one sense every
one of us may be asked the question which Jehu returned
to Joram: "What hast thou to do with peace?" since our life
must be a perpetual warfare, dominated by the fighting
spirit.   The physician, like the Christian, has three great
foes—ignorance, which is sin; apathy, which is the world;
and vice, which is the devil.   There is a delightful Arabian
proverb two lines of which run: "He that knows not, and
knows not that he knows not, is a fool.   Shun him.   He
that knows not, and knows that he knows not, is simple.
Teach him."   To a large extent these two classes represent
the people with whom we have to deal.   Teaching the
simple and suffering the fools gladly, we must fight the wilful
ignorance of the one and the helpless ignorance of the other,
not with the sword of righteous indignation, but with the

skilful weapon of the tongue. On this ignorance the charlatan and the quack live, and it is by no means an easy matter
to decide how best to conduct a warfare against these wily
foes, the oldest and most formidable with whom we have to
deal. As the incomparable Fuller remarks: "Well did the
poets feign Aesculapius and Circe brother and sister, . . .
for in all times (in the opinion of the multitude) witches, old
women, and impostors have had a competition with
doctors." Education of the public of a much more systematic and active kind is needed. The congress on quackery
which is announced to take place in Paris, with some twenty-
five subjects for discussion, indicates one important method
of dealing with the problem. The remarkable exhibit held
last year in Germany of everything relating to quacks and
charlatans did an immense good in calling attention to the
colossal nature of the evil. A permanent museum of this
sort might well be organized in Washington in connexion
with the Department of Hygiene. It might be worth while
to imitate our German brethren in a special national exhibit,
though I dare say many of the most notorious sinners would
apply for large space, not willing to miss the opportunity for
a free advertisement! One effective measure is enforced in
Germany: any proprietary medicine sold to the public must
be submitted to a government analyst, who prepares a
statement (as to its composition, the price of its ingredients,
etc.), which is published at the cost of the owner of the
supposed remedy in a certain number of the daily and
weekly papers.

By far the most dangerous foe we have to fight is apathy
—indifference from whatever cause, not from a lack of
knowledge, but from carelessness, from absorption in other
pursuits, from a contempt bred of self-satisfaction. Fully
25 per cent. of the deaths in the community are due to this

accursed apathy, fostering a human inefficiency, and going far to counterbalance the extraordinary achievements of the past century. Why should we take pride in the wonderful railway system with which enterprise and energy have traversed the land, when the supreme law, the public health, is neglected? What comfort in the thought of a people enjoying great material prosperity when we know that the primary elements of life (on which even the old Romans were our masters) are denied to them? What consolation does the 'little red school-house' afford when we know that a Lethean apathy allows toll to be taken of every class, from the little tots to the youths and maidens? Western civilization has been born of knowledge, of know-ledge won by hard, honest sweat of body and brain, but in many of the most important relations of life we have failed to make that knowledge effective. And, strange irony of life, the lesson of human efficiency is being taught us by one of the little nations of the earth, which has so far bettered our instruction that we must again turn eastward for wisdom. Perhaps in a few years our civilization may be put on trial, and it will not be without benefit if it arouses the individual from apathy and makes him conscious of the great truth that only by earnest individual human effort can knowledge be made effective, and if it arouses communities from an apathy which permits mediaeval conditions to prevail without a protest.

Against our third great foe—vice in all its forms—we have to wage an incessant warfare, which is not less vigorous because of the quiet, silent kind. Better than any one else the physician can say the word in season to the immoral, to the intemperate, to the uncharitable in word and deed. Personal impurity is the evil against which we can do most good, particularly to the young, by showing the possibility of the pure life and the dangers of immorality. Had I time, and were this the proper occasion, I would like to rouse the profession to a sense of its responsibility toward the social evil—the black plague which devastates the land. I can but call your attention to an important society, of which Dr. Prince Morrow, of New York, is the organizer, which has for one of its objects the education of the public on this important question. I would urge you to join in a crusade quite as important as that in which we are engaged against tuberculosis.

CONCORD

Unity promotes concord—community of interests, the same aims, the same objects give, if anything can, a feeling of comradeship, and the active co-operation of many men, while it favours friction, lessens the chances of misunderstanding and ill will. One of the most gratifying features of our professional life is the good feeling which prevails between the various sections of the country. I do not see how it could be otherwise. One has only to visit different parts and mingle with the men to appreciate that everywhere good work is being done, everywhere an earnest desire to elevate the standard of education, and everywhere the same self-sacrificing devotion on the part of the general practitioner. Men will tell you that commercialism is rife, that the charlatan and the humbug were never so much in evidence, and that in our ethical standards there has been a steady declension. These are the Elijahs who are always ready to pour out their complaints, mourning that they are not better than their fathers. Few men have had more favourable opportunities than I have had to gauge the actual conditions in professional private life, in the schools, and in the medical societies, and as I have seen them in the past twenty years I am filled with thankfulness for the present and with hope for the future.   The little rift within the lute is the absence in many places of that cordial professional harmony which should exist among us. In the larger cities professional jealousies are dying out. Read Charles Caldwell's *Autobiography* if you wish for spicy details of the quarrels of the doctors in this country during the first half of the last century.   I am sorry to say the professors have often been the worst offenders, and the rivalry between medical schools has not always been friendly and courteous.   That it still prevails to some extent must be acknowledged, but it is dying out, though not so rapidly as we could wish.   It makes a very bad impression on the public, and is often a serious stumbling-block in the way of progress.   Only the other day I had a letter from an intelligent and appreciative layman who is interested in a large hospital scheme about which I had been consulted.   I quote this sentence from it in sorrow, and I do so because it is written by a strong personal friend of the profession, a man who has had long and varied experience with us: "I may say to you that one of the distressing bewilderments of the layman who only desires the working out of a broad plan is the extraordinary bitterness of professional jealousy between not only schoolmen and non-schoolmen, but between schoolmen themselves, and the reflections which are cast on one another as belonging to that clique, which makes it exceedingly difficult for the layman to understand what way there is out of these squabbles."

The national and special societies, and particularly the American Medical Association, have brought men together and have taught them to know each other and to appreciate the good points which at home may have been overlooked. As Dr. Brush said yesterday in his address, it is in the smaller towns and country districts that the conditions are most favourable for mutual misunderstandings. Only those of us who have been brought up in such surroundings can appreciate how hard it is for physicians to keep on good terms with each other. The practice of medicine calls equally for the exercise of the heart and the head; and when a man has done his best, to have his motives misunderstood and his conduct of a case harshly criticized not only by the family, but by a colleague who has been called in, small wonder, when the opportunity arises, if the old Adam prevails and he pays in kind. So far as my observation goes there are three chief causes for the quarrels of doctors. The first is lack of proper friendly intercourse, by which alone we can know each other. It is the duty of the older man to look on the younger one who settles near him not as a rival, but as a son. He will do to you just what you did to the old practitioner, when, as a young man, you started—get a good many of your cases; but if you have the sense to realize that this is inevitable, unavoidable, and the way of the world, and if you have the sense to talk over, in a friendly way, the first delicate situation that arises, the difficulties will disappear and recurrences may be made impossible. The young men should be tender with the sensibilities of their seniors, deferring to their judgment and taking counsel with them. If young graduates could be taken more frequently as assistants or partners, the work of the profession would be much lightened, and it would promote amity and good fellowship. A man of whom you may have heard as the incarnation of unprofessional conduct, and who has been held up as an example of all that is pernicious, may be, in reality, a very good fellow, the victim of petty jealousies, the mark of the arrows of a rival faction; and you may, on acquaintance, find that he loves his wife and is

devoted to his children, and that there are people who
respect and esteem him.   After all, the attitude of mind is
the all-important factor in the promotion of concord.   When
a man is praised, or when a young man has done a good bit
of work in your special branch, be thankful—it is for the
common good.   Envy, that pain of the soul, as Plato calls,
it, should never for a moment afflict a man of generous
instincts who has a sane outlook in life.   The men of rival
schools should deliberately cultivate the acquaintance of
each other and encourage their students and the junior
teachers to fraternize.   If you hear that a young fellow just
starting has made mistakes or is a little "off colour," go out
of your way to say a good word to him, or for him.   It is the
only cure; any other treatment only aggravates the malady.

The second great cause is one over which we have direct
control.   The most widespread, the most pernicious of all
vices, equal in its disastrous effects to impurity, much more
disastrous often than intemperance, because destructive
of all mental and moral nobility as are the others of bodily
health, is uncharitableness—the most prevalent of modern
sins, peculiarly apt to beset all of us, and the chief enemy
to concord in our ranks.   Oftentimes it is a thoughtless
evil, a sort of tic or trick, an unconscious habit of mind
and tongue which gradually takes possession of us.   No
sooner is a man's name mentioned than something slighting
is said of him, or a story is repeated which is to his disadvantage, or the involuntary plight of a brother is ridiculed,
or even his character is traduced.   In chronic and malign
offenders literally "with every word a reputation dies."
The work of a school is disparaged, or the character of the
work in a laboratory is belittled; or it may be only the
faint praise that damns, not the generous meed from a full
and thankful heart.   We have lost our fine sense of the

tragic element in this vice, and of its debasing influence on
the character.   It is interesting that Christ and the Apostles
lashed it more unsparingly than any other.   Who is there
among us who does not require every day to lay to heart
that counsel of perfection: "Judge not according to the
appearance, but judge righteous judgment?"   One of
the apostles of our profession, Sir Thomas Browne, has a
great thought on the question:

While thou so hotly disclaimest the devil, be not guilty of diabolism.
Fall not into one name with that unclean spirit, nor act his nature whom
thou so much abhorrest—that is, to accuse, calumniate backbite, whisper,
detract, or sinistrously interpret others.   Degenerous depravities, and
narrow-minded vices! not only below St. Paul's noble Christian, but
Aristotle's true gentleman.   Trust not with some that the Epistle of St.
James is apocryphal, and so read with less fear that stabbing truth, that in
company with this vice thy religion is in vain.   Moses broke the tables
without breaking the law; but where charity is broke the law itself is
shattered, which cannot be whole without love, which is the fulfilling of it.
Look humbly upon thy virtues; and though thou art rich in some, yet
think thyself poor and naked without that crowning grace, which thinketh
no evil, which envieth not, which beareth, hopeth, believeth, endureth all
things.   With these sure graces, while busy tongues are crying out for a
drop of cold water, mutes may be in happiness, and sing the Trisagion in
heaven.

And the third cause is the wagging tongue of others who
are too often ready to tell tales and make trouble between
physicians.   There is only one safe rule—never listen to a
patient who begins with a story about the carelessness and
inefficiency of Dr. Blank.   Shut him or her up with a snap,
knowing full well that the same tale may be told of you a
few months later.   Fully half of the quarrels of physicians
are fomented by the tittle-tattle of patients, and the only
safeguard is not to listen.   Sometimes it is impossible to
check the flow of imprecation and slander; and   then
apply the other rule—perfectly safe, and one which   may
be commended as a good practice—never believe what a

patient tells you to the detriment of a brother physician, even though you may think it to be true.

To part from the profession of this country and from this old Faculty, which I have learned to love so dearly, is a great wrench, one which I would feel more deeply were it not for the nearness of England, and for the confidence I feel that I am but going to work in another part of the same vineyard, and were it not for the hope that I shall continue to take interest in your affairs and in the welfare of the medical school to which I owe so much. It may be that in the hurry and bustle of a busy life I have given offence to some—who can avoid it? Unwittingly I may have shot an arrow o'er the house and hurt a brother—if so, I am sorry, and I ask his pardon. So far as I can read my heart I leave you in charity with all. I have striven with none, not, as Walter Savage Landor says, because none was worth the strife, but because I have had a deep conviction of the hatefulness of strife, of its uselessness, of its disastrous effects, and a still deeper conviction of the blessings that come with unity, peace, and concord. And I would give to each of you, my brothers—you who hear me now, and to you who may elsewhere read my words— to you who do our greatest work labouring incessantly for small rewards in towns and country places—to you the more favoured ones who have special fields of work—to you teachers and professors and scientific workers—to one and all, through the length and breadth of the land—I give a single word as my parting commandment:

"It is not hidden from thee, neither is it far off. It is not in heaven, that thou shouldest say, 'Who shall go up for us to heaven, and bring it unto us, that we may hear it, and do it?' Neither is it beyond the sea, that thou shouldest say, 'Who shall go over the sea for us, and bring it unto us, that we may hear it, and do it?' But the word is very nigh unto thee, in thy mouth and in thy heart, that thou mayest do it"—CHARITY.

XXII
L'ENVOI

"I am a part of all that I have met."

(*Ulysses.*)

TENNYSON.

XXII

L'ENVOI[1]

I AM sure you all sympathize with me in the feelings which naturally almost overpower me on such an occasion. Many testimonials you have already given me of your affection and of your regard, but this far exceeds them all, and I am deeply touched that so many of you have come long distances, and at great inconvenience, to bid me Godspeed in the new venture I am about to undertake. Pardon me, if I speak of myself, in spite of Montaigne's warning that one seldom speaks of oneself without some detriment to the person spoken of. Happiness comes to many of us and in many ways, but I can truly say that to few men has happiness come in so many forms as it has come to me. Why I know not, but this I do know, that I have not deserved more than others, and yet, a very rich abundance of it has been vouchsafed to me. I have been singularly happy in my friends, and for that I say "God be praised." I have had exceptional happiness in the profession of my choice, and I owe all of this to you. I have sought success in life, and if, as some one has said, this consists in getting what you want and being satisfied with it, I have found what I sought in the estimation, in the fellowship and friendship of the members of my profession.

I have been happy too in the public among whom I have worked—happy in my own land in Canada, happy here among you in the country of my adoption, from which I

[1] Remarks at farewell dinner given by the profession of the United States and Canada, New York, May 2, 1905.

cannot part without bearing testimony to the nobility and the grace of character which I have found here in my colleagues. It fills me with joy to think that I have had not only the consideration and that ease of fellowship which means so much in life, but the warmest devotion on the part of my patients and their friends.

Of the greatest of all happiness I cannot speak—of my home. Many of you know it, and that is enough.

I would like to tell you how I came to this country. The men responsible for my arrival were Samuel W. Gross and Minis Hays of Philadelphia, who concocted the scheme in the *Medical News* office and asked James Tyson to write a letter asking if I would be a candidate for the professorship of Clinical Medicine in the University of Pennsylvania. That letter reached me at Leipsic, having been forwarded to me from Montreal by my friend Shepherd. So many pranks had I played on my friends there that, when the letter came, I felt sure it was a joke, so little did I think that I was one to be asked to succeed Dr. Pepper. It was several weeks before I ventured to answer that letter, fearing that Dr. Shepherd had perhaps surreptitiously taken a sheet of University of Pennsylvania notepaper on purpose to make the joke more certain. Dr. Mitchell cabled me to meet him in London, as he and his good wife were commissioned to "look me over," particularly with reference to personal conditions. Dr. Mitchell said there was only one way in which the breeding of a man suitable for such a position, in such a city as Philadelphia, could be tested:— give him cherry pie and see how he disposed of the stones. I had read of the trick before and disposed of them genteelly in my spoon—and got the Chair!

My affiliations with the profession in this country have been wide and to me most gratifying. At the University of

Pennsylvania I found men whom I soon learned to love and esteem, and when I think of the good men who have gone— of Pepper, of Leidy, of Wormley, of Agnew, of Ashhurst—I am full of thankfulness to have known them before they were called to their long rest.   I am glad to think that my dear friends Tyson and Wood are here still to join in a demonstration to me.

At Johns Hopkins University I found the same kindly feeling of friendship and my association with my colleagues there has been, as you all know, singularly happy and delightful.

With my fellow workers in the medical societies—in the American Medical Association, in the Association of American Physicians, in the Pediatric, Neurological and Physiological Societies—my relations have been most cordial and I would extend to them my heartfelt thanks for the kindness and consideration shown me during the past twenty years.

With the general practitioners throughout the country my relations have been of a peculiarly intimate character. Few men present, perhaps very few men in this country, have wandered so far and have seen in so many different sections the doctor at work.   To all of these good friends who have given me their suffrage I express my appreciation and heartfelt thanks for their encouragement and support.

And lastly, my relations with my students—so many of whom I see here—have been of a close and most friendly character.   They have been the inspiration of my work, and I may say truly, the inspiration of my life.

I have had but two ambitions in the profession: first, to make of myself a good clinical physician, to be ranked with the men who have done so much for the profession of this country—to rank in the class with Nathan Smith,

Bartlett, James Jackson, Bigelow, Alonzo Clark, Metcalfe, W. W. Gerhard, Draper, Pepper, DaCosta and others. The chief desire of my life has been to become a clinician of the same stamp with these great men, whose names we all revere and who did so much good work for clinical medicine.

My second ambition has been to build up a great clinic on Teutonic lines, not on those previously followed here and in England, but on lines which have proved so successful on the Continent, and which have placed the scientific medicine of Germany in the forefront of the world. And if I have done anything to promote the growth of clinical medicine it has been in this direction, in the formation of a large clinic with a well organized series of assistants and house physicians and with proper laboratories in which to work at the intricate problems that confront us in internal medicine. For the opportunities which I have had at Johns Hopkins Hospital to carry out these ideas, I am truly thankful. How far I have been successful, or not, remains to be seen. But of this I am certain:—If there is one thing above another which needs a change in this country, it is the present hospital system in relation to the medical school. It has been spoken of by Dr. Jacobi but cannot be referred to too often. In every town of fifty thousand inhabitants a good model clinic could be built up, just as good as in smaller German cities, if only a self-denying ordinance were observed on the part of the profession and only one or two men given the control of the hospital service, not half a dozen. With proper assistants and equipment, with good clinical and pathological laboratories there would be as much clinical work done in this country as in Germany.

I have had three personal ideals. One to do the day's work well and not to bother about to-morrow. It has been urged that this is not a satisfactory ideal. It is; and there is not one which the student can carry with him into practice with greater effect. To it, more than to anything else, I owe whatever success I have had—to this power of settling down to the day's work and trying to do it well to the best of one's ability, and letting the future take care of itself.

The second ideal has been to act the Golden Rule, as far as in me lay, towards my professional brethren and towards the patients committed to my care.

And the third has been to cultivate such a measure of equanimity as would enable me to bear success with humility, the affection of my friends without pride and to be ready when the day of sorrow and grief came to meet it with the courage befitting a man.

What the future has in store for me, I cannot tell—you cannot tell. Nor do I care much, so long as I carry with me, as I shall, the memory of the past you have given me. Nothing can take that away.

I have made mistakes, but they have been mistakes of the head not of the heart. I can truly say, and I take upon myself to witness, that in my sojourn among you:——

> "I have loved no darkness,
> Sophisticated no truth,
> Nursed no delusion,
> Allowed no fear."

BED-SIDE LIBRARY FOR MEDICAL STUDENTS.

A LIBERAL education may be had at a very slight cost of time and money. Well filled though the day be with appointed tasks, to make the best possible use of your one or of your ten talents, rest not satisfied with this professional training, but try to get the education, if not of a scholar, at least of a gentleman. Before going to sleep read for half an hour, and in the morning have a book open on your dressing table. You will be surprised to find how much can be accomplished in the course of a year. I have put down a list of ten books which you may make close friends. There are many others; studied carefully in your student days these will help in the inner education of which I speak.

I. Old and New Testament.
II. Shakespeare.
III. Montaigne.[1]
IV. Plutarch's *Lives*.[1]
V. Marcus Aurelius.[2]
VI. Epictetus.[2]
VII. *Religio Medici*.[2]
VIII. *Don Quixote*.
IX. Emerson
X. Oliver Wendell Holmes—Breakfast-Table Series.

[1] The Temple Classics, J. M. Dent & Co.
[2] Golden Treasury Series, Macmillan & Company, Ltd.